MASTER
MEDICINE

Medical Pharmacology

A clinical core text for integrated curricula with self-assessment

PETER WINSTANLEY
MD FRCP DTM&H

Professor of Clinical Pharmacology
University of Liverpool;
Honorary Consultant Physician
Royal Liverpool University Hospital

TOM WALLEY
MD FRCP FRCPI

Professor of Clinical Pharmacology
University of Liverpool;
Honorary Consultant Physician
Royal Liverpool University Hospital

SECOND EDITION

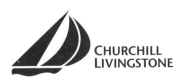

CHURCHILL
LIVINGSTONE

EDINBURGH   LONDON   NEW YORK   PHILADELPHIA   SYDNEY   TORONTO   2002

CHURCHILL LIVINGSTONE
An imprint of Elsevier Limited

© Pearson Professional Limitied 1996
Assigned to Harcourt Brace and Company 1998
© 2002, Elsevier Limited. All rights reserved.

First edition 1996
Second edition 2002
 Reprinted 2005

ISBN 0 443 07055 5

British Library Cataloguing in Publication Data
A catalogue record for this book is available from the British Library

Library of Congress Cataloging in Publication Data
A catalog record for this book is available from the Library of Congress

Notice
Medical knowledge is constantly changing. Standard safety precautions
must be followed, but as new research and clinical experience broaden
our knowledge, changes in treatment and drug therapy may become
necessary or appropriate. Readers are advised to check the most current
product information provided by the manufacturer of each drug to be
administered to verify the recommended dose, the method and duration
of administration, and contraindications. It is the responsibility of the
practitioner, relying on experience and knowledge of the patient, to
determine dosages and the best treatment for each individual patient.
Neither the Publisher nor the editors/contributor assumes any liability
for any injury and/or damage to persons or property arising from this
publication.

The Publisher

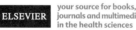
ELSEVIER your source for books,
journals and multimedia
in the health sciences
www.elsevierhealth.com

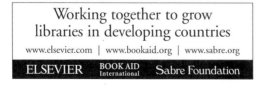
Working together to grow
libraries in developing countries

www.elsevier.com | www.bookaid.org | www.sabre.org

ELSEVIER   BOOK AID
International   Sabre Foundation

The
Publisher's
policy is to use
**paper manufactured
from sustainable forests**

Printed in Spain by Graphos

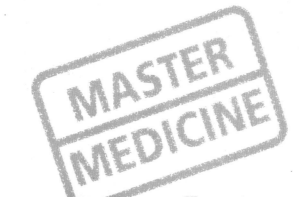

Medical Pharmacology

Commissioning Editor: Timothy Horne
Project Development Manager: Barbara Simmons
Project Manager: Frances Affleck
Designers: Judith Wright, George Ajayi

Contents

Using this book

Philosophy of the book

What drugs are used for hypertension? How do they work? What adverse effects do they have, and who should *not* receive them? This book will help you with these, and similar, questions with the general aims of passing the examination *and* retaining an understanding of pharmacology for your future career.

Drugs have always been, and remain, one of the main ways of treating and preventing disease. Broadly, the discipline of *pharmacology* is concerned with how drugs work and how they reach their site of action, while *therapeutics* is concerned with their clinical use. Most doctors have expertise in therapeutics—they use it every day of practice. However, detailed expertise in pharmacology is not needed by all doctors, but most retain a degree of 'background knowledge', which renders their therapeutic use of drugs more rational.

Your aim should be to develop an understanding of the principles which govern the clinical use of drugs.

Layout of the book

This book is organised along clinical, rather than strictly pharmacological, lines to render it more accessible to medical students. Consequently the chapters focus on anatomical systems (e.g. the cardiovascular system) or the therapy of specific diseases (e.g. cancer chemotherapy) rather than on mechanisms of drug action. In each chapter we have tried to set out mechanisms and principles, rather than lists, and have tried to link together sections of the book where the same topic is dealt with from different angles.

The chapters are subdivided into sections, each dealing with a therapeutic area (e.g. the cardiovascular chapter includes sections on hypertension, angina and arrhythmias) and we have tried to construct these in a reasonably uniform way. Each section starts with a brief description of the clinical context: there would be little point learning about antiepileptic drugs, for example, if you did not understand the nature of epilepsy. Many diverse drugs may be relevant to the therapy used to treat the same condition: we have grouped similar drugs under the same class heading (e.g. the benzodiazepines). For each drug class we describe:

- mode of action: at the molecular, cellular, organ and whole-body levels where relevant
- examples and clinical pharmacokinetics: there are usually several drugs of each class in common use, we describe the commoner examples and contrast their pharmacokinetic properties
- therapeutic uses: a drug class can be used for several indications (e.g. although beta-blockers are described in the ischaemic heart disease section of Chapter 3, they are also used for hypertension, anxiety and migraine)
- adverse effects: are described in detail under subheadings and, because some subgroups of the population are at particular risk from certain drugs (e.g. beta-blockers precipitate asthma), these *contraindications* are listed
- interactions: patients often take more than one drug at a time: potential adverse interactions, and their clinical consequences, are described.

The final section of each chapter allows self-assessment; we have tried to set questions that require thought rather than recollection of facts. The questions are in the form of patient management problems (which require short answers), multiple choice and essays. The answer is given along with a detailed explanation in each case. Some aspects of a topic may be covered for the first time in this section of the book.

Approach to examinations

There is no correct way to revise for an exam and, by this stage in your career, you have already passed many, so your own system cannot be too bad. However, your performance may be improved by reading the brief notes below.

Before starting to prepare for the exam, you need to know:

- the scope of the syllabus in your medical school (these vary quite widely): consult the list of lectures/tutorials given, or the study guides presented at the start of the course
- the format of the examination (consult past papers if you can)
- how many examinations you will be sitting at once (your revision plan will need to divide time between subjects).

The *notes* you made during lectures, tutorials or group sessions are probably the ideal revision material; the subject was described by, or your reading was guided by, those who set the exam, and reading your notes should stimulate your memory. Large *textbooks of clinical pharmacology* are useful as a reference source during revision, as they were during the course, but you should not try to read them from cover to cover. Furthermore, it is probably unwise to buy more than one reference text; different books may cover the same topic in differing ways, causing confusion. Condensed 'crammers' which rely heavily on lists are probably best avoided: they encourage retention of facts rather than understanding and, on the whole, pharmacology does not lend itself to lists. The present book covers most, but not all, of the topics likely to crop up in undergraduate examinations, and may be used to complement your own notes.

Tips on methods of examination

Multiple choice questions (MCQs)

For the most part, these test your recall of facts. Read the stem of the question with care, paying attention to words such as *only, rarely, usually, never* and *always*.

The most common forms of MCQs involve *either* choosing the most appropriate answer from a list (usually one out of five) *or* answering true/false to each part of the question.

Remember to check the marking system—many MCQ exams employ negative marking.

Short notes

The examiners will have decided on a marking system for each important fact. You should set out your knowledge in a concise manner—no marks will be gained for superfluous information.

Patient management problems

This type of question may be designed to test both recall of factual knowledge and its application to a clinical therapeutic problem. Formats vary, but a common form is an evolving case history, with information being presented sequentially and responses to specific questions (e.g. on choice of drug or anticipated adverse effects). As with '*Short notes*' you should aim to be concise.

Extended matching items questions

In these questions you must choose the option from the list provided that best fits the given statement or question. This type of question, not normally associated with negative marking, is used in United States licensing examinations and similar exams for other bodies, and is used by several undergraduate schools. These questions can easily be adapted to fit multi-disciplinary ('integrated') assessments.

1 Basic principles

Overview

A drug can be taken to mean any molecule used to alter body functions to prevent or treat disease. Though a drug generally produces the same *type* of effect in different people, there can be wide variation in the *degree* of that effect. The factors underlying such *interindividual variation in drug response* have obvious clinical importance and are the main theme of this chapter. Pharmacodynamics describes the physiological and biochemical effects of drugs in the whole animal and at the tissue and molecular level. Most drugs exert their effects by interacting with macromolecular 'targets', which may be receptors, enzymes or structural proteins. Pharmacokinetics is the description of processes affecting the amount of a drug reaching its target location (e.g. rates of absorption and distribution) and its ultimate fate (e.g. metabolism and excretion).

Learning objectives

You should:

- be able to classify the ways in which drugs work at the molecular level

- be able to describe the main forms of regulatory *receptors*, the secondary processes that are usually initiated within the cell and the role of 'second messengers'

- be able to define the terms *agonist* and *antagonist*

- know the mechanisms underlying interindividual responses to drugs

- be able to describe the relationships between drug concentration and response or toxic effects

- be able to define the term therapeutic index and list some drugs with small and large indices.

1.1 Pharmacodynamics

Most drugs exert their effects on the body by interacting with macromolecules, which are usually on the surface of, or within, cells. Variation in these macromolecule targets (such as the number available and the concentration of other compounds competing for binding to the target) is one cause of interindividual variability in drug response. The processes underlying these concepts are termed pharmacodynamics.

Clinical sketch

A 70-year-old man has been taking beta-blockers for many years for his angina. He develops intermittent claudication, and his doctor stops the beta-blocker suddenly. His angina worsens within days, and he is admitted to hospital with a myocardial infarction.

Comment: it is likely that receptor numbers are increased ('upregulated') in the presence of prolonged 'blocking'. Sudden withdrawal of the drug can produce marked effects, as here.

Clinical sketch

A 45-year-old woman with asthma takes both salbutamol and aminophylline for her wheeze.

Comment: both these drugs act via the same 'second messenger', cyclic AMP. Salbutamol increases cyclic AMP production by interacting with a G-protein-linked receptor, while aminophylline 'blocks' the enzyme that metabolises cyclic AMP.

Drug action at the tissue and molecular level

The target macromolecules may be regulatory **receptors**, enzymes or structural proteins. A few drugs can interact directly with transport mechanisms and some can exert direct physical effects (e.g. the osmotic diuretic mannitol).

Target macromolecules

Receptors

Regulatory molecules have evolved to allow endogenous chemical signals (including neuronal and hormonal activity) to affect the internal function of cells; these are termed receptors (Fig. 1). Some receptors are **intracellular**, for example those for glucocorticoids and thyroid hormone. Clearly, in these cases, the drug must be lipid soluble in order to cross the cell membrane. Where the drug–receptor complex influences DNA transcription, the resultant mRNA encodes for the synthesis of a new protein that alters cell function: such complicated processes are slow.

Many receptors are situated in the cell membrane and act in various ways to pass the message to the cell interior.

Transmembrane enzymes. These may have a drug (or hormone) binding site lying outside the cell membrane (e.g. the receptor for insulin) and an enzyme moiety at the intracellular end; insulin receptors work in this way. Binding of hormone (or drug) to the receptor causes the enzyme to become active, catalysing a reaction.

Other transmembrane receptors act via G-protein. Binding of hormone (or drug) to the extracellular receptor causes interaction with a G-protein on the inside aspect of the cell membrane. The G-protein may 'amplify' the initial signal (because the G-protein may remain 'active' long after the receptor has dissociated from the agonist molecule) and interacts with an intracellular enzyme, the product of which (a **second messenger**) changes cell function. Such second messengers include cyclic AMP, inositol polyphosphates and cyclic GMP. Clinical examples of such receptors include β-adrenoceptors and

angiotensin, histamine H_2, 5-hydroxytryptamine (5-HT, or serotonin) and muscarinic acetylcholine receptors.

Ion channels. These transmembrane proteins have a central channel down which selected ions may flow when the channel is open. They permit more rapid responses needed for neuronal function, and the cardiac conducting system. These receptors bridge the lipid bilayer and, when activated, open to allow the passive diffusion of specific ions. Diffusion of the ion along a concentration gradient changes the transmembrane potential, which elicits further intracellular responses. Clinical examples include sodium channels in heart muscle (see cardiac arrhythmia in Ch. 4).

Other target macromolecules

Enzymes. Lipid-soluble drugs often alter cell function by impairing enzyme activity. The drug may resemble the enzyme's natural substrate, with which it may compete for binding. Alternatively, the drug may bind irreversibly to the active site of the enzyme. Examples of enzymes that may be inhibited by drugs are numerous and include dihydrofolate reductase (methotrexate), xanthine oxidase (allopurinol) and monoamine oxidase (selegiline).

Structural proteins. An example of a drug targeting structural proteins is the binding of colchicine (used for gout) to tubulin. Drug binding inhibits tubulin polymerisation and, therefore, interferes with the migration and mitosis of cells of the immune system.

Transport mechanisms. Living cells maintain internal concentrations of ions such as Na^+, K^+, Cl^- and Ca^{2+} that differ from external concentrations. Therefore, the passive entry of ions via specific channels must be opposed by active pumping in the reverse direction to maintain

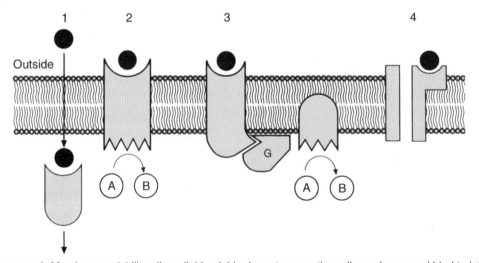

Fig. 1 Drug receptors. **1.** Membrane solubility allows lipid-soluble drugs to cross the cell membrane and bind to intracellular receptors. **2.** Transmembrane proteins bind the drug at the extracellular side of the cell membrane and binding activates an intracellular enzyme site. **3.** The transmembrane protein is linked to an enzyme via a G-protein. **4.** The receptor is a transmembrane ion channel.

gradients. Such pumps are usually enzyme systems that consume energy in the form of ATP. Examples include NA^+/K^+-ATPase (which is inhibited by digoxin) and H^+/K^+-ATPase (which is inhibited by omeprazole).

Drugs with physicochemical effects

Some drugs have direct physiochemical effects, for example antacids (used for dyspepsia), resins (such as those used for hypercholesterolaemia) and osmotically active compounds (such as mannitol).

Relationship between dose and response

Agonists

Agonists are compounds that bind to receptors and stimulate them. In in vitro systems, the relationship between concentration and response resembles that in Figure 2. The maximum drug effect is often termed E_{max} and the concentration of drug required for half the maximum effect is termed EC_{50} ('effective concentration 50%'). Agonists can be subdivided into *full* agonists (Fig. 3, compound A), which induce a maximal response when all receptors are occupied, and *partial* agonists, which produce a submaximal response even when all receptors are occupied (Fig. 3, compound B). Compound A in Figure 3 has greater **efficacy** than compound B. The term **potency** refers to the relative concentration (or dose) of a drug needed to produce a given response. In Figure 3, drugs A and B are equipotent even though A is more efficacious; drug C has greater potency than either A or B (i.e. drug C achieves the same effect at a lower dose). The *shape* of the curve also has clinical significance: drugs A and D have similar E_{max} and EC_{50} values, but drug D has a much steeper curve; this may have clinically important consequences if undesirable

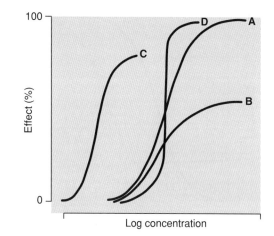

Fig. 3 Full and partial agonists and the concepts of efficacy and potency. Drug A is a full agonist while drug B is a partial agonist. Drugs A and B are equipotent even though A is more efficacious, while drug C has greater potency than either A or B. Drug D has similar potency to drug A and is equally efficacious, but it has a steeper dose–response curve.

effects (like coma) are seen at the higher concentrations. Drug D may have a narrow **therapeutic window**.

Therapeutic window

Clinicians use drugs to achieve a particular result, which is termed therapeutic. If the dose of any drug is increased sufficiently, unwanted or toxic effects invariably develop. In a given population, the dose of drug required to produce a desired effect varies, usually yielding a bell-shaped curve when plotted, a so-called normal distribution; the same is usually true for undesired effects (Fig. 6). The 'gap' between the dose needed to produce the desired effect in 50% of the population and that needed for the undesired effect is termed the therapeutic window or index. Drugs with broad therapeutic windows (like penicillins, β_2-agonists and thiazide diuretics) are generally safe and easy to use. Those with narrow therapeutic windows (like digoxin, theophyllines, lithium and phenytoin) can be difficult to use unless plasma concentrations are measured frequently: this is called **therapeutic drug monitoring**.

Antagonists

Antagonists bind to receptors *without* stimulating them; by occupying the receptors they prevent access by agonists. **Competitive** antagonists (for example, beta-blockers; Ch. 3) form bonds with receptor molecules that are rapidly reversible, just like those of the agonist. As the antagonist concentration rises, progressively more receptors become occupied; however, the effects of a competitive antagonist may be abolished by increasing the agonist concentration so that the agonist competes with the antagonist for the binding site

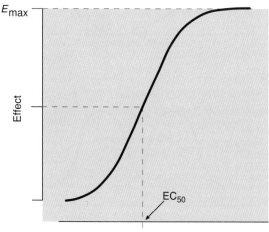

Fig. 2 A dose–response curve.

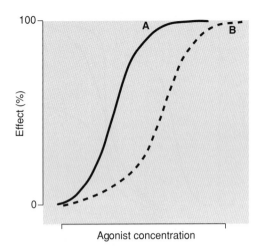

Fig. 4 Competitive antagonist. Curve A is the agonist effect in the absence of antagonist. Curve B is its effect in the presence of a fixed concentration of antagonist. The antagonist effect is abolished at high concentrations of agonist.

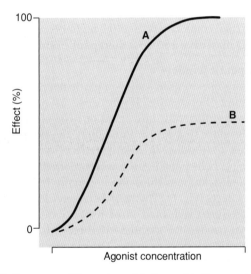

Fig. 5 Non-competitive antagonist. Curve A is the agonist effect in the absence of agonist. Curve B is its effect in the presence of a fixed concentration of antagonist. The antagonist effect cannot be overcome entirely, in contrast to the competitive antagonist.

(Fig.4). **Non-competitive** antagonists (e.g. omeprazole) form bonds with the receptor, usually at sites other than the 'natural' agonist-binding site, that are near-irreversible; in some cases, they may be covalent. When covalent bonding occurs, the inhibition of effect cannot be overcome entirely no matter how high the agonist concentration is raised (Fig. 5). The duration of action of such antagonists is determined by the rate of receptor turnover.

How drugs work at the 'level' of the intact animal

Clinical sketch

A patient with infective endocarditis is treated with high-dose penicillin and gentamicin. The concentration of penicillin is not monitored, but that of gentamicin is monitored frequently.

Comment: infective endocarditis is fatal if improperly treated. Penicillin has a very large therapeutic window and, so long as the patient is not allergic, serious toxicity from penicillin is unusual. In contrast, the therapeutic index of gentamicin is very small: unless concentrations are carefully monitored, patients develop ototoxicity and nephrotoxicity.

Clinical sketch

A 40-year-old man has been abusing diamorphine (heroin) for many years. Gradually, the dose needed to achieve the desired effect has increased. He is found dead in his flat.

*Comment: there is downregulation of opiate receptors in individuals who take the drug for long periods, and greater doses are needed to achieve euphoria (**tolerance**). Unfortunately, diamorphine is a respiratory depressant, and there is less tolerance to this effect.*

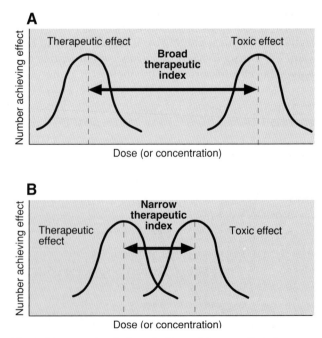

Fig. 6 Therapeutic window. **A.** A broad therapeutic index, where there is a wide gap between the desired effect and toxic effects. **B.** A narrow therapeutic index.

Pharmacodynamic causes of interindividual variation in drug response

There are two main pharmacodynamic reasons for the variation between individuals in their response to drugs.

Variation in concentration of endogenous agonists

The concentration of endogenous agonists, like catecholamines, can vary between individuals and within the same person. Predictably therefore, specific antagonists or agonists administered against this varying background produce variable responses.

Variation in receptors

Continued stimulation/inhibition of living systems tends to induce compensatory processes, and the area of receptor–agonist/antagonist interactions is no exception. Consequently, individuals continually exposed to an agonist/antagonist predictably require larger doses to achieve a given effect than would a drug-naive subject. For example, people continually exposed to gamma-aminobutyric acid (GABA) agonists (like benzodiazepine sedatives) need bigger doses to achieve an effect. This **tolerance** is thought, in part, to result from a decrease in receptor numbers, or **downregulation**. The opposite may also occur; in patients on long-term beta-blocker therapy, it is thought that catecholamine receptor numbers are increased – **upregulation**. This explains the tendency to a marked rise in blood pressure if the drug is stopped suddenly (rebound hypertension). In addition to changes in the numbers of a receptor, changes can also occur in receptor sensitivity to an agonist. Sensitivity can decrease with constant exposure although it is not fully understood how this occurs. There may also be genetic variation in the sensitivity of a receptor to a drug, with individual patients showing varying responses, e.g. responses of β-adrenoceptors.

1.2 Pharmacokinetics

Learning objectives

You should:

- appreciate that most drugs act systemically and need to be absorbed; a proportion of a topical drug may also be absorbed

- be able to describe the Henderson–Hasselbach equation and follow its relevance to drug disposition

- appreciate that most drugs are partially bound to plasma proteins but it is the unbound drug fraction that is active

- be aware of the influence of disease on plasma protein binding

- appreciate that biotransformation usually converts drugs into inactive water-soluble compounds for elimination in urine or bile

- be aware that biotransformation is very prone to interindividual variation (caused by genetic and environmental factors)

- know that drugs can be excreted in bile and by the kidneys

Clinical response to a drug can sometimes be directly measured with accuracy, like the effect of insulin on blood sugar or warfarin on clotting, and this measurement alone can be enough to predict how *much* drug is needed and *how often*. More usually such direct measurements are impossible and an indirect approach (using drug concentrations, and their rates of change) can be used to predict the magnitude and duration of action of a drug. Variation in drug concentration and their rates of change (because of differences in absorption, distribution, metabolism or excretion) is the other major cause of interindividual variability in drug response: the underlying concepts are termed *pharmacokinetics*.

Clinical sketch

A man with angina pectoris has not understood instructions on the use of glyceryl trinitrate tablets. He swallows them instead of putting them under his tongue. There is no therapeutic benefit.

Comment: this drug is subject to extensive first-pass metabolism.

Clinical sketch

A patient with extensive burns is given intramuscular opiate for the pain. His blood pressure is very low. Adequate pain relief is not achieved for over half an hour.

Comment: muscle blood flow is reduced by shock, and the rate of drug absorption can be affected.

Absorption

Most drugs require absorption for activity. Topical drugs may also be absorbed, giving rise to unwanted effects.

Factors affecting the rate and degree of absorption

Lipid solubility

Drugs must cross lipid cell membranes in order to be absorbed. The lipid solubility of a drug is largely determined by factors such as molecular weight and structure. However, lipid solubility of an individual drug is variable: only the *unionised* fraction of the drug is lipid soluble. Most drugs are weak acids or bases, and their degree of ionisation is determined by the surrounding pH and their pK_a (the pK_a is the pH at which the drug is 50% ionised). The Henderson–Hasselbach equation allows the unionised fraction to be calculated:

for acids: pH = pK_a + log (ionised conc./unionised conc.)

for bases: pH = pK_a + log (unionised conc./ionised conc.).

Thus, weak bases are predictably better absorbed from the small bowel. Weak acids might be expected to be absorbed from the stomach, but factors such as surface area influence this.

Surface area

The greater the surface area, the faster absorption takes place. The surface area of the small bowel exceeds that of the stomach to such a degree that even acidic drugs will usually be more extensively absorbed from this site. So if given orally, the rate of absorption of most drugs is greatly influenced by the rate of gastric emptying. Small bowel surface area can be reduced by diseases.

Other factors

The drug must spend an adequate time at the absorption site. Short transit time (e.g. during gastroenteritis) may reduce the degree of absorption. Blood flow is another important factor. For example, in severe hypotension, blood flow to muscle may be low and intramuscular (i.m.) drugs may be absorbed slowly.

Bioavailability

Bioavailability refers to the fraction of the dose which proceeds *unaltered* from the site of administration to the systemic circulation. When a drug is given intravenously (i.v.), 100% of the dose enters the systemic circulation, and bioavailability is 1.0. While incomplete absorption often accounts for low bioavailability, there are other possible explanations (Fig. 7):

- it may be broken down by acid conditions in the gut, e.g. benzylpenicillin
- it may be metabolised by enzymes in the gut wall or liver before reaching the systemic venous blood (e.g. glyceryl trinitrate). This is termed the **first pass** effect.

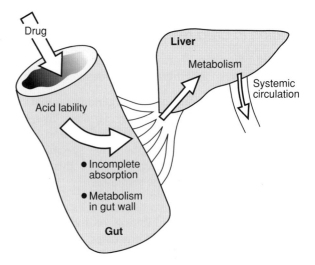

Fig. 7 Causes of incomplete bioavailability.

Distribution

Clinical sketch

A man takes phenytoin for his epilepsy. Unknown to him, his plasma albumin falls markedly over the next few weeks, without the dose of phenytoin being changed. He develops marked ataxia.

Comment: the clinical relevance of plasma protein binding is often much less clear cut than in this example. Here, the patient's ataxia has resulted from an increase in the free concentration of phenytoin.

Clinical sketch

A patient with meningitis is treated with gentamicin. The organism is very sensitive to the antibiotic in vitro, but the patient shows no improvement.

Comment: this would be very unacceptable clinical practice and the patient may well die. Gentamicin does not readily cross the blood–brain barrier.

Plasma protein binding

Most drugs travel in the plasma partly in solution in the plasma water and partly bound to plasma proteins—the ratio of one to the other varies between drugs. Binding is reversible and the bound and unbound drug fractions are always in a state of dynamic equilibrium. Only the *unbound* drug fraction is available to cross membranes and produce an effect. Acidic drugs mainly bind to albumin, while basic drugs bind more avidly to α_1-acid glycoprotein. Plasma protein binding can be clinically important when, because of a disease state (see Ch. 20), plasma protein concentrations fall (e.g. albumin concen-

A

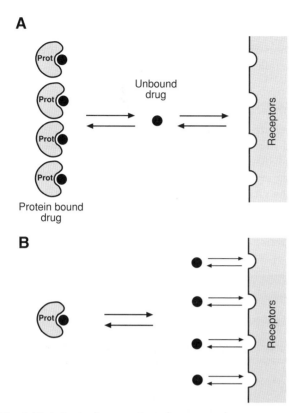

Fig. 8 Variation in plasma protein concentration. **A.** High levels of plasma proteins; **B.** reduced levels of plasma proteins.

trations in liver cirrhosis) or rise (e.g. α_1-acid glycoprotein in acute infection) (Fig. 8). Warfarin and diazepam are examples of drugs extensively bound to proteins (90% or more). Examples of drugs with less extensive protein binding include digoxin and gentamicin.

Tissue distribution

Most drugs have their effects in the tissues. The degree to which a given drug is likely to accumulate in a tissue can be predicted (without accuracy) from knowledge of its lipophilicity and the blood flow of the tissue. A highly lipophilic drug crosses membranes readily even in the presence of tight junctions between endothelial cells (e.g. into the central nervous system (CNS)); the principal determinant of tissue distribution is organ blood flow. For example, the anaesthetic thiopental is highly lipophilic and accumulates to a greater degree in brain than in muscle because of the much higher blood flow to the former. In contrast, a hydrophilic drug (like gentamicin) crosses membranes poorly. The principal determinant of tissue distribution will, therefore, be the degree of 'leakiness' of the capillary endothelium. For example, gentamicin accumulates to a greater degree in muscle than in brain because of the leaky nature of muscle capillaries.

Biotransformation (or drug metabolism)

Most biotransformation takes place in the liver (other sites include the gut wall (e.g. contraceptive steroids) and plasma (succinylcholine)). The chemical processes involved are numerous and are broadly classified into phase I and II reactions, which (confusingly) does not mean that phase I necessarily precedes or is followed by phase II. **Phase I** processes include oxidation, reduction and hydrolysis. Of these, oxidation reactions are most common and are often catalysed by one of the family of cytochrome P450 enzymes. Phase I usually results in:

- introduction or exposure of a polar group
- increased water solubility
- abolition of pharmacological activity.

However, this is not invariable: the phase I products of some drugs have pharmacological activity while the parent compound does not (the so-called **prodrugs**, e.g. enalapril, see Ch. 31) while in other cases the phase I products are highly toxic, for example in paracetamol poisoning (see Ch. 7). **Phase II** processes (often termed conjugation) involve the attachment to the drug of an endogenous substance, such as glucuronate, sulphate or acetyl groups. The resulting conjugate is almost invariably polar, water soluble and without pharmacological activity (morphine is an exception, see Ch. 7).

Variation in biotransformation

Genetic factors (genetic polymorphisms)
Genetically differences have profound effects on the levels of certain drugs in the body. For example, several drugs are eliminated by **acetylation**, e.g. isoniazid (Ch. 13), procainamide (Ch. 3) and hydralazine (Ch. 3). 'Slow acetylators' are at risk of toxicity from these drugs. (The proportions of fast and slow acetylators vary between ethnic groups.) Other genetically determined variations include poor metabolisers of the muscle relaxant succinylcholine (Ch. 8).

Disease-induced factors
Diseases affecting the liver are particularly important in drug metabolism, for example metabolism of opioids is slower in patients with liver disease (see Ch. 20).

Induction and inhibition of cytochrome P450 enzymes
Some drugs can increase the rate of synthesis of cytochrome P450 enzymes and this enzyme induction can enhance the clearance of other drugs. Usually such induction requires exposure to the inducing agent for over a week before effects are seen. Examples of inducing agents are:

- rifampicin
- carbamazepine
- phenobarbital
- phenytoin.

Other drugs can inhibit cytochrome P450 enzymes (usually by competing for the enzyme's active site). This is usually seen rapidly after drug exposure (within a couple of days). Examples of enzyme-inhibiting agents are:

- cimetidine
- erythromycin
- ciprofloxacin
- isoniazid.

Concentration-dependent biotransformation
Most drugs are metabolised by concentration-independent mechanisms: in other words there is always excess enzyme 'capacity' irrespective of drug concentration. Consequently, the proportion of drug metabolised in a set time is constant. However, some drugs can saturate a rate-limiting enzyme within the therapeutic range. Under these circumstances (some-

times called zero-order processes) the proportion of drug metabolised in a set time diminishes as its concentration rises. A good clinical example of this is the antiepileptic drug phenytoin (Ch. 6).

Excretion

Some drugs (e.g. aminoglycosides, atenolol, gliclazide and digoxin) are mainly excreted without metabolism; renal disease will cause such drugs to accumulate. Most drug metabolites are inactive, hence biotransformation is the vital step in terminating drug action. If, however, metabolites are active (e.g. the principal metabolite of diazepam), drug action may only be terminated by excretion.

Clinical sketch

A patient with congestive cardiac failure is being treated with loop diuretics. She has severely impaired renal function. The diuresis obtained by enormous doses of furosemide (frusemide) is modest.

Comment: we tend to think of renal excretion as a terminator of drug action. In the case of the loop diuretics, the drug works on ion transporters in the luminal membrane. Therefore, drug action correlates with glomerular filtration rate, and furosemide (frusemide) tends to work poorly in patients with renal failure.

Clinical sketch

A patient is given digoxin for atrial fibrillation. He has impaired renal function. No measurements of digoxin concentration are made, and the patient develops complete heart block.

Comment: digoxin is eliminated unchanged, and accumulates in renal impairment. Therapeutic drug monitoring is mandatory, and this case illustrates a very low standard of clinical practice.

Renal excretion

Glomerular filtration
Renal blood flow is about 1.5 l/min, and about 10% of this, by volume, appears as glomerular filtrate. Only unbound drug may be filtered since protein molecules are too large.

Tubular secretion
Cells of the proximal convoluted tubule can actively secrete some compounds, mostly relatively strong acids and bases, into the lumen of the nephron (e.g. peni-

cillin). Under these circumstances and assuming that no reabsorption occurs, the rate of excretion of a drug exceeds its rate of filtration.

Tubular reabsorption

Active reabsorption has evolved to help to conserve nutrients. Certain drugs too may be extensively reabsorbed: such compounds tend to be lipid soluble and unionised at urine pH (see the Henderson–Hasselbach equation on p. 8). This is of most importance in drug poisoning. For example, in aspirin overdose:

- aspirin is an acid with a pK_a of 3.5
- if the urinary pH is 2.5 then the ratio of ionised:unionised drug is 0.1 (antilog of -1), i.e. 90% of the drug is unionised, it crosses membranes readily and will be reabsorbed
- if the urine pH were 5.5 then the same ratio is 100 (antilog of 2), i.e. only 1% of the drug is unionised and it crosses membranes poorly.

This is the basis of 'alkaline diuresis' (see Ch. 17).

Other routes of excretion

Biliary

Parent drugs and metabolites with molecular weights greater than 350 may be actively excreted into the bile; examples include many drug conjugates (products of phase II metabolism). This process may be followed by loss of the drug in the faeces. However, drug conjugates may be broken down by gut bacteria, releasing the parent drug, which may be reabsorbed. The resulting **enterohepatic circulation** may have important clinical consequences, for example with oral contraceptive steroids.

Minor routes

Drugs may be excreted in saliva, sweat, tears and expired air, but none of these is a major route. Lactating mothers excrete some drugs in breast milk, with potentially important consequences for the breast-fed infant.

1.3 Pharmacokinetic parameters

Learning objectives

You should:

- be able to describe the phases of the concentration versus time curves of a drug after oral administration
- appreciate that, to make useful clinical predictions, drug disposition must be 'reduced' to numerical parameters, such as half-life, clearance and apparent volume of distribution
- be aware that pharmacokinetic parameters allow predictions to be made regarding the duration of drug action and the effects of disease states, interindividual variation and other drugs on drug disposition.

Clinical sketch

A patient with moderately severe renal failure needs gentamicin for septicaemia. The clinical team consults Appendix 3 of the BNF and is advised to give the drug at reduced dose and longer dose interval.

Comment: gentamicin is eliminated by the kidney and its half-life is longer in patients with renal failure.

Clinical sketch

A patient is admitted after a large overdose of amitriptyline. The clinical team consults the local poisons unit and is told that haemodialysis would not contribute to management.

Comment: amitriptyline has a large volume of distribution (around 18 l/kg). This indicates that most of the drug is in the tissues. Therefore, only a small proportion of the drug in the body would pass through the haemodialysis machine.

Pharmacokinetics allows predictions to be made regarding the activity of a drug in the body; to be useful, these predictions must be reduced to numerical parameters such as half-life, clearance and volume of distribution (VD).

Half-life

Half-life is the easiest pharmacokinetic parameter to envisage and is the time taken for concentration to fall to half its original value; the unit of measurement is hours. Drug concentration data are usually plotted against time, as illustrated in Figure 9. When concentration data are plotted arithmetically (Fig. 9A), an exponential curve results, and the data are often easier to handle if the vertical scale is logarithmic (Fig. 9B). Half-life is the main determinant of dose frequency (Fig. 10). A drug achieves 50% of its steady-state concentration after one half-life, 75% after two half-lives, 88% after three, 94% after four and 97% after five half-lives.

Area under the curve

The area under the curve (AUC) refers to the area under a concentration versus time curve for a drug and is used

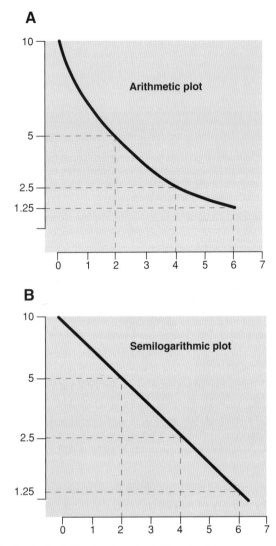

Fig. 9 The half-life of a drug. **A.** Arithmetic plot.
B. Semilogarithmic plot.

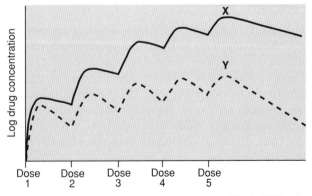

Fig. 10 Two drugs given at the same interval. The half-life of drug X is half that of drug Y, and drug X, therefore, accumulates to a greater degree.

in the calculation of most other parameters. In Figure 11, which represents data obtained after an oral dose, AUC

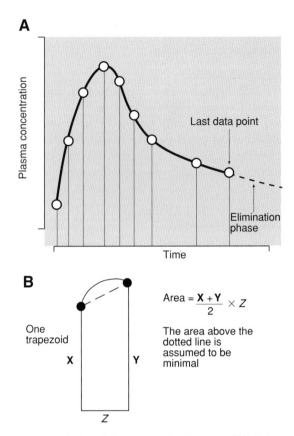

Fig. 11 Calculation of the area under the curve (AUC) from summation of trapezoids. **A.** Data from multiple oral doses. **B.** One trapezoid.

can be calculated from the time of dosing to the last data point by summation of the trapezoids. Extrapolation of the elimination phase (the dotted line in Fig. 11A) allows calculation of the AUC to infinity; the unit of measurement is of the form grams per litre per hour (g/l per h).

Clearance

For the majority of drugs the rate of elimination E is directly proportional to the drug concentration c. In other words: $E = kc$, where k is a constant. This constant is termed clearance (C) and can be envisaged as the *volume* of plasma that is 'cleared' completely of the drug per unit time; the unit of measurement is, therefore, of the form litres per hour (l/h).

Apparent volume of distribution

Once in the tissue, most drugs bind to macromolecules: some of this binding mediates drug action, while other binding is 'inert'. Some drugs, like aspirin, mainly stay in the circulation and undergo little tissue binding whereas others, like the tricyclic antidepressants, are so extensively bound in the tissues (mostly in an 'inert'

A

B

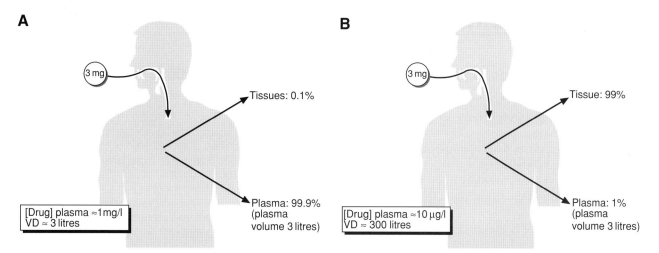

Fig. 12 Apparent volume of distribution (VD). **A.** A drug that is minimally tissue bound would have, for example, 0.1% in the tissues and 99.9% left in the plasma; For a 3 mg dose, this would leave 2.997 mg in the plasma. In a 70 kg adult with a plasma volume of 3 litres, the plasma concentration would be 0.999 mg/l. VD is the drug in the body divided by that in the plasma, i.e. 3 ÷ 0.999 = 3.003l. This is roughly equal to the plasma volume. **B.** An extremely tissue-bound drug might have 99% in the tissues and in this case a 3 mg dose will give a plasma concentration of 10 μg l^{-1} and VD of 300 litres.

manner) that plasma concentrations are small. Figure 12 shows the effect of tissue binding on the plasma concentration of the drug and on its VD. VD is calculated from the amount of drug in the body, divided by the plasma concentration. Where drugs have minimal tissue binding (Fig. 12A) the VD is close to the plasma volume. Where tissue binding is high, the apparent VD is high, 300 litres in Figure 12B. In the real world, we never know precisely how much drug is in the tissues of a living subject—it cannot be measured—but VD gives an *indirect* measure of the degree of tissue distribution. The units of measurement are those of volume (millilitre or litre) and are often adjusted for body weight. VD values range from about 0.1 l/kg body weight (e.g. for salicylate or warfarin), through 1–10 l/kg (e.g. digoxin or propranolol) to 20 l/kg (e.g. tricyclics).

Self-assessment: questions

Multiple choice questions

1. Regarding drug receptors:
   a. A drug usually binds to only one receptor type
   b. Cellular responses to receptors that are ion channels are usually fast
   c. Cellular responses are slow if the mode of action involves modification of DNA transcription
   d. G-proteins amplify the effect of receptor stimulation
   e. Receptors are continually being synthesised and destroyed by the cell

2. Antagonists:
   a. Do not themselves bind to receptors but interfere with the binding of agonists
   b. Bind to receptors but do not stimulate them
   c. May bind covalently to receptors
   d. Usually bind to receptors for very short periods (fractions of a second)
   e. If competitive, can be overcome by increasing the agonist concentration

3. The following statements describe pharmacodynamic concepts:
   a. All drugs act by binding to cell macromolecules
   b. Drug A is said to be more potent than drug B if drug A's maximal effect is greater than that of drug B
   c. A partial agonist is a drug that binds to a receptor without stimulating it
   d. The expression therapeutic index refers to the difference between the concentration of a drug required to produce its effects and that required to produce toxicity
   e. Drug A is said to be more efficacious than drug B if drug A produces its maximum effect at a lower concentration than drug B

4. The following statements describe pharmacokinetic concepts:
   a. Only the unbound (free) drug fraction has pharmacological effects
   b. All drug metabolism takes place in the liver
   c. All drugs must first be metabolised before they can be excreted
   d. Only the unionised drug fraction may cross intact cell membranes
   e. Drug metabolites invariably lack pharmacological effects

Case history questions

Case history 1

> A 40-year-old man is on salbutamol for his asthma. His doctor finds that he is hypertensive and starts him on atenolol.

1. How do salbutamol and atenolol work?
2. Is this good prescribing?
3. What will the likely outcome be to this man's hypertension and asthma?

Case history 2

> You are the expert witness for the prosecution in a case of alleged medical negligence.
>
> A young woman on a low-dose combined oral contraceptive pill went on holiday to St Petersburg with her boyfriend. She had read that many people catch gastroenteritis in this destination and sought advice from her doctor. He prescribed doxycycline and advised her to take this throughout her 3-week stay. Upon her return, she became concerned that she may be pregnant and did a pregnancy test: it was positive.

1. What may have happened?
2. Do you think she has a case?
3. What concerns might there be for the fetus?

Short note questions

Write short notes on the following:

1. A new drug is being developed and its manufacturers want to know its oral bioavailability:
   a. What clinical reasons are there for determining oral bioavailability?
   b. Should bioavailability be tested with only fasted subjects? If your answer is no, explain why
   c. How would you go about measuring bioavailability in a group of 12 healthy subjects?

2. An antihypertensive drug is given to 12 volunteers; the concentration of the drug is measured in the plasma, and its effects on blood pressure are recorded. As seen in Figure 13, the drug had a very

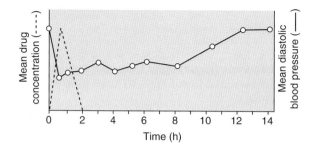

Fig. 13 Plasma concentration of the antihypertensive drug and changes in blood pressure.

short half-life (about 30 minutes) and was detectable for only 2 hours. However, as can also be seen in Figure 13, the effect on diastolic blood pressure was maximal 30 minutes after dosing and returned to predose values after 12 hours. Give two possible explanations for these findings.

3. Consider the following model of drug disposition: water is flowing into a washbasin at a rate of 10 l/min; there is a plug, but it has a 5 mm diameter hole in it.

a. just after the tap is switched on, is the rate of flow through the hole equal to, greater than or less than that from the tap?
b. If the tap is left running at 1 l/min, what will eventually happen to the level of water in the basin?
c. If the tap is left running at 1 l/min but the diameter of the hole is halved, what will happen to the level of water in the basin?
d. If the rate of flow is now gradually reduced, what will happen to the level of water in the basin?
e. In this model, is clearance best represented by the rate of flow through the drain, or by the diameter of the hole?

4. A new drug is found to be eliminated entirely by renal excretion, with no prior metabolism. Its renal clearance (found from plasma and urine concentration data) in an experiment on six healthy subjects is found to be about 200 ml/min; the mean glomerular filtration rate of the six volunteers is about 125 ml/min. What do these data tell you about the mode of excretion of the drug?

Self-assessment: answers

Multiple choice answers

1. a. **False**. We often classify a drug by the type of receptor relevant to its pharmacological effect, but drugs probably bind to far more cell macromolecules than documented. Some of these interactions produce adverse effects, but many produce no obvious effect.
   b. **True**. The influx of ions induced by receptor activation rapidly changes conditions within the cell.
   c. **True**. Such a mechanism explains the slow response to corticosteroids.
   d. **True**. Once activated, many G-proteins remain active for longer than the receptor is occupied by the drug; the second message is dependent upon active G-protein, not occupied receptors, so the signal is amplified.
   e. **True**. Receptors have a variable life-span; the cell can up- or downregulate receptor numbers by increasing/decreasing their rate of synthesis/destruction.

2. a. **False**. Antagonists bind to receptors without stimulating them; they, therefore, occupy receptors that would otherwise be occupied by agonist. This has the effect of reducing the effect of the agonist.
   b. **True**.
   c. **True**. Non-competitive (irreversible) antagonists may do this; there are few clinically used examples, e.g. the alpha-antagonist phenoxybenzamine.
   d. **True**. Competitive antagonists (the group in most common clinical use) usually bind for milliseconds and hence can be displaced by raising the concentration of the agonist.
   e. **True**. As agonist concentrations rise, receptor occupancy by agonist molecules becomes more likely at any given moment. Eventually the effect of the antagonist may be nearly completely overcome.

3. a. **False**. Some drugs act via physical effects, for example osmotic diuretics.
   b. **False**. This is the definition of efficacy.
   c. **False**. A partial agonist binds to a receptor and stimulates it; however, the maximal achievable response is lower than that seen with a full agonist. A partial agonist is also a partial antagonist!
   d. **True**.
   e. **False**. This is the definition of potency.

4. a. **True**. Only the unbound fraction is available to diffuse across membranes to reach its site of action.
   b. **False**. Other sites include lung, gut wall, plasma and kidney.
   c. **False**. Some polar compounds, like gentamicin and digoxin, are excreted unchanged.
   d. **True**. The unionised fraction is lipid soluble and therefore can pass through the membrane.
   e. **False**. Many drugs act entirely via the effects of their metabolites, for example enalapril and zidovudine.

Case history answers

Case history 1

1. Salbutamol is an agonist at β_2-adrenoceptors while atenolol is a β-adrenoceptor antagonist with greater affinity for β_1- than for β_2-adrenoceptors. Even so, its use here carries the strong risk of antagonising the effects of the salbutamol.
2. This is very poor prescribing. In essence, the atenolol is being used for the long-term prevention of cardiovascular risk, such as stroke. There are many alternative drugs that could have been used.
3. Salbutamol will have no deleterious effects on control of blood pressure but atenolol will probably worsen the patient's asthma.

Case history 2

1. Oral contraceptive steroids are given in very low dose to avoid adverse effects. Reliance is placed on enterohepatic circulation. The tetracyclines, by killing gut bacteria, interrupt this circulation and may cause drug failure.
2. The court will decide but, on the face of it, she does. The doctor should have been aware of the interaction (see Appendix 1 of the BNF) and ought to have advised her to use alternative contraceptive precautions.
3. Tetracyclines cross the placenta and may damage developing bone and teeth.

Short note answers

1. a. The new drug must have been shown to have desired pharmacological effects in vitro and also probably in an animal model to get this far.

However, unless the drug gets into the human body, it cannot produce its effects. Bioavailability can vary markedly between species, and even between individuals; this is of obvious importance in deciding dose size.

b. Food can affect bioavailability, and this needs to be examined since the drug will, in due course, be in general use. In many cases, food reduces bioavailability, for example penicillins, cephalosporins, rifampicin, isoniazid and captopril, but in some cases it is increased (e.g. propranolol, metoprolol, griseofulvin and hydralazine).

c. This is usually determined from the AUC of the drug after oral dosing divided by that (in the same subject, but on a different occasion) after i.v. dosing. So in Figure 14, the two AUC values for drug A are about the same: this drug has a bioavailability of about 1.0. Drug B, however, has a much smaller AUC when it is given orally, and also a lower bioavailability.

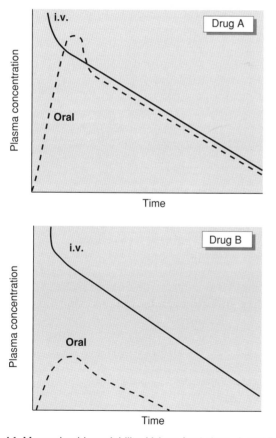

Fig. 14 Measuring bioavalability. Values for 2 days, A and B, given as an oral dose (---) or as an i.v. dose (—).

2. a. This could be a prodrug, which produces its effects through an unidentified metabolite; as shown in Figure 15, the metabolite may have a much longer half-life than the parent compound.

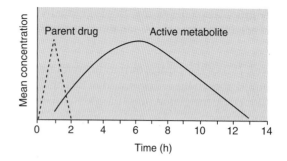

Fig. 15 Plasma concentration for parent drug (---) and active metabolite(—).

b. The drug could be a non-competitive antagonist, which binds irreversibly to its receptor. Drug effects would be terminated by receptor turnover, rather than drug elimination from the plasma.

3. This may seem a poor model for drug disposition, but the two have much in common. Soon after the tap is switched on, the rate of drainage from the basin is much less than the rate of entry, and water accumulates in the basin until the two are equal. Analogous with this is the period immediately after drug dosing (phase A in Fig. 16): the rate of drug absorption exceeds that of elimination, and the plasma concentration rises. Because the rate of elimination is proportional to drug concentration, a time will come when the two are equal (point B in Fig. 16). In the model, narrowing the hole in the plug will reduce the rate of drainage, causing further accumulation of water in the basin until a new equilibrium is reached. The diameter of the hole represents the constant termed **clearance**. Finally, if the tap is gradually turned off over the next half hour or so, the level of water in the basin will fall. The same happens to a finite drug dose: as the proportion of the dose unabsorbed falls, the rate of

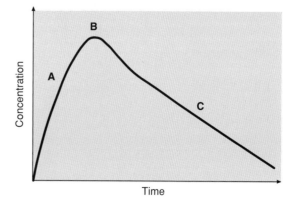

Fig. 16 Clearance of a drug.

absorption also falls, so that this is gradually exceeded by the rate of elimination (phase C in Fig. 16).

4. About 25% of the cardiac output (therefore about 1.2 l/min^{-1}) goes to the kidneys, and of this about 10% is filtered by the glomerulus (the glomerular filtration rate; GFR). The maximum clearance of a drug by this route is, therefore, equal to the GFR; in fact most drugs have much lower filtration rates since only unbound drug can be filtered. The renal clearance of this new drug *exceeds* the GFR; the likeliest explanation is that it is extensively *secreted* by the renal tubules.

2 The autonomic nervous system

Overview

Many drugs have their effects, or adverse effects, by working on the autonomic nervous system. In this chapter the basic anatomy and physiology of the system is described, with the classes of drug that affect it.

The autonomic system can be separated into sympathetic and parasympathetic divisions and the roles of these are described.

2.1 Structure and function

Learning objectives

You should:

- be able to describe the anatomical layout of the sympathetic and parasympathetic systems

- be able to list the neurotransmitter substances released by preganglionic and postganglionic fibres of both systems

- be able to describe the classification, relevant structure and function of the various receptors found in both systems

- be able to describe the mechanisms that terminate neurotransmitter 'activity'.

Many drugs produce their effects by working on the autonomic system, for example antihypertensives and bronchodilators, and the same mechanisms explain the adverse effects of many others, for example some neuroleptics and the antiarrhythmics. The autonomic nervous system regulates visceral functions, such as cardiac output, gut motility, endocrine and exocrine gland func-

tion and blood vessel tone, and is not under conscious control. It is separated on anatomical and physiological grounds into **sympathetic** and **parasympathetic** divisions. It is useful to think of stimulation by the sympathetic division inducing conditions for *flight* or *fight*, such as increased heart rate and stroke volume, dilatation of the pupils, increased blood sugar, cutaneous vasoconstriction and contraction of sphincters, while stimulation by the parasympathetic system usually, but not always, has the opposite actions.

Structure of the sympathetic system

The sympathetic system is controlled by centres in the hypothalamus and brainstem. 'Outflow' from the brain is via the **descending reticular system** of synapsing neurones. Nerve fibres finally leave the spinal cord with the nerve roots, between T1 and L2, and pass into the **sympathetic trunk** where most synapse. The 'first-order neurones' are referred to as **preganglionic**. **Postganglionic** fibres then pursue a lengthy course (Fig. 17) finally reaching such structures as the heart, blood vessels, bronchi, pupillary muscle and gut. One exception to this general pattern is innervation of the

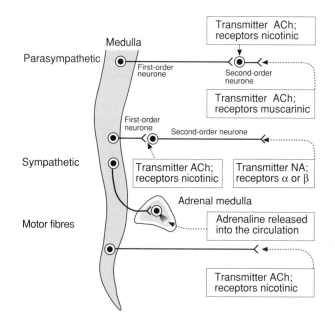

Fig. 17 Anatomy of the autonomic nervous system. ACh, acetylcholine; NA, noradrenaline.

adrenal medulla, where first-order neurones travel directly to the organ and synapse with modified neurones in the medulla, which secretes adrenaline (epinephrine) into the circulation.

Structure of the parasympathetic system

The parasympathetic system is also controlled within the hypothalamus and brainstem, by a series of specific nuclei. Preganglionic fibres leave the CNS with the cranial nerves (especially the vagus nerve) and sacral nerve roots. Unlike sympathetic ganglia, those of the parasympathetic system are very close to their destination, and postganglionic fibres are short (Fig. 17).

Function

Neurotransmitters

The term neurotransmitter is given to any molecule, released by neurones, that causes depolarisation of the membrane of another cell (another neurone, a muscle fibre or a gland). There are antagonists to specific receptors, described below.

Preganglionic neurotransmitters. Neurones of both parasympathetic and sympathetic systems release acetylcholine, as do somatic nerve fibres.

Postganglionic neurotransmitters. Second-order neurones of the parasympathetic system release acetylcholine. In contrast, fibres of the sympathetic system release noradrenaline. There are two exceptions to this: (a) the sympathetic transmitter at sweat glands is acetylcholine, and (b) certain postganglionic sympathetic fibres release dopamine, for example those to the renal/ splanchnic vasculature.

Termination of neurotransmitter action

The action of acetylcholine in synaptic clefts is terminated very rapidly by the local enzyme acetylcholinesterase (Fig. 18).

The action of noradrenaline (norepinephrine) is partly terminated by diffusion away from the cleft but mainly by cellular absorption. Absorption into the presynaptic cell (**uptake 1**) leads to metabolism of noradrenaline (norepinephrine) by mitochondrial monoamine oxidase (MAO). Absorption into the postsynaptic cell (**uptake 2**) leads to metabolism by catechol-*O*-methyltransferase (COMT) (Fig. 18).

Receptors

Receptors are divided into groups based on the neurotransmitter involved. They can be further subdivided by their response to agonists and knowledge of these subgroups and the effects of their stimulation has been used in the design of drugs for a desired effect.

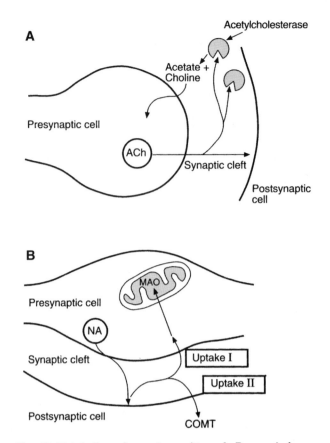

Fig. 18 Metabolism of neurotransmitters. **A.** Removal of acetylcholine (ACh) from the cholinergic synaptic cleft, which terminates its activity. **B.** In adrenergic synaptic clefts, noradrenaline (NA) (norepinephrine) is absorbed into the cells where it is metabolised by monoamine oxidase (MAO) or by catechol-*O*-methyltransferase (COMT).

Cholinergic receptors

Receptors on postganglionic fibres and effector cells differ in their structure, and this explains the selectivity of many of the drugs dealt with below.

Postganglionic receptors. In *both* sympathetic and parasympathetic divisions, receptors on the postganglionic cell membranes, as well as responding to acetylcholine, can be stimulated by the agonist nicotine. They are, therefore, termed **nicotinic**. The receptor is an ion channel for Na^+ and K^+, and activation of the receptor causes depolarisation of the postganglionic fibre.

Receptors on effector cells of the parasympathetic system. These are found in such tissues as smooth muscle and glands. They can be stimulated by muscarine and are, therefore, termed **muscarinic**. The cellular events that occur after stimulation of muscarinic receptors are complex: intracellular cyclic GMP levels rise, inositol phospholipid turnover accelerates and adenyl cyclase is inhibited, but the role of each second messenger is not established.

Adrenergic receptors

The adrenergic receptors (adrenoceptors) respond to catecholamines.

The α₁-adrenoceptors. These are *postsynaptic* and are found especially on smooth muscle. At a cellular level, stimulation causes release of inositol trisphosphate and an increase in intracellular Ca^{2+}. At an organ level, stimulation causes contraction of smooth muscle.

The α₂ adrenoceptors. *Outside the CNS,* these are *presynaptic,* occurring at peripheral adrenergic nerve terminals. At a cellular level, stimulation causes inhibition of adenyl cyclase and reduction of intracellular cyclic AMP; this leads to inhibition of release of further noradrenaline (norepinephrine) from the terminal. Stimulation of α₂-adrenoceptors, therefore, acts as 'feedback' control of noradrenaline release. In contrast, *inside the CNS,* α₂-adrenoceptors are *postsynaptic,* and are the main adrenoceptors of the CNS components of the sympathetic system.

The β₁-adrenoceptors. These are mainly located in the heart. At a cellular level, stimulation causes activation of adenyl cyclase and an increase in intracellular cyclic AMP. At an organ level, stimulation produces an increase in heart rate (positive chronotropic effect) and contractility (positive inotropic effect).

The β₂-adrenoceptors. These are widely distributed, but sites of particular importance include the smooth muscle of blood vessels, bronchi and uterus. The cellular mechanisms are the same as for β₁-adrenoceptors. At an organ level, stimulation of β₂-adrenoceptors produces smooth muscle relaxation.

Dopamine receptors. These are most numerous within the CNS, but they are also important in control of renal blood flow. Stimulation produces renal vasodilatation.

2.2 Cholinergic drugs

Learning objectives

You should:

- be able to distinguish drugs that are true agonists from those that block acetylcholine metabolism (anticholinesterases)
- be able to outline the organ specific effects of cholinergic agonists and their clinical uses
- appreciate that the anticholinergics in therapeutic use all act at the muscarinic receptor, and that there are no antinicotinics in common use
- be able to list some antimuscarinic drugs and describe their clinical use
- be able to list the organ-specific effects of atropine.

Clinical sketch

A woman develops a painful red eye. The ophthalmologist diagnoses acute closed-angle glaucoma and plans surgery to correct this. To reduce the intraocular pressure immediately, pilocarpine eye drops are prescribed.

Comment: Pilocarpine is a direct-acting cholinergic agonist. It causes pupillary constriction, thereby opening up the angle between the iris and the cornea. This enhances drainage of the aqueous humour.

Cholinergic agonists

True cholinergic agonists have their effect by a direct interaction with the cholinergic receptor, indirect agonists act by prolonging the life of acetylcholine.

True agonists

Pilocarpine is a muscarinic agonist applied topically to cause pupillary constriction (miosis) in the treatment of glaucoma (Fig. 19).

Bethanechol is another muscarinic agonist. It can be used to increase smooth muscle tone in the bladder when treating postoperative urinary retention. Bethanechol is contraindicated in patients with asthma, bradycardia and urinary/gut outflow obstruction.

Indirect agonists

Anticholinesterases act by inhibiting acetylcholinesterase, thereby prolonging the duration of acetylcholine action (see Ch. 8).

Cholinergic antagonists (anticholinergics)

Cholinergic antagonists can be classified as antimuscarinic or antinicotinic depending on the subgroup of receptor affected. Only antagonists acting at muscarinic receptors are in common clinical use.

Antimuscarinic drugs

The classical example of an antimuscarinic drug is *atropine,* a naturally occurring alkaloid that is a non-selective reversible muscarinic antagonist. All the other examples described below have structural similarities with atropine. The effects of atropine on various organs is as follows:

- eye: pupillary dilatation (mydriasis)
- CNS: in standard doses, it causes mild sedation and in high doses, agitation, seizures, hallucinations and

coma; anti-Parkinsonian effects (see Ch. 6) can result from its action in basal ganglia

- gut: reduced secretion and motility, causing constipation
- heart: tachycardia (the vagus nerve is blocked)
- bronchi: bronchodilatation
- bladder: relaxation of the walls, which may lead to urinary retention
- sweat glands: reduced secretion.

Clinical sketch

A man develops parkinsonism from the neuroleptic drugs that he takes for schizophrenia; he takes trihexyphenidyl (benzhexol) for this (see Ch. 6). He becomes depressed and takes an overdose of trihexyphenidyl. On admission, he is confused and has a narrow-complex tachycardia of around 160 beats/min; his blood pressure is low.

Comment: trihexyphenidyl is very like atropine, and causes these features in overdose. Acetylcholine 'agonists', such as physostigmine, may be helpful.

Muscarinic receptors in these sites vary slightly in their drug affinities and this has led to a system of classification as subgroups. Detailed knowledge of this classification is of limited value, but the point to remember is that some drugs bind better at some muscarinic receptors than others, and this explains their selectivity.

Examples of antimuscarinic drugs

Atropine. Atropine is given intravenously (i.v.) to increase heart rate in patients with symptomatic bradycardias and during asystolic cardiac arrest. It may also be used topically in iritis as a mydriatic agent, to prevent the formation of adhesions between the iris and the cornea. Derivatives such as *tropicamide* are more commonly used in this setting.

Pirenzipine. This is a second-line drug for peptic ulcer (Ch. 11).

Trihexyphenidyl (benzhexol). Used for parkinsonism (see Ch. 6).

Ipratropium. Unlike the other examples, this molecule is polar and poorly absorbed from most sites. It is used topically for asthma.

Adverse effects

Adverse effects are dose related and include dryness of the mouth, urinary retention, constipation, raised intraocular pressure, tachycardia and confusion. In severe poisoning, there may be tachyarrhythmias, coma and seizures. Some drugs used for other indications have **antimuscarinic side effects**, notably tricyclic antidepressants (Ch. 6), neuroleptics (Ch. 6) and disopyramide and quinidine (Ch. 3).

Contraindications

Glaucoma. Antimuscarinic agents induce mydriasis, which narrows the angle between the iris and the cornea, thereby reducing drainage of aqueous humour into the canal of Schlemm (Fig. 19).

Prostatic hypertrophy. Urinary retention is worsened.

Clinical sketch

A woman with closed angle glaucoma presents with severe asthma; her doctors wonder whether it would be safe to use nebulised ipratropium.

Comment: glaucoma is a relative contraindication to the use of this atropine-like drug. However, exacerbation of glaucoma is uncommon, and the benefits may exceed the risks in a case such as this.

Antinicotinic drugs

Antagonists at skeletal muscle nicotinic receptors (which are not part of the autonomic system) are widely used in anaesthesia as muscle relaxants (Ch. 8). Autonomic antinicotinic drugs (the 'ganglion blockers') were used in the past for hypertension but are now obsolete.

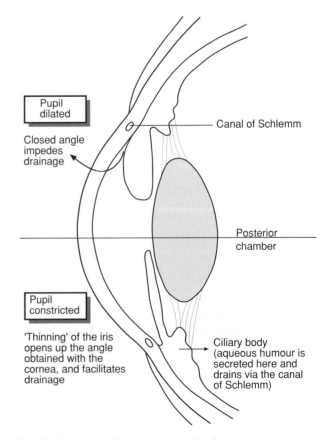

Pupil dilated

Canal of Schlemm

Closed angle impedes drainage

Posterior chamber

Pupil constricted

'Thinning' of the iris opens up the angle obtained with the cornea, and facilitates drainage

Ciliary body (aqueous humour is secreted here and drains via the canal of Schlemm)

Fig. 19 Use of miotics in closed-angle glaucoma.

2.3 Drugs acting on the sympathetic nervous system

Learning objectives

You should:

- be able to list the main adrenergic agonists and describe the effects of each agonist on specific tissues and the whole animal

- be able to list the receptor subtypes that each agonist binds to

- be able to describe the clinical uses of adrenergic agonists.

Adrenergic agonists (sympathomimetics)

Different endogenous and synthetic sympathomimetics have different affinities for the subtypes of adrenoceptors. From these, their effects can be predicted.

Noradrenaline (*norepinephrine*) binds to α_1-, α_2-and β_1-adrenoceptors. Injected i.v., noradrenaline (norepinephrine) tends to cause marked *vasoconstriction* and an increase in myocardial contractility: blood pressure, therefore, rises. Although a positive chronotropic effect would be expected, this is usually overcome by vagal homeostatic mechanisms.

Adrenaline (*epinephrine*) binds to α_1-, α_2-, β_1-and β_2-adrenoceptors. The net effect of an i.v. injection of adrenaline (epinephrine) is usually unchanged vascular resistance (vascular resistance increases markedly in some vascular beds, while decreasing in others; this reflects local distribution of receptor types), increased myocardial contractility, increased heart rate, increased systolic blood pressure and little or no change in diastolic pressure.

Isoprenaline binds to β_1-and β_2-adrenoceptors. The net effect of an i.v. injection is increased heart rate, increased myocardial contractility and decreased vascular resistance; blood pressure may fall.

Dobutamine. This is selective for β_1-adrenoceptors, it causes increased heart rate and contractility. Blood pressure rises. Like dopamine, dobutamine at high concentration activates α_1-adrenoceptors, causing unwanted vasoconstriction.

Salbutamol. This is selective for β_2-adrenoceptors. It causes relaxation of vascular and bronchial smooth muscle. At higher concentrations, salbutamol becomes less selective, binding to β_1-adrenoceptors, which causes tachycardia.

Ephedrine. A non-selective sympathomimetic with a similar spectrum to adrenaline (epinephrine).

Therapeutic uses

Anaphylaxis. This syndrome of shock (secondary to vasodilatation) and bronchospasm in response to an allergen (Ch. 10) is treated with subcutaneous epinephrine (adrenaline), which induces bronchodilatation, vasoconstriction and raises blood pressure.

Asthma. Inhaled, oral or parenteral β_2-agonists such as salbutamol are drugs of first choice (Ch. 10).

Cardiogenic shock. This is caused by an acute reduction in myocardial contractility, usually after a massive myocardial infarction. Dobutamine, by its β_1-effects, increases stroke volume and heart rate and improves the perfusion of vital structures; however, if the concentration rises too high, dobutamine causes vasoconstriction through α-agonist activity.

Asystole. Adrenaline (epinephrine) may be given i.v. during resuscitation from asystole.

Reduction of local blood flow. The local anaesthetic lidocaine is formulated in combination with adrenaline (epinephrine) for certain procedures. Local vasoconstriction reduces the rate of removal of the anaesthetic from the site and prolongs its effect, while at the same time reducing blood loss. This drug combination must not be used when anaesthetising extremities (e.g. fingers) because of the risk of gangrene.

Nasal decongestants. Ephedrine is given orally to reduce nasal congestion; it is often present in proprietary cough mixtures.

Drug interactions

Non-selective, older, monoamine oxidase inhibitors (MAOI) are still sometimes used for depression (see Ch. 6). Ingestion of sympathomimetics (usually in cough mixtures) may cause severe hypertension.

Adrenergic antagonists (alpha- and beta-blockers)

These drugs are also known as alpha-blockers and beta-blockers and are considered in Chapter 3.

Clinical sketch

A man is admitted to the coronary care unit after a massive myocardial infarction. He is in sinus rhythm (rate of 100 beats/min) and is well-hydrated but his blood pressure is unrecordable and his urine output is very low. The doctors start a constant rate infusion of dobutamine.

Comment: dobutamine is a β_1-agonist, which increases myocardial contractility. It can help in 'cardiogenic shock', as described here.

Clinical sketch

An asthmatic uses salbutamol to get rid of wheeze.

Comment: salbutamol is a β_2-agonist, which dilates bronchi.

Self-assessment: questions

Multiple choice questions

1. The following statements are true:
   a. Salbutamol given i.v. causes tachycardia
   b. Dobutamine i.v. is indicated for shock secondary to gastrointestinal haemorrhage
   c. Isoprenaline i.v. causes bronchodilatation
   d. Noradrenaline (norepinephrine) i.v. causes bronchodilatation
   e. Dobutamine i.v. dilates renal arterioles

2. The action of noradrenaline:
   a. Is terminated by its uptake from the synapse
   b. Is potentiated by inhibitors of monoamine oxidase B
   c. Is potentiated by tricyclic antidepressants
   d. Includes vasodilatation in some arteriolar beds
   e. Is potentiated by cocaine

3. Atropine:
   a. Is a direct agonist at autonomic acetylcholine receptors
   b. Slows the heart rate
   c. Causes a dry mouth
   d. Bronchodilates
   e. Raises intraocular pressure

Case history questions

Case history 1

A 6-year-old girl is brought to casualty because of collapse at home. She had been playing unsupervised in a local wood and had been well previously. She is semi-conscious and confused, her pupils are dilated, her skin is dry and her pulse rate is 200 beats/min.

1. What may be the cause of her problem?
2. What should be done?
3. How is the autonomic nervous system involved?

Case history 2

A farmer is brought as an emergency after an accident with crop-spraying equipment, during which he was copiously sprayed with insecticide. He is salivating profusely and has difficulty breathing; his pulse rate is 40 beats/min.

1. What is the mechanism of the poisoning?
2. What should be done?

Case history 3

A 70-year-old man takes disopyramide (see Ch. 3) as prophylaxis against cardiac arrhythmias. He also has parkinsonism for which his doctor has put him on benztropine (see Ch. 6). He becomes constipated and, within 2 days of starting the latter drug, he is admitted in acute retention of urine.

What has happened?

Short note question

Write short notes on the relevance of the autonomic nervous system to clinical pharmacology and therapeutics, using clinical examples to illustrate your answer.

Self-assessment: answers

Multiple choice answers

1. a. **True**. Salbutamol has higher affinity for β_2- than for β_1-adrenoceptors; however, binding to the latter does occur, causing tachycardia.
   b. **False**. Dobutamine dilates splanchnic vessels, including those to the stomach/duodenum and could worsen bleeding.
   c. **True**. Isoprenaline binds to both β_1- and β_2-adrenoceptors.
   d. **False**. Noradrenaline (norepinephrine) has little activity at β_2-adrenoceptors.
   e. **False**. Dobutamine is a specific β_1-agonist and has little effect on splanchnic vessels.

2. a. **True**. Noradrenaline is taken up presynaptically (uptake I) and postsynaptically (uptake II).
   b. **False**. Monoamine oxidase A metabolises noradrenaline and 5-HT, while monoamine oxidase B metabolises dopamine.
   c. **True**. Tricyclic antidepressants inhibit uptake I.
   d. **False**. Noradrenaline (norepinephrine) binds to α_1-, α_2- and β_1-adrenoceptors.
   e. **True**. Cocaine interferes with uptake of noradrenaline from the synapse; unlike lidocaine, cocaine need not be formulated with epinephrine (adrenaline) for this reason.

3. Atropine:
   a. **False**. Atropine is an antagonist at these receptors.
   b. **False**. The vagus nerve carries acetylcholinergic parasympathetic fibres to the sinoatrial node, and stimulation slows the heart rate. By blocking this, atropine is positively chronotropic.
   c. **True**. Parasympathetic fibres are secretomotor to the salivary glands.
   d. **True**. See Chapter 10.
   e. **True**. By causing pupillary dilatation, atropine closes the angle between the cornea and the iris, opposing drainage of aqueous humour and raising intraocular pressure.

Case history answers

Case history 1

1. This patient has features of anticholinergic poisoning; she may have eaten deadly nightshade berries or fungi. She is confused because the alkaloid has crossed her blood–brain barrier.

2. Her airway should be protected and her stomach emptied (even if poisoning was some time ago as anticholinergics delay gastric emptying). Supportive care with attention paid to maintenance of breathing and the circulation, and termination of seizures (usually with diazepam), is indicated. The nearest National Poisons Centre should be phoned. Anticholinesterases (Ch. 8) may be useful to potentiate acetylcholine: physostigmine is then the drug of first choice since it crosses the blood–brain barrier.

3. Secretomotor fibres to her salivary and sweat glands have been blocked, as have parasympathetic fibres of the vagus.

Case history 2

1. Organophosphorus insecticides are potent and long-acting anticholinesterases: overactivity at parasympathetic receptors is responsible for the clinical features, and his breathlessness may be caused by bronchospasm.

2. Contaminated clothes should be removed, and he should be washed in copious water—the compound can cross the skin. Bronchospasm should be treated according to asthma guidelines (Ch. 10), and he should be given frequent doses of i.v. atropine for its antimuscarinic effects. Pralidoxime is a specific antidote capable of regenerating active cholinesterase by releasing it from covalent binding to the insecticide.

Case history 3

Benztropine is an antimuscarinic, and disopyramide has antimuscarinic side effects. Both tend to increase the tone of the bladder sphincter, decrease the tone of the bladder wall and cause urinary retention. Both can also cause constipation. In addition, disopyramide can occasionally *cause* tachyarrhythmias through its antimuscarinic activity (though this complication has not happened here).

Short note answers

Many drugs produce their effects by working on the autonomic system, and the same mechanisms explain the adverse effects of many others. Dealing with such drugs (which include antihypertensives, antiarrhythmics, bronchodilators, neuroleptics) as agonists and antagonists at autonomic receptors allows better understanding of their therapeutic use, and adverse effects.

1. Define what you mean by agonists and antagonists.

2. Deal with cholinergic receptors.

   a. *Nicotinic agonists*: none in regular clinical use; mention 'indirect agonists', i.e. the anticholinesterases
   b. *Nicotinic antagonists*: none in regular clinical use (ganglion blockers are obsolete)
   c. *Muscarinic agonists*: for example, pilocarpine, which causes pupillary constriction and is used in glaucoma, or bethanechol, which causes increased muscle tone in the bladder
   d. *Muscarinic antagonists*: for example, atropine (also list several other antimuscarinics and their uses). Give the adverse effects of antimuscarinic drugs. Mention drugs that either achieve their effect through antagonism of muscarinic receptors (e.g. pirenzipine, benztropine and ipratropium) or that produce adverse effects by the same mechanism (e.g. quinidine, disopyramide, tricyclic antidepressants).

3. Deal with adrenergic receptors: cover the effects of stimulation of α_1-, α_2-, β_1- and β_2-adrenoceptors and describe their anatomical locations.

4. Describe the clinical use of the agonists salbutamol, adrenaline (epinephrine), noradrenaline (norepinephrine), isoprenaline, dobutamine and dopamine.

5. Describe the clinical use of the antagonists propranolol, atenolol, prazosin and phenoxybenzamine.

3

Drugs in cardiovascular disease 1: prevention

Clinical sketch

A 57-year-old man has smoked 40 cigarettes per day for the past 40 years. His blood pressure is 186/106 mmHg and total cholesterol to serum HDL ratio is 5. He has recently been diagnosed as suffering from non-insulin-dependent diabetes.

Comment: This man illustrates how risk factors accumulate in individual patients to put them at high risk of a cardiovascular event. Work out this patient's cardiovascular risk, i.e. the risk of a cardiovascular event over the next 10 years from the risk tables in Figure 20.

Overview

Major risk factors for cardiovascular and cerebrovascular disease may be non-modifiable (age, gender, family and personal history) or modifiable (smoking, hyperlipidaemia, hypertension and diabetes). These factors will combine to put a person at high or low risk of cardiovascular or cerebrovascular events. Patients are considered to be at high risk if they have established ischaemic heart disease, a combination of risk factors that makes their risk of a cardiovascular event greater or equal to 30% over 10 years, severe hypertension or hyperlipidaemia. For these, drug treatment may be necessary to lower the risk. The major classes of drug to treat hypertension are thiazide diuretics, beta-blockers, drugs acting on the renin–angiotensin–aldosterone system and calcium channel blockers. The major drugs used to treat hyperlipidaemia are the 3-hydroxy-3-methylglutaryl-CoA reductase inhibitors ('statins').

3.1 Clinical aspects and cardiovascular risk factors

Learning objectives

You should:

- be able to list the major non-modifiable and modifiable risk factors
- understand the interaction of these factors to produce overall cardiovascular risk
- be able to identify patients at high risk of cardiovascular disease
- advise on general and specific measures to decrease that risk.

Cardiovascular disease (such as angina, myocardial infarction) and cerebrovascular disease are among the most common causes of death. The presence of cardiovascular risk factors puts a person at higher or lower risk of these conditions. These risk factors may be non-modifiable (e.g. age, gender, family or personal history) or modifiable (smoking, hyperlipidaemia, hypertension). Diabetes mellitus is a further risk factor that is partially modifiable by better control of diabetes. Many of these risk factors are asymptomatic until they cause disease, and so it may be wise to screen apparently healthy people to detect them.

In general, many risk factors can be treated by lifestyle changes that could be almost universally recommended (better diet, stopping smoking, more exercise). Some modifiable risk factors may require pharmacological intervention (hyperlipidaemia, hypertension and, for some patients, stopping smoking—see Ch. 18).

In deciding whether to treat these conditions, it is generally helpful to consider the patient's overall risk. In patients with more non-modifiable risk factors, it is important to treat the modifiable risks more aggressively.

Primary prevention is intended to stop the disease from becoming established, e.g. in a patient with many risk factors. Secondary prevention is limiting further damage in patients who already have the disease (e.g. patients who have had a myocardial infarction).

Level of risk

Patients are at high risk of coronary and cerebrovascular disease if they have:

- a previous history of ischaemic heart disease
- evidence of end-organ damage caused by hypertension (e.g. cardiac enlargement)

- diabetes mellitus
- multiple risk factors giving an overall risk of 30% or more of having a cardiovascular event over the next 10 years.

The relative risk of an event can be calculated from epidemiological data. An easy to use way to assess risk in practice is a series of graphs based on this epidemiological data (Fig. 20). These graphs do not apply to patients who have already had ischaemic heart disease and may not apply well to some very high-risk populations such as Asians resident in the UK.

Sometimes a single risk factor is so important or severe that it requires treatment on its own, even if the patient's overall risk is less than 30%.

3.2 Hypertension

Learning objectives

You should:

- be able to identify patients whose blood pressure requires treatment
- be able to advise on general measures

- be able to describe each of the four major classes of antihypertensive drug and give examples
- be able to describe how these drugs might be used in practice
- know the management of hypertensive emergencies.

Clinical sketch

A 72-year-old woman has a blood pressure of 180/84 mmHg. Her doctor is aware of this but is reluctant to treat her because this blood pressure is normal for her age.

Comment: Blood pressure does tend to rise with increasing age, but this is associated with an increased risk of stroke, which can be reduced by treating the hypertension. This pressure is definitely not 'normal' for her age although it is fairly common. The target in such a patient will be a systolic of less than 140 mmHg. This may be difficult to achieve without causing unacceptable adverse effects and this must be balanced against the potential benefits to the patient of successfully lowering her blood pressure to this target. This patient has lone systolic hypertension—once not considered a cardiovascular risk but now known also to be associated with an increased risk of storke.

A NO DIABETES

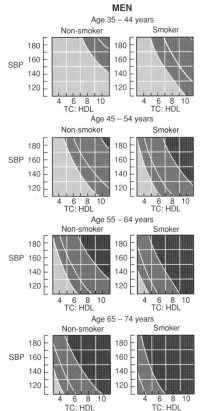

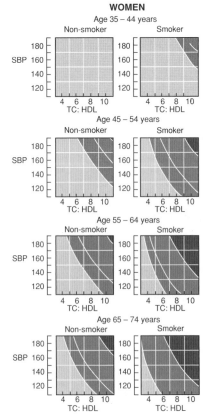

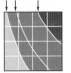

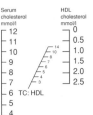

Fig. 20 *see page 29 for caption*

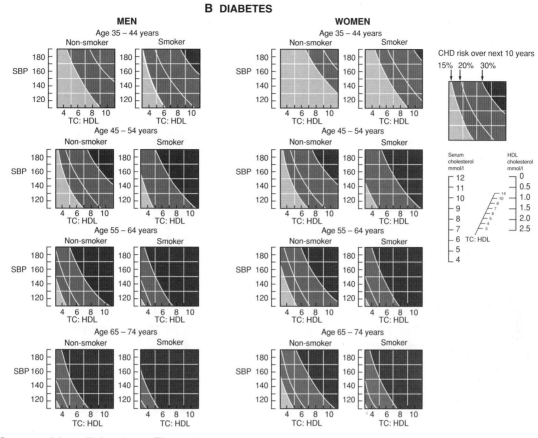

B DIABETES

Fig. 20 Coronary risk prediction charts. These charts are used to estimate risk of coronary heart disease (CHD: non-fatal myocardial infarction and coronary death) for individuals who have not developed symptomatic CHD or other major, atherosclerotic disease. SBP, systolic blood pressure (mmHg); TC: HDL, ratio JOF serum total cholesterol to high density lipoprotein cholesterol. (Modified with permission from Heart 1998; S1–S29. © The University of Manchester.)

Hypertension refers to high blood pressure, which can damage blood vessels and predispose to the development of atheromatous disease. In severe cases, it can also cause heart and renal failure. Treating hypertension reduces mortality and morbidity from these conditions, particularly from cerebrovascular disease but also from ischaemic heart disease.

Causes of hypertension

The cause of hypertension is usually unknown ('primary hypertension'), but about 5–10% of cases are secondary, resulting from alcohol abuse, coarctation of the aorta, phaeochromocytoma (a tumour that secretes catecholamines), primary hyperaldosteronism (Conn's syndrome), Cushing's syndrome (excessive glucocorticoids, either endogenous or iatrogenic), or renal disease (including renal artery stenosis).

Diagnosis

Blood pressure is a continuous variable and it is a little arbitrary where it becomes 'hypertension'. The British

Hypertension Society guidelines for when to start treatment are shown in Figure 21. These take account of both the severity of the blood pressure alone and also the overall cardiovascular risk.

Blood pressure should usually be measured on three or more occasions, while the patient is sitting comfortably, over a period of several weeks before deciding to treat, although very high blood pressure with complications may require immediate treatment. Systolic blood pressure is more important than diastolic.

Treatment

Urgent lowering of blood pressure is rarely necessary (but see Box 1, below). Non-pharmacological treatment should be the first approach in mild-to-moderate hypertension, including weight loss, alcohol and salt restriction, perhaps behavioural therapy, and mild exercise. Other cardiovascular risk factors should be considered also, such as smoking, hyperlipidaemia, etc. If this fails to improve the blood pressure substantially over a period of months, or sooner in patients with more severe hypertension, drug therapy should be considered.

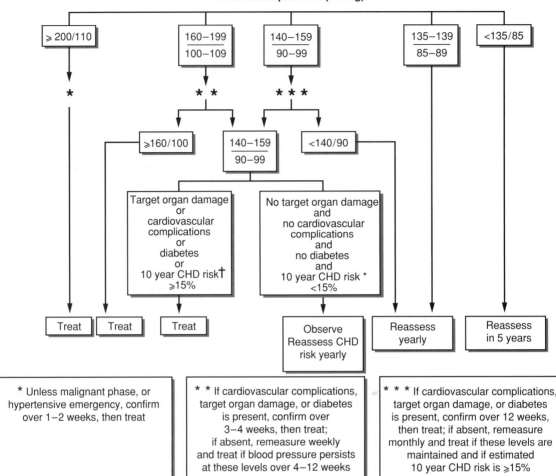

Fig. 21 The British Hypertension Society guidelines for when to start treatment in hypertension.

The target blood pressure is usually a systolic pressure of less than 150 mmHg or a fall of at least 10 mmHg, and a diastolic pressure of 80–85 mmHg, but these figures, like the level at which to begin treatment, depend on consideration of the patient's risk—diabetic patients for instance should be treated to achieve 140/80 mmHg.

Drugs in hypertension

There are four major classes of drug used in the treatment of hypertension:

- thiazide and other diuretics
- beta-blockers
- drugs that affect the renin–angiotensin–aldosterone system
- calcium-channel blockers.

Thiazides and other diuretics

Diuretics promote the excretion of water. They can act at different sites in the nephron and in different ways. There are three major groups:

- thiazides
- loop diuretics
- potassium-sparing diuretics.

Thiazides

Thiazides act by inhibiting the absorption of Na^+ in the distal convoluted tubule. Water is lost with the Na^+. More Na^+ reaches the distal tubule, where it is exchanged for K^+, and the thiazides also cause K^+ loss. Magnesium is also lost, while Ca^{2+} is retained (Fig. 22). The major effect in hypertension, however, is a vasodilatory effect, and little effect comes from the diuresis.

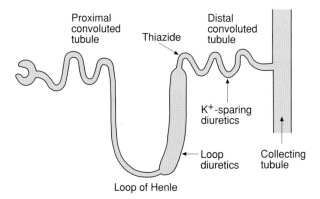

Fig. 22 Sites of action of diuretics.

The maximal hypotensive response to thiazides is reached at relatively low doses, In the past, thiazides were used in excessively high doses with no better anti-hypertensive effect and a higher incidence of adverse effects.

Example

Bendroflumethiazide (bendrofluazide) is well absorbed after oral administration and causes a diuresis in about 1–2 hours, which lasts for up to 12 hours.

Therapeutic uses

- Hypertension
- Congestive cardiac failure.

Adverse effects

- Dehydration: a risk in all diuretic use, especially in the elderly
- Hypokalaemia: usually mild and not requiring treatment
- Hyperuricaemia/gout
- Impaired glucose tolerance/diabetes mellitus
- Hypercholesterolaemia: in short-term therapy, but probably not seen in long-term use
- Impotence
- Hypercalcaemia.

Contraindications

- Gout
- Renal disease.

Loop diuretics

Loop diuretics (*furosemide* (frusemide) or *bumetamide*) are generally used in hypertension only in combination with other drugs or in renal failure. They are discussed in the section on heart failure in Chapter 4.

Potassium-sparing diuretics

Potassium-sparing diuretics are a chemically diverse group that, unlike other diuretics, retain K^+. They act in the distal convoluted tubule where K^+/Na^+ exchange occurs and are only weak diuretics. Their major use is in treating or preventing hypokalaemia caused by thi-azides or loop diuretics. In the past, K^+ supplements were widely used, but very high doses are required, reducing patient compliance. It is not often necessary to prevent or treat diuretic-induced hypokalaemia, but if this is required, K^+-sparing diuretics should be used.

Examples

Spironolactone is an aldosterone antagonist. Aldosterone causes Na^+ retention and K^+ loss, and spironolactone does the reverse. It can be used in treating hypertension caused by primary hyperaldosteronism (Conn's syndrome). It is also used in heart failure and in other conditions with fluid retention.

Triamterene and *amiloride* interfere with Na^+/K^+ exchange.
All are administered orally.

Adverse effects

- Hyperkalaemia
- Gynaecomastia (spironolactone only).

Drug interactions

The action of thiazides and loop diuretics is inhibited by non-steroidal anti-inflammatory drugs. Lithium (Ch. 6) excretion may be reduced by diuretics and this can lead to serious toxicity.

Potassium-sparing diuretics can interact with K^+ supplements or angiotensin-converting enzyme (ACE) inhibitors to cause dangerous hyperkalaemia.

Loop diuretics can be combined with K^+-sparing diuretics to reduce K^+ loss, or with ACE inhibitors in heart failure or hypertension.

Beta-blockers

The beta-blockers competitively block the β-adrenoceptors in the heart and thereby reduce the noradrenaline- and adrenaline-induced production of cyclic AMP. The β-adrenoceptors in the heart are mostly $β_1$-adrenoceptors but $β_2$-adrenoceptors are also present. Beta-blockers can be non-selective (act on both types of receptor) or selective (mainly affect $β_1$-adrenoceptors).

Beta-blockers improve oxygen availability by:

- decreasing oxygen demand
  —slowing the heart
  —reducing its force of contraction
- increasing oxygen supply by lengthening diastole, during which most blood flows in the coronary arteries.

They are, thus, effective in treating angina (see Ch. 4) and also lower blood pressure in patients with angina and other patients. The exact mechanism of this lowering of blood pressure is not known.

Beta-blockers must be avoided (even the relatively selective $β_1$-blockers) in patients dependent on β-stimulation, e.g. asthmatics.

Some beta-blockers have partial agonist (stimulating) activity (also known as intrinsic sympathomimetic activity) at the β-adrenoceptor in addition to beta-blocking properties. These drugs may cause less bradycardia and peripheral vasoconstriction than other beta-blockers.

When blocked by prolonged use of a beta-blocker, the β-adrenoceptor may undergo upregulation, i.e. the number and sensitivity of the receptors increase. This may make sudden withdrawal of beta-blockers dangerous in patients with ischaemic heart disease, as the patient may suffer a rebound worsening of angina.

Examples
Beta-blockers may be lipophilic (penetrate lipids and cell membranes well and are metabolised by the liver) or hydrophilic (do not penetrate lipids and membranes so well and are excreted unchanged by the kidney rather than metabolised). The three beta-blockers most widely used are:

propranolol: a lipophilic non-selective beta-blocker
atenolol: a hydrophilic β$_1$-selective blocker
metoprolol: a lipophilic β$_1$-selective blocker.

Therapeutic uses
- Hypertension
- Angina pectoris
- Myocardial infarction (both acute treatment and to reduce risk of recurrence)
- Antiarrhythmic
- Heart failure
- Anxiety (reduces manifestations of anxiety such as tremor).

Chapter 4 gives more details of therapeutic uses.

Adverse effects
- Bradycardia, including heart block
- Bronchospasm
- Peripheral vasoconstriction: cold hands and feet
- Fatigue, depression, vivid dreams (especially the lipophilic drugs).

Contraindications
- Asthma or any obstructive airway disease
- Raynaud's phenomenon or peripheral vascular disease
- Heart block of any degree
- Insulin-dependent diabetes mellitus—may decrease awareness of hypoglycaemia by masking somatic effects.

Drugs affecting the renin–angiotensin–aldosterone system

The renin–angiotensin–aldosterone system (Fig. 23) is vital in maintaining blood volume and renal blood supply. In some hypertensives, this system is relatively

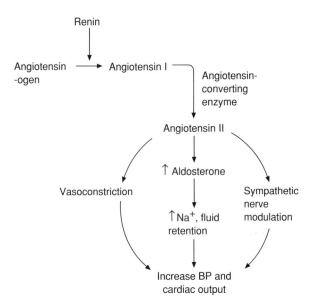

Fig. 23 The renin–angiotensin–aldosterone axis.

overactive. ACE inhibitors are particularly effective in hypertension if used with a diuretic; this increases dependence on the renin–angiotensin system, which is then blocked. Angiotensin II has other effects in tissues, resulting in new tissue formation. In some situations this may be harmful.

ACE inhibitors
ACE inhibitors prevent the formation of angiotensin II, preventing its vasoconstrictor effects as well as decreasing aldosterone production and fluid retention. ACE also breaks down a number of inflammatory peptides, such as bradykinin, and the potentiation of these may contribute to its antihypertensive effect.

Examples
Captopril is given orally and is cleared by the kidney. It is given two or three times per day.

Enalapril is also given orally. It is a prodrug and is activated to the active compound, enalaprilat, by the liver. It is cleared by the kidneys. Enalapril is given once per day.

Ramipril is given orally usually twice per day.

Therapeutic uses
- Hypertension
- Cardiac failure: ACE inhibitors clearly reduce mortality (Ch. 4)
- After myocardial infarction
- In reducing cardiac risk in high-risk patients; one very good trial suggests a benefit in these patients independent of any effect on blood pressure
- Reducing progression to renal failure in diabetic patients with microalbuminuria (whether hypertensive or not).

These last three uses may relate to preventing inappropriate new tissue development.

Adverse effects

- Severe hypotension: especially in renal artery stenosis, or in patients with heart failure, on the first dose, or in patients on high-dose diuretics; the dose of diuretic should be reduced as much as possible before starting ACE inhibitors
- Hyperkalaemia: because K^+-losing effects of aldosterone are blocked
- Impairment of renal function: through decrease in renal perfusion and intrarenal haemodynamics
- Cough: very common but not serious, probably occurs through potentiation of bradykinin
- Angioedema: more serious and possibly also caused by potentiation of bradykinin
- Occasionally worsening of asthma.

Contraindications

- Renal artery stenosis, which is often asymptomatic but should be suspected in a patient with hypertension and peripheral vascular disease
- Other forms of renal disease: ACE inhibitors should be used cautiously because they may precipitate a reduction in renal function.

Drug interactions

- With K^+-sparing diuretics or K^+ supplements: a risk of dangerous hyperkalaemia.

Angiotensin II receptor antagonists

Drugs can block the receptor at which angiotensin II acts rather than blocking its production. Their effects are broadly similar to those of ACE inhibitors, but because they will not affect bradykinin, cough is rare. They are only used at present in hypertension but may in time be used for the wider range of indications, as for ACE inhibitors, as new evidence becomes available.

Examples

Losartan (short acting); *valsartan* (longer acting).

Calcium-channel blockers

In cardiac muscle or vascular smooth muscle, a change in membrane potential causes Ca^{2+} to enter the cell through voltage-dependent calcium channels. Calcium is essential in the interaction between actin and myosin filaments causing muscle contraction. Calcium-channel blockers inhibit the voltage-dependent calcium channels, and reduce Ca^{2+} entry. They reduce smooth muscle contraction and cause vasodilation and hence are useful in hypertension and in angina. They also reduce the force of contraction of the heart, and slow the heart rate in vitro. They have no effect on skeletal muscle, which is less dependent on exogenous Ca^{2+}.

Examples

There are three types of calcium-channel blocker, which bind to different but related receptor sites on the calcium channel and have different effects in different tissues.

Dihydropyridines. This group (e.g. *nifedipine*, *amlodipine*) mainly cause intense arterial vasodilatation and lower the blood pressure and the afterload (i.e. the load against which the heart must eject blood) on the heart. Because of the vasodilatation, a sympathetic reflex occurs, which increases the heart rate and force of contraction (in isolated hearts without sympathetic reflexes, nifedipine behaves like other calcium-channel blockers and tends to slow the heart and decrease the force of contraction). Nifedipine is well absorbed orally and is metabolised by the liver.

Verapamil. Unlike nifedipine, verapamil tends to have more effect on the heart, slowing the heart and reducing force of contraction, and less effect on the peripheral circulation. It also slows conduction through the atrioventricular (AV) node (where the action potential is largely dependent on Ca^{2+}) and has a special role in treating supraventricular tachycardia. Verapamil can be given orally or i.v. It is metabolised by the liver, and there is extensive first-pass metabolism.

Diltiazem has more effect on the heart than nifedipine, and more effect on the peripheral circulation than verapamil. Diltiazem is metabolised by the liver.

Therapeutic uses

All the calcium-channel blockers are used for hypertension and angina. Nifedipine is also used for Raynaud's phenomenon and verapamil is also used for supraventricular tachycardia.

Adverse effects

These mainly result from smooth muscle relaxation and vasodilatation.

nifedipine. facial flushing and ankle swelling, headaches and dizziness
verapamil: headaches and dizziness, constipation, heart block and bradycardia
diltiazem: constipation, ankle oedema, flushing, headache.

Drug interactions

Nifedipine can be combined with beta-blockers in angina or hypertension; rarely, the combination may precipitate heart failure. The combination of verapamil with beta-blockers can be dangerous (especially if verapamil is given i.v.) and causes severe hypotension and bradycardia.

Other drugs used in hypertension

Other drugs used in hypertension include alpha-blockers and some drugs used in special circumstances, which are considered below. Other drugs are largely obsolete: they include hydralazine, an arterial vasodilator, and methyl-dopa, which still has a role in treating hypertension in pregnancy.

Alpha-blockers

The alpha-blockers (e.g. *prazosin*, *doxazosin*) vasodilatate by blocking the α_1-adrenoceptor in peripheral blood vessels. Adverse effects include postural hypotension (particularly a risk after the first dose), headache, urinary frequency and tachycardia. There is some concern that these drugs may not reduce mortality despite lowering blood pressure.

Choice of drug in hypertension

All the four major classes have been shown to reduce mortality from stroke and (in some cases) from myocardial infarction. The oldest drugs, the thiazides, have particularly strong evidence and are inexpensive, which is important considering the large numbers of hypertensive patients.

In the past, the general approach was the use of 'stepped care', i.e. step 1 a thiazide or a beta-blocker; step 2, a thiazide and a beta-blocker; step 3, a thiazide, a beta-blocker and a vasodilator. This approach is still often applied but today a more 'tailored care' approach is favoured, i.e. tailoring the choice of drug to the individual patient taking into account the total risk factor profile.

There is debate over whether patients who fail to respond to the first antihypertensive drug should have a second drug added to the first or substituted instead of the first. In this scheme, drugs might be used as follows.

Clinical sketch

A patient presents with high blood pressure which is sustained on repeated readings. The doctor initiates treatment with bendroflumethiazide (bendrofluazide) and although this lowers blood pressure slightly, it is still unsatisfactory. The doctor then adds in a second drug, atenolol, which again achieves some lowering of blood pressure, but this remains unsatisfactory. The doctor adds in a third drug, a calcium channel blocker, amlodipine. Satisfactory blood pressure is achieved on this.

Comment: Many patients need multiple drug therapy to achieve satisfactory blood pressure levels. This increases the risk of adverse effects. Some patients may have apparently uncontrollable hypertension, not because their blood pressure is genuinely poorly controlled but because the patient may be poorly compliant with antihypertensive medications, or because the patient has the phenomenon of white coat hypertension, i.e. the blood pressure goes up whenever it is measured. Failure to recognise this condition can lead to overtreatment. It is best detected by 24 hour ambulatory blood pressure monitoring.

Thiazides. The first choice for most patients, especially the elderly; they are inexpensive, effective and proved to prevent strokes. But not suitable for patients with hypercholesterolaemia, renal disease or gout.

Beta-blockers. These are also a reasonable first choice, especially in younger patients or patients with angina pectoris. Not suitable for patients with asthma, heart failure or peripheral vascular disease.

ACE inhibitors. First choice in diabetics but best avoided in renal disease; they need close monitoring of renal function.

Calcium-channel blockers. These tend to have a higher rate of adverse effects, but this is improved by the use of slow-release preparations. Useful in patients with angina, hyperlipidaemia or renal disease. Expensive.

Alpha-blockers. These are considered a second-line drug in patients who do not tolerate other drugs; possibly suitable particularly for hyperlipidaemics or patients with urinary hesitancy.

Combinations. No more than 50–60% of patients will respond to any one drug; many patients will need more than one. Appropriate combinations include thiazide plus beta-blocker; thiazide plus ACE inhibitor; beta-blocker plus calcium-channel blocker; ACE inhibitor and calcium-channel blocker.

In coexisting disease. Some patients who have hypertension and other diseases might be considered more suitable for certain drugs:

- with asthma or chronic obstructive pulmonary disease (COPD): diuretics or calcium-channel blockers
- with heart failure: diuretics and ACE inhibitors
- with angina: beta-blockers or calcium-channel blockers
- with diabetes mellitus: ACE inhibitors.

Monitoring

Patients treated for hypertension need regular monitoring of their blood pressure and for adverse effects and review of their cardiovascular risk. Patient education on the need for antihypertensives and of the use of their medication is very important.

Treatment of hypertension in special circumstances

Box 1 gives the treatment of hypertensive emergencies.

Resistant hypertension

Failure to respond to triple therapy with standard drugs should be fully investigated to exclude secondary hypertension. Poor compliance with treatment or 'white coat' hypertension are common and may give the appearance of resistance.

Urgent lowering of blood pressure is only indicated in patients with hypertensive encephalopathy, or hypertension-induced renal or heart failure. These conditions are rare.

High blood pressure readings alone in the absence of these conditions do not warrant urgent blood pressure reduction, which may be dangerous by reducing cerebral or coronary perfusion.

If urgent treatment is needed, the patient should be admitted to hospital for rest and very careful monitoring. Oral therapy with beta-blockers, ACE inhibitors or calcium channel blockers may be adequate.

In rare cases where parenteral therapy is necessary, *sodium nitroprusside* is used by i.v. infusion but only in an intensive care ward: it is a very powerful arterial and venous vasodilator. It acts very rapidly and has a very short duration of action: blood pressure rises within a minute of the infusion being stopped. It allows control of the blood pressure while other slower-acting drugs are introduced. If used for prolonged periods (>24 hours), cyanide, a toxic metabolite, may form. *Labetalol*, a combined alpha-and beta-blocker can also be given i.v.

Minoxidil is used in resistant hypertension. It is a vasodilator that causes fluid retention and tachycardia and should be used only with diuretics and a beta-blocker for that reason. A peculiar side effect is the stimulation of male pattern hair growth, and hence it is generally avoided in women.

Hypertension in pregnancy
This is covered in Chapter 19.

3.3 Hyperlipidaemia

Learning objectives

You should:

● be able to identify patients who require treatment for hyperlipidaemia

● be able to describe the drugs used in the treatment of hyperlipidaemia and their practical use.

Hyperlipidaemia refers to high levels of fats in blood. There are two major fractions of fats in blood: cholesterol and triglycerides.

Cholesterol is derived from the diet and also manufactured in all cells but mainly by the liver. It is essential for the formation of lipid membranes, steroid hormones and many other vital bodily functions. Triglycerides are used as an energy source.

A 62-year-old man had a myocardial infarction but has now recovered. His serum cholesterol is 5.8 mmol/l despite diet. His medications include aspirin and atenolol. He wonders if his cholesterol should be treated.

Comment: This is secondary prevention, i.e. the treatment of a patient who has already had an event to try to prevent further events. Patients who have had an event have already declared themselves to be at very high risk, and the risk tables do not apply to such patients. The risk tables only apply to primary prevention. Other examples of patients worthy of secondary prevention include patients with established angina or peripheral vascular disease. Such patients need rigorous lowering of their serum cholesterol, ideally to a serum cholesterol of less than 5 mmol/l. This is likely to require the prescribing of a drug such as simvastatin.

Absorbed cholesterol is taken from the intestine in chylomicrons to the liver. Cholesterol and triglyceride are then transported in the blood from the liver in association with lipoproteins, as very low density lipoproteins (VLDL). VLDL are broken down by lipoprotein lipase in peripheral tissues to low density lipoproteins (LDL). LDL carry cholesterol to the cells, and these are cleared by specific receptors on the cells and especially in the liver. LDL cholesterol is particularly associated with atheroma and cardiovascular disease. High density lipoproteins (HDL) carry cholesterol from the tissues back to the liver (reverse transport) and seem to be protective against atheroma. The ratio of LDL cholesterol to HDL cholesterol is used in measuring cardiovascular risk.

Triglycerides are less important than cholesterol in causing atherosclerosis. High triglyceride concentrations are associated with pancreatitis.

Some forms of hypercholesterolaemia are inherited either as a single gene (usually severe), or more commonly as polygenic traits (less severe). Hypercholesterolaemia may occur as an isolated abnormality or in association with rises in triglycerides. Isolated hypertriglyceridaemia can also occur.

The exact cholesterol concentration requiring treatment depends on the patient's overall cardiovascular risk. In high-risk patients, such as those who have established ischaemic heart disease, treating a total cholesterol level above 5.0 mmol/l would be appropriate, while in otherwise healthy patients, patients might be better treated on the basis of their overall cardiovascular risk (≥ 30% over 10 years). The target cholesterol is less than 5.0 mmol/l or a 30% reduction.

In patients with a family single gene inherited hyperlipidaemia, more aggressive treatment should be undertaken even in the absence of other risk factors. These patients often have very high cholesterol levels (> 8.0 mmol/l).

Lowering cholesterol concentrations by drug therapy (with statins) reduces mortality from ischaemic heart disease either in secondary prevention or in high-risk patients in primary prevention. It may also reduce the risks of stroke although this is less certain.

Underlying diseases that may cause hyperlipidaemia, such as hypothyroidism or liver disease, should be excluded. At least two readings of cholesterol should be obtained over 2–3 months.

Treatment

The first line of treatment for hyperlipidaemia should always be diet, although in many patients this will be ineffective, sometimes because of poor compliance. Drug therapy may be needed in patients who do not respond to diet alone after several months. Drugs may take several weeks to achieve their effects and frequent changes of drug are not advised.

Drugs in hypercholesterolaemia

The statins: 3-hydroxy-3-methylglutaryl-CoA reductase inhibitors

3-Hydroxy-3-methylglutaryl (HMG)-CoA reductase is an enzyme that controls the rate-limiting step in the synthesis of cholesterol in the liver. If inhibited, the hepatocyte cannot manufacture cholesterol and responds by increasing its uptake of LDL from the blood. This does not interfere with the production of steroid hormones. Drugs that inhibit this enzyme are the most effective cholesterol-lowering drugs and reduce plasma LDL by as much as 50% depending on the dose used. In patients treated with these drugs, the relative risk of cardiovascular disease falls by about 25–30%.

Examples
Simvastatin and *pravastatin*, both taken once a day.

Therapeutic use
Hypercholesterolaemia, with or without hypertriglyceridaemia, which may also be lowered.

Adverse effects

- Headache
- Abdominal pain
- Transient minor elevations of liver function tests or of creatine phosphokinase are common and usually resolve spontaneously despite continued therapy
- Myositis
- Simvastatin can interfere with the metabolism of warfarin.

Other drugs

Fibrates (e.g. *gemfibrozil*, *bezafibrate*, *fenofibrate*) mainly lower triglycerides, and to a lesser extent LDL cholesterol, while increasing HDL cholesterol. Their exact actions are unclear but may include inhibition of HMG-CoA reductase (see above) and activation of lipoprotein lipase. They are heavily protein bound and this may interfere with other drugs, e.g. warfarin.

Gemfibrozil is proven to lower mortality from ischaemic heart disease.

Their adverse effects include myositis, gastrointestinal upset and increased gallstone formation.

Bile acid sequestrants (e.g. *colestyramine*) are taken orally and are not absorbed but bind to bile acids in the intestines. The bile acids are lost in the faeces, breaking their enterohepatic circulation and reducing the bile acid pool. The liver cells take up more cholesterol from LDL, lowering LDL serum concentrations, to increase its production of bile salts. Many patients find them unpleasant to take as they cause constipation and abdominal discomfort and compliance may be poor. They are not often used today.

Self-assessment: questions

Multiple choice questions

1. Drugs used in treating hypertension include:
   a. Diuretics
   b. Levodopa
   c. Oral nitrates
   d. ACE inhibitors
   e. Naproxen

2. In hypertension:
   a. A curable cause is found in most cases
   b. Treatment reduces the risks of stroke
   c. The choice of drug is often dictated by the patient's overall condition
   d. Non-drug therapy has no role
   e. A blood pressure reading of 210/120 mmHg with no complications requires urgent i.v. therapy

3. Calcium-channel blockers:
   a. Are negatively inotropic
   b. Are all highly selective for vascular smooth muscle
   c. Nifedipine may sometimes cause angina
   d. Sublingual nifedipine may be used in hypertensive crisis
   e. They are proven to reduce the risk of stroke when used to treat hypertension

4. With regard to hypercholesterolaemia:
   a. Patients with an average serum cholesterol are not at risk of myocardial infarction
   b. Lowering serum cholesterol by drugs improves life expectancy
   c. Hyperthyroidism may cause hypercholesterolaemia in patients without overt ischaemic heart disease
   d. Cholesterol is a vital part of cell membranes
   e. High HDL cholesterol is associated with an increased risk of atherosclerosis

5. Considering the drugs used to treat hyperlipidaemia:
   a. Simvastatin inhibits drug-metabolising enzymes
   b. Gemfibrozil may cause gallstones
   c. Simvastatin has a long safety record and can be recommended as first-line therapy
   d. Statins can be used for mixed hyperlipidaemia
   e. Colestyramine depletes the bile acid pool

6. The following drugs are correctly paired with their adverse effects:
   a. Gemfibrozil and abdominal pain
   b. Beta-blockers and cold hands
   c. Verapamil and diarrhoea
   d. Simvastatin and Addison's syndrome (adrenocortical failure)
   e. Thiazides and hypothyroidism

Case history questions

Case history 1

A 54-year-old man is a non-insulin-dependent diabetic and obese. He smokes 20 cigarettes per day. His blood pressure is 160/100 mmHg and his serum cholesterol is 6.4 mmol/l.

1. What is his risk of a cardiovascular event over the next 10 years?
2. What advice should he be given about his life-style?
3. What drug therapies might be considered for his hypertension?
4. What target would you set for his blood pressure control?
5. What drug therapies might be considered for his hypercholesterolamia?

Case history 2

A 55-year-old woman is found to have a blood pressure of 180/110 mmHg on several occasions. No cause is found, although she is obese.

1. She asks why she should be bothered about her blood pressure; what will you tell her?
2. What other cardiovascular risk factors need to be considered?
3. What drug therapy might be considered as a first line?

Her blood pressure is still not controlled.

4. What factors might you need to reconsider?
5. What drug therapy might be tried next?

Case history 3

A 45-year-old man who has had a myocardial infarction is found to have a serum cholesterol of 6.4 mmol/l.

1. Is this cause for concern?

> His triglycerides are normal and the LDL cholesterol is the fraction raised. He is given a low-cholesterol diet but his serum cholesterol does not improve over the next 3 months.

2. What treatment should be considered now?
3. What adverse effects should he be warned of?
4. What other drugs might he need to take?
5. Will lowering the patient's serum cholesterol substantially reduce the risk of further episodes of ischaemic heart disease?

Short note questions

Write short notes on the following:

1. Describe the management of a patient presenting to his GP with a blood pressure of 170/110 mmHg, with no other symptoms or signs of organ damage.
2. Two patients are found to have a serum cholesterol of 6.0 mmol/l and total cholesterol to HDL ratio of 4.2. The first is a 52-year-old man who has angina and smokes. The second is a 36-year-old woman who is normotensive (systolic blood pressure of 128 mmHg) and a non-smoker. She is not diabetic. How would you treat each of these two patients?

Extended matching items question

Theme: the cardiovascular system: prevention
Options

A. Doxazosin
B. Irbesartan
C. Hydralazine
D. Bendroflumethiazide (bendrofluazide)
E. Diazepam
F. Amiodarone
G. Moxonidine
H. Minoxidil
I. Atenolol
J. Diltiazem
K. Isosorbide mononitrate
L. Enalapril
M. Nifedipine
N. Methyldopa

For each of the patients in 1–4 who have mild hypertension, select the *most* appropriate drug therapy from options A–N to lower the blood pressure. Each option may be used once, more than once or not at all.

1. A 40-year-old woman who has asthma and who uses salbutamol and beclometasone inhalers.
2. A 50-year-old man who has been an insulin-dependent diabetic for 30 years and who has significant proteinuria.
3. A 70-year-old man with a previous history of gout.
4. A 60-year-old woman, a heavy smoker despite your advice, who also has COPD (chronic obstructive pulmonary disease) and angina.

Self-assessment: answers

Multiple choice answers

1. a. **True.** Thiazides are the main diuretics used but in patients with resistant hypertension or renal disease, loop diuretics are used.
   b. **False.** Levodopa is used to treat Parkinson's disease (see Ch. 6). Methyldopa is sometimes used to treat hypertension.
   c. **False.** Oral nitrates have little effect in hypertension.
   d. **True.** This is their most common use.
   e. **False.** Naproxen is a non-steroidal anti-inflammatory drug, many of which can cause fluid retention and exacerbate hypertension.

2. a. **False.** Only in 5–10% of cases is an underlying and treatable cause found.
   b. **True.** This is the main justification for treating hypertension.
   c. **True.** This is the essence of 'tailored care'.
   d. **False.** Although how effective non-drug therapy is, is often debated.
   e. **False.** Blood pressure is often overtreated in this situation. Oral therapy is probably adequate.

3. a. **True.** They reduce the force of contraction and may cause cardiac failure. Nifedipine may increase the force of contraction by sympathetic reflex; however, if the patient is taking beta-blockers, this is prevented and the negative inotropic effects of nifedipine may become more apparent.
   b. **False.** Hence adverse effect like constipation, caused by smooth muscle relaxation in the gastrointestinal tract.
   c. **True.** A paradox, because although used for treating angina, nifedipine may cause a tachycardia and can bring on angina. Nifedipine is, therefore, not first choice for exercise-induced angina, for which beta-blockers should be used.
   d. **False.** This was a popular treatment that lowered the blood pressure but can cause stroke or myocardial infarction because of the speed with which the blood pressure falls. Urgent treatment in hypertension is rarely necessary, so oral preparations are best used (including long-acting preparations of nifedipine).
   e. **True.** For some specific calcium-channel blockers (e.g. nitrendapine, a derivative of nifedipine) and presumably also for other calcium-channel blockers.

4. a. **False.** Cholesterol is only one risk factor and, in the UK, the average concentration is associated with ischaemic heart disease.
   b. **True.** Both in secondary prevention and in high-risk patients.
   c. **False.** Hypothyroidism causes hypercholesterolaemia.
   d. **True.**
   e. **False.** High HDL cholesterol concentrations seem to be protective against ischaemic heart disease. High LDL cholesterol concentrations are associated with increased risk. The ratio of HDL to LDL cholesterol is the favourite measure of cholesterol for assessing cardiac risk.

5. a. **True.** It can interfere with the metabolism of warfarin—an effect not found with pravastatin.
   b. **True.** A well-recognised adverse effect.
   c. **True.** Simvastatin has an established safety record and is proved to reduce overall mortality in hypercholesterolaemic patients with ischaemic heart disease.
   d. **True.** Not all statins are licenced for this use.
   e. **True.** This causes the liver to take up cholesterol from the blood.

6. a. **True.** Because of gastrointestinal upsets and gall stones.
   b. **True.** They block vasodilatory β_2-adrenoceptors (even the β_1-adrenoceptor-selective drugs).
   c. **False.** On the contrary, constipation is a problem.
   d. **False.** If simvastatin blocks cholesterol synthesis, it might be expected to have an effect on cholesterol-based hormonal production, such as cortisol. In fact, this is not a problem.
   e. **False.** There is no association.

Case history answers

Case history 1

1. His risk of an ischaemic event over the next 10 years is greater than 30%, so he merits aggressive treatment of all his risk factors.
2. He needs to stop smoking, lose weight and ensure good control of his diabetes.
3. The antihypertensive drug of first choice in this man would be an ACE inhibitor but thiazides or beta-blockers would be a reasonable alternative. Beta-blockers might be avoided if he requires insulin. There is uncertainty over whether calcium-channel

blockers should be used in diabetics. Some studies have suggested that calcium-channel blockers cause poorer outcomes than other drugs in diabetics, but other studies have rejected this view.

4. The blood pressure target for this man is 140/80 mmHg. This is a rigorous target and many patients will require combination therapy to achieve it.

5. His hyperlipidaemia is probably of a mixed type, i.e. both raised triglycerides and cholesterol, so either a statin (simvastatin is best for this) or a fibrate would be reasonable.

Case history 2

1. Blood pressure at this level increases her risk of stroke and myocardial infarction substantially—probably by a factor of about 2. Her absolute risk of a cardiovascular event (i.e. either stroke or myocardial infarction) is probably around 10–20% over the next 10 years. So she can be told that drug therapy can be expected to reduce risks of such events.

2. The other risk factors that might be considered are her cholesterol, her family history and her menopausal state: the risk of cardiovascular disease rises after the menopause, and it is not certain that hormone replacement therapy can prevent this rise (see Ch. 12).

3. There are several reasonable choices: thiazides, beta-blockers, calcium-channel blockers or ACE inhibitors are the most widely used. Thiazides or beta-blockers are the first choice both on grounds of the weight of evidence for their use and also of cost.

4. Is she complying with drug and other treatment, does she have white coat hypertension, could she have secondary hypertension? Has the blood pressure been measured properly, e.g. large cuff in an obese patient? Always ask about adverse effects of drugs, which a patient may not volunteer but which may result in poor adherence to the prescribed drugs.

5. One would consider adding a second drug, e.g. thiazides with a beta-blocker, or a trial of substitution, for instance swapping a thiazide for a beta-blocker or vice versa.

Case history 3

1. Yes: this cholesterol is raised and is probably a contributory factor in such a young patient having an infarct. If persistently elevated above 5.0 mmol/l, it should be treated with drug therapy. Other risk factors such as smoking etc. should also be considered. Note that this is secondary prevention, i.e. the patient has already had an event. The

guidelines in Figure 21 do not apply to these patients, who need more aggressive treatment of all risk factors.

2. Drug treatment with simvastatin or pravastatin should be the first choice.

3. Serious but rare adverse effects include hepatitis and myositis. More common and less severe are headache and abdominal pain, and sometimes (simvastatin) nightmares.

4. A patient like this will probably also be on low-dose aspirin, a beta-blocker and possibly an ACE inhibitor.

5. Yes, and it will reduce mortality risk (by around 30%).

Short note answers

1. The management of this patient should follow the broad guideline laid out in Figure 21. The patient should have the blood pressure measurement repeated on a number of occasions over 1 month, but if found to be sustained the patient is going to need treatment. Non-pharmacological treatment is indicated, such as weight loss, increased exercise and also addressing general cardiovascular risk factors, such as smoking etc. If the patient needs antihypertensive therapy, this should be tailored to the particular patient's needs. You should list some of the more commonly used drugs and which kinds of patient you would or would not use them in.

2. The first patient is a case for secondary prevention where rigorous lowering of his cholesterol is required. The second patient is a case of possible primary prevention and her data can be put into the risk tables. This demonstrates that, in fact, she is at fairly low risk of a cardiovascular event; therefore, at present she would not be a priority for cholesterol-lowering therapy, the risks of which might outweigh the benefits for her. (The 10-year risk for cardiovascular event in the first patient is of the order of 45% to 50%.)

Extended matching items answer

1. D is best but M is also acceptable. Of the main classes of antihypertensive, this patient is clearly unsuitable for a beta-blocker. ACE inhibitors are not ideal in asthmatics either, although they might be used with caution: their potentiation of bradykinin might exacerbate asthma, and their propensity to cause cough (especially in women, where it occurs in about 15–20%) can give rise to diagnostic problems. Thiazides are effective, inexpensive, have the longest experience and are proven to prevent stroke. Consequently, they are an ideal first choice. A long-acting calcium channel blocker would also be a

reasonable choice, e.g. sustained-release nifedipine or possibly diltiazem. The other listed antihypertensives should be reserved drugs for patients who fail to respond to the first line suggested.

2. L is the best choice. ACE inhibitors have been shown to reduce proteinuria in diabetics and this seems to slow developing nephropathy. This effect seems to be over and above any benefit in slowing nephropathy achieved just by lowering the blood pressure. Angiotensin receptor antagonists such as irbesartan (B) would probably have a similar effect, although this is the subject of ongoing trials at present. Calcium channel blockers have a weaker and less certain effect. Beta-blockers should probably be avoided in insulin-taking diabetics: they might mask some of the early symptoms of hypoglycaemia. Neither beta-blockers nor thiazides are shown to benefit proteinuria.

3. I would be best but L or M are also reasonable. Clearly a thiazide would not be a good choice here as it would be likely to exacerbate his gout. Other reasonable alternatives are, therefore, calcium channel blockers, ACE inhibitors and beta-blockers. This case and the others illustrate the importance of tailoring the medication to the patient's profile.

4. M or J would be best. Here we are using an antihypertensive which also has antianginal actions to try to achieve better control of two problems. Lowering the blood pressure alone might improve the angina but it seems reasonable to try to improve both with specific medication if possible. Beta-blockers would probably be the most effective for both but are excluded by her COPD. Isosorbide mononitrate is widely used in angina but has no useful antihypertensive effect.

Overview

This chapter reviews the drugs used in the treatment of established heart disease. The most common such disease is ischaemic heart disease, which often presents with angina or with myocardial infarction. Angina is treated with drugs that decrease the workload of the heart. Acute myocardial infarction is also treated with such drugs, together with thrombolytic agents to remove the clot that has blocked a coronary artery. Cardiac failure is the end result of other processes damaging the heart muscle, such as ischaemic heart disease or hypertension. It is mainly treated by 'offloading' the heart using ACE inhibitors, and by reducing fluid overload by using diuretics. Cardiac arrhythmia may complicate ischaemic heart disease but may also occur for other reasons. Drugs used to treat such arrhythmias are often negatively inotropic and may themselves cause arrhythmias.

4.1 Ischaemic heart disease

Learning objectives

You should:

- be able to explain the pathophysiology of atheromatous disease, angina and myocardial infarction
- be able to describe the drugs used in the treatment of angina pectoris and how these drugs are used in practice
- be able to describe the drugs used in the treatment of acute myocardial infarction
- know the emergency management of acute myocardial infarction
- be able to list the drug therapy that might be used in a patient after recovery from acute myocardial infarction.

Ischaemic heart disease is usually caused by atherosclerosis, with narrowing of the coronary arteries. Risk factors are described in Chapter 3. The most frequent manifestations of ischaemic heart disease are sudden death, angina pectoris or myocardial infarction.

Angina pectoris

Angina pectoris ('stable' angina) occurs when there is an imbalance between the oxygen supply (reduced by the narrowed vessels caused by atheroma or, in some patients, by spasm of a coronary artery) and oxygen demand (typically during exercise) and presents most commonly as an intermittent chest pain of short duration (Fig. 24). It is typically provoked by exertion or stress and is eased by rest.

Unstable angina is when a patient experiences repeated attacks with little or no provocation over a short period of time. It is caused by unstable atheromatous plaque and platelet aggregation. It is a medical emergency since many of these patients may go on to have a myocardial infarction.

Management of stable angina

The management of stable angina involves:

1. Treating a single acute attack:

- rest
- *glyceryl trinitrate* (GTN) tablets or spray

Clinical sketch

A 70-year-old man gets chest pain on exertion. This has been diagnosed as angina but has been stable for some time. One day he gets severe chest pain while sitting down, which is typical of his angina. He uses his GTN spray, which gives transient relief but the pain recurs within a matter of a few minutes. He uses the GTN spray again, but gets little relief.

Comment: This patient had previously stable angina but it now seems to be unstable, since it is occurring at rest. It has also failed to respond to GTN spray. This patient should seek medical attention immediately, either by contacting his GP or by going to the local A&E department, possibly by ambulance. He may be in the early stages of a myocardial infarction. He will require urgent hospital admission, investigation and stabilisation.

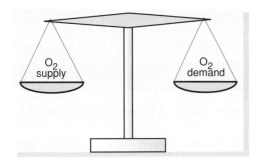

Decreased by:
Coronary artery
disease
Anaemia

Increased by:
Nitrates
Calcium-channel blockers
Beta-blockers

Increased by:
Exercise
Tachycardia
Hypertension

Decreased by:
Nitrates
Calcium-channel blockers
Beta-blockers

Fig. 24 The balance of oxygen demand and supply in the heart.

- medical attention for patients whose attacks do not respond within minutes to a first or second GTN tablet (they may be in the early stages of a myocardial infarction).

2. Prophylactic therapy: this should be taken regularly and involves three types of drug:

  - beta-blockers
  - calcium-channel blockers
  - oral nitrates.

  Each drug acts in a different way and they can often usefully be combined in the same patient. In general for patients with exercise-induced angina, a beta-blocker should be first choice.

3. Aspirin is also used, provided there are no contraindications, to reduce the risk of serious thrombotic complicatiᵒons. In patients who have had

Clinical sketch

A patient with angina is treated initially with a beta-blocker and GTN as required. His angina gradually deteriorates and a calcium channel blocker is added. This leads to initial improvement, but again over a period of 12 months there is a deterioration and a long-acting oral nitrate is added.

Comment: Antianginal drugs are often used in combination, although the evidence that such combinations are more effective than single or at the most two drugs is very weak. Patients with difficult to control angina (and many would advocate all patients) should have angiography to see if they are suitable for surgery. Patients also need their cardiovascular risk factors assessed and treated and this patient should probably also be on aspirin and, if his cholesterol is raised, on a lipid-lowering agent.

a previous myocardial infarction, aspirin may reduce the risks of further infarcts.

4. Correct risk factors where possible.

5. Many patients may benefit from interventions to relieve blockages in coronary vessels. Selection of patients for this depends on investigation, including treadmill exercise testing and angiography.

Management of unstable angina

Unstable angina is treated with antiplatelet agents such as oral aspirin in all patients and also with glycoprotein IIb/IIIa receptor inhibitors in high-risk patients. These drugs, e.g. *tirofiban* are given i.v. and act by binding to the receptor that is responsible for the final activation of platelet aggregation. They reduce the risks of subsequent myocardial infarction by about 40%. Patients with unstable angina are also treated with low-molecular-weight heparin. Other treatment is to initiate prophylactic antianginals immediately, especially beta-blockers. Patients whose pain does not settle quickly may need a procedure to relieve blockages.

Myocardial infarction

Myocardial infarction happens when thrombosis occurs on a ruptured atherosclerotic plaque, occluding a coronary artery so that part of the myocardium has no blood supply and dies. The patient usually suffers severe chest pain. Apart from loss of myocardium (which may lead to heart failure), the patient is also at risk from potentially fatal arrhythmias. Prompt action may reduce the loss of myocardium and improve survival.

Management of an acute myocardial infarction with ST elevation on ECG

Management is described in Box 2.

Box 2 Management of an acute myocardial infarction

1. Sublingual glyceryl trinitrate (it may be a severe attack of angina, and not a myocardial infarction)

2. Pain relief – use i.v. opiates (usually with an antiemetic)

4. Aspirin (if there is no contraindication) orally

5. Thrombolytic drugs (if there is no contraindication) (see Ch. 5)

6. Other treatments can also decrease mortality but are less widely used, including i.v. atenolol.

Treatment after myocardial infarction

All of these drugs have been proven to reduce mortality after myocardial infarction; they are often used in combination:

- beta-blockers
- ACE (angiotensin-converting enzyme) inhibitors

- aspirin
- lipid-lowering therapy.

Drugs to treat ischaemic heart disease

Nitrates

At a cellular level, nitrates are converted in the body to nitric oxide (NO), which combines with sulphydryl (–SH) groups to form nitrosothiols. These activate the enzyme guanyl cyclase to produce the second messenger cyclic GMP. Cyclic GMP causes smooth muscle relaxation and vasodilatation (Fig. 25).

In the body, nitrates dilate blood vessels in three areas: the venous circulation, which decreases venous return and the preload on the heart; the arterioles, reducing peripheral resistance and the afterload (both of these reduce the stress on the myocardial wall and lower oxygen demand); and the coronary arteries, especially if there is coronary spasm (this improves oxygen supply). The reduction in preload is probably the major effect.

Nitrate tolerance

Many patients become tolerant to the antianginal effects of nitrates if they receive them for prolonged periods (>24 hours) as a result of depletion of the essential –SH groups. When prescribing, a nitrate-free period should be built into the regimen. For example, *isosorbide dinitrate* taken at 8 a.m. and 2 p.m. provides cover for daytime exertion and leaves the patient free of nitrates overnight, preventing tolerance. The best regimen must be worked out for each patient.

Examples

Glyceryl trinitrate is well absorbed when given sublingually; if taken orally, it is broken down by first-pass metabolism in the liver. GTN is volatile, and the tablets should be kept in a sealed dark container; tablets from an opened container will lose their effect after about 4 weeks. A GTN spray is more expensive but keeps longer. It acts very rapidly after sublingual use, within 1–2 minutes and the effects last for 30–60 minutes. It can also be given i.v. or in the form of GTN ointment or transdermal patches as it can be absorbed through the skin. All patients with angina should carry either GTN tablets or spray with them at all times to treat any acute attacks.

Isosorbide dinitrate is taken sublingually, orally or i.v. It is absorbed more slowly but has a longer action. It is partly metabolised by the liver to isosorbide mononitrate, and both the dinitrate and mononitrate contribute to its effects. Its half-life is 2–4 hours. Isosorbide mononitrate can also be given orally. It is not metabolised by the liver, and so more reliable plasma nitrate concentrations are obtained after mononitrate than dinitrate—this is usually of little practical importance.

Therapeutic uses

- Angina pectoris—acute treatment and prophylaxis
- Congestive cardiac failure (see below).

Adverse effects

These result from vasodilatation and include headache (from vasodilatation of cerebral blood vessels) and facial flushing (very common).

Nicorandil

Nicorandil has dual actions, partly nitrate-like and partly those of a potassium-channel opener (similar effects to a calcium-channel blocker). It is as effective as other drugs in monotherapy but its role in combinations is uncertain.

Other drugs

See Chapter 3 for:

- beta-blockers
- calcium-channel blockers
- ACE inhibitors.

See Chapter 5 for:

- aspirin
- low-molecular-weight heparin
- thrombolytic agents.

4.2 Cardiac failure

Learning objectives

You should:

- be able to list the causes of heart failure
- be able to describe the pathophysiology of heart failure including the role of the renin–angiotensin–aldosterone system
- know the drugs used in the treatment of heart failure and the use of these drugs in practice.

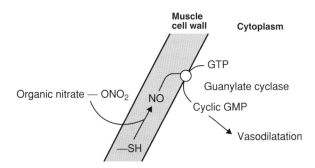

Fig. 25 The actions of nitrates.

Cardiac failure is usually the result of damage to the myocardium, from ischaemic heart disease, myocarditis or cardiomyopathy. Other causes include poorly controlled hypertension or damage to the valves of the heart, fluid overload, metabolic disease such as thyrotoxicosis, or drugs. Cardiac failure may result in poor perfusion of tissues or vital organs (forward failure) and congestion of the lungs or periphery with excessive fluid (backward failure, causing pulmonary or peripheral oedema). Treatment of acute pulmonary oedema is described in Box 3.

Box 3 Treatment of acute pulmonary oedema

Oxygen, usually in high concentration

Morphine with antiemetic i.v.

Loop diuretic i.v.

Consider nitrates to reduce preload if no rapid response

If hypotensive and still in pulmonary oedema, consider possible cardiogenic shock—may need positive inotropes

Consider underlying causes, e.g. ischaemic heart disease, arrhythmia, etc.

The renin–angiotensin–aldosterone axis

Reduced perfusion of vital organs prompts counter-regulatory mechanisms to restore perfusion. The sympathetic nervous system causes peripheral vasoconstriction and stimulates the heart directly. The renin–angiotensin–aldosterone system, a physiological means of controlling blood pressure and fluid balance, is activated. Renin is secreted by the juxtaglomerular apparatus in the kidney in response to a fall in renal perfusion. Renin converts angiotensinogen, a protein produced by the liver, to angiotensin I, and ACE converts this to the active angiotensin II. Angiotensin II acts at specific receptors (AT receptors) to cause direct vasoconstriction, raising blood pressure (Fig. 26). It also stimulates release of aldosterone from the adrenal gland, which in turn promotes Na^+ and fluid retention and enhances the actions of the sympathetic system by promoting noradrenaline release.

In cardiac failure, all of these are useful in the short term, but in the long term they increase the load on the failing heart and are ultimately detrimental. Heart failure tends to progress. The New York Heart Association Classification of Heart Failure and likely drugs used at each stage are shown in Table 1.

Treatment of chronic cardiac failure involves reducing fluid retention with diuretics and reducing the preload or afterload on the heart by using vasodilators, particularly the ACE inhibitors, which will also block the renin–angiotensin–aldosterone system (Fig. 26). Drugs that increase the force of contraction of the heart (positive inotropic drugs) have only a minor role and may be harmful.

Clinical sketch

A male patient aged 75 has previously had a myocardial infarction. He now finds that he gets progressively shorter and shorter of breath when he exerts himself. His ankles tend to swell. He feels generally tired, but has no chest pain.

Comment: The commonest cause of cardiac failure in the Western world is ischaemic heart disease, leading to left ventricular dysfunction. The aim of treating acute myocardial infarction is to prevent loss of myocardium; however, as more patients survive myocardial infarctions and grow older, the incidence of heart failure is rising. This patient is probably suffering from cardiac failure, but we cannot exclude chronic obstructive pulmonary disease as the cause of his symptoms. He should have an echocardiogram; given his previous history of myocardial infarction, heart failure is likely. He will probably need treatment with an ACE inhibitor and a diuretic. When stable he might also benefit from a beta-blocker.

The patient presents to hospital with palpitations and shortness of breath. On examination he is found to be in atrial fibrillation.

Comment: Atrial fibrillation is probably the commonest pathological cardiac arrhythmia. It can compromise cardiac function in two ways. First, the loss of the atrial 'push' (which may account for 20 to 25% of total cardiac output) and, second, and more important, the rapid heart rate can lead to poor filling of the left ventricle with even more loss of cardiac output. Treatment should be, if possible, to get the patient out of atrial fibrillation (this may require electrical cardioversion). If this is not possible or feasible then controlling the rate with digoxin would be the usual treatment. The patient will need a loading dose of digoxin over 24 to 48 hours in hospital followed by a lower maintenance dose. The patient should also be considered for warfarin therapy to reduce the risk of embolic phenomena from the atrial fibrillation. The cause of the atrial fibrillation should be investigated and treated if necessary.

The patient is treated with a standard dose of digoxin and his atrial fibrillation comes under control. Subsequently he develops chronic renal failure with a decrease in his creatinine clearance. He presents at the A&E department with a heart rate of 30 beats/min.

Comment: Digoxin is cleared by filtration. In patients with impaired renal function, accumulation of digoxin with adverse effects such as profound bradycardia can occur. The maintenance dose needs to be reduced in patients with impaired renal function. It is important to monitor plasma concentrations of digoxin and adjust the dose as well, but the patient response is always more important than plasma concentration.

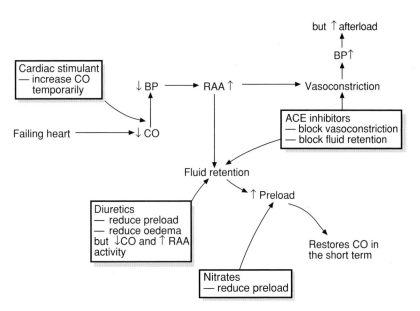

Fig. 26 Treating heart failure. BP, blood pressure; CO, cardiac output; RAA, renin–angiotensin–aldosterone axis.

Table 1 New York Heart Association Classification of Heart Failure

Grade	Description	Typical drugs
I	Left ventricle dysfunction detectable but asymptomatic	ACE inhibitor
II	Dyspnoeic on mild-to-moderate exertion	ACE inhibitor and diuretic
III	Dyspnoeic on mild exertion	ACE inhibitor and diuretic and spironolactone
IV	Dyspnoeic at rest	ACE inhibitor and diuretic and spironolactone

Drugs to treat congestive cardiac failure

The main types of drug used are:

- diuretics
- ACE inhibitors
- nitrates
- beta-blockers
- inotropic drugs.

Diuretics

Thiazides may be used alone in mild heart failure. For moderate-to-severe heart failure, loop diuretics will be used. In very severe heart failure with extensive resistant oedema, thiazides may be used cautiously with loop diuretics to achieve a very profound diuresis.

Loop diuretics

The loop diuretics act by inhibiting the resorption of Cl^- in the ascending limb of the loop of Henle. This causes loss of Cl^- and its main cation, Na^+, and water follows the electrolytes.

The response to loop diuretics is dose related. They have a greater diuretic effect than the thiazides.

When used i.v. in acute pulmonary oedema, the loop diuretics also cause venodilatation and reduce preload before diuresis can start. Like the thiazides, the loop diuretics cause K^+ loss, but unlike them, they also cause Ca^{2+} loss.

Examples

Furosemide (frusemide) or *bumetamide* act within 10 minutes of an i.v. dose. After oral administration, their effects peak at about 1 hour and last about 4–6 hours.

Therapeutic uses

- Congestive heart failure
- Oedema for other reasons
- Hypertension (only in combination with other drugs or if renal failure present; Ch. 3).

Adverse effects

- Hypokalaemia
- Renal impairment: resulting from dehydration and from prerenal failure and a direct toxic effect on the kidney
- Ototoxicity, i.e. deafness (furosemide only).

Drug interactions

These are as for thiazides (Ch. 3).

Potassium-sparing diuretics

The K^+-sparing diuretics are a chemically diverse group that, unlike other diuretics, retain K^+. They act in the distal convoluted tubule where K^+/Na^+ exchange occurs and are only weak diuretics. Their major use is in treating or preventing hypokalaemia caused by thiazides or loop diuretics. In the past, K+ supplements were widely used, but very high doses are required, reducing patient compliance. It is often not necessary to prevent or treat diuretic-induced hypokalaemia, but if this is required, K+-sparing diuretics should be used. This is not usually necessary and may be dangerous (possible severe hyperkalaemia) in patients taking ACE inhibitors as well as diuretics.

Examples

Spironolactone is an aldosterone antagonist. Aldosterone causes Na+ retention and K+ loss, and spironolactone does the reverse.

Triamterene and *amiloride* interfere with Na+/K+ exchange.
All are administered orally.

Therapeutic uses

Spironolactone:

- severe congestive heart failure (usually with loop diuretics and with ACE inhibitors): in these patients it reduces mortality probably by ensuring the maximum blockade of the renin–angiotensin–aldosterone system
- primary hyperaldosteronism (Conn's syndrome)
- ascites resulting from liver disease
- diuretic-induced hypokalaemia.

Triamterene/amiloride:

- diuretic-induced hypokalaemia
- oedema.

Adverse effects

- Hyperkalaemia
- Gynaecomastia (spironolactone only).

Drug interactions

Combinations with K+ supplements or ACE inhibitors may lead to dangerous hyperkalaemia.

Other diuretics

Osmotic diuretics (e.g. *mannitol*) are filtered by the glomerulus and retain water in the tubule by their osmotic effects, causing diuresis. They are rarely used, but when they are, it is most often to lower intracranial pressure and in glaucoma. The carbonic anhydrase inhibitor *acetazolamide* causes mild diuresis and severe hypokalamia—it is used to treat glaucoma.

ACE inhibitors

The ACE inhibitors are described in Chapter 3. In heart failure, they have been shown to reduce mortality by about 25%, to ease symptoms and to reduce hospitalisation. They should be used in all grades of heart failure if tolerated. Even in the mildest failure, they reduce the risk of further deterioration.

Nitrates

Nitrates are venodilators and, therefore, reduce preload on the heart. This is very effective in acute heart failure where i.v. isosorbide dinitrate may be used. In chronic heart failure, nitrates may be used as venodilators but the combined arterial and venous vasodilatation achieved by ACE inhibitors is more effective.

Beta-blockers

Some beta-blockers (*carvedilol*, *bisoprolol* and *metoprolol*) have been shown to reduce mortality and hospitalisations when given to patients with stable heart failure (i.e. not within 2–3 months of any deterioration or hospital admission). They may do this by protecting the myocardium from excessive sympathetic stimulation, from ischaemia or from arrhythmias. Beta-blockers are negatively inotropic so they must be used cautiously under expert guidance.

Inotropic drugs

The inotropic drugs are cardiac stimulants. *Digoxin* is discussed below. Other positive inotropes such as **dobutamine** (stimulates β_1-adrenoceptors) can be used in acute cardiogenic shock (i.e. severe acute heart failure with hypotension). Attempts to use other positive inotropes (e.g. milrinone) in the long term have been abandoned as they increased mortality.

Digoxin and other digitalis glycosides

At a cellular level, the digitalis compounds block the exchange of intracellular Na+ for extracellular K+ by inhibiting Na+/K+-ATPase in the cell membrane; this increases intracellular Na+ and encourages its exchange for Ca^{2+}, raising intracellular Ca^{2+} and causing a positive inotropic effect (Fig. 27). These effects cause characteristic changes in the electrocardiograph (ECG) ('reverse tick').

In the body, digitalis compounds also stimulate the vagus and increase vagal tone. This is its mode of action in its main clinical use, which is to slow the heart in atrial fibrillation. The positive inotropic effect may be useful in heart failure, even if the patient is in sinus rhythm.

Examples

Digoxin can be given orally (well absorbed) or parenterally and is excreted unchanged by the kidneys. Its half-life is 1.5 days but is greatly prolonged in renal impairment. Digoxin has a narrow therapeutic range, and it is useful to monitor plasma digoxin levels. If a rapid effect is required, it is useful to give a loading dose initially, followed by a maintenance dose daily because of the long half-life.

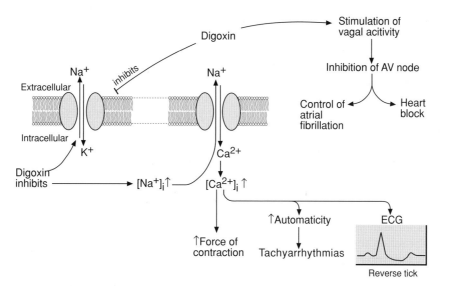

Fig. 27 Actions of digoxin. AV, atrioventricular.

Digitoxin has a longer half-life, about 6 days, and is metabolised by the liver.

Therapeutic uses

- Atrial fibrillation (to slow the ventricular response)
- Congestive heart failure (even in patients in sinus rhythm).

Adverse effects

- Note hypokalaemia or hypercalcaemia increases the risk of digitalis toxicity
- Hypothyroidism or old age increases sensitivity to standard doses
- Gastrointestinal effects: anorexia, nausea, vomiting, occasionally diarrhoea
- Neurological effects: malaise, fatigue, depression, confusion, insomnia, altered colour vision (yellow/green predominance)
- Cardiovascular effects: any cardiac arrhythmia may occur, especially ventricular bigeminy and bradycardias including complete heart block; the ECG may show first-degree heart block at an early stage, but serious arrhythmias may occur without warning
- Others: gynaecomastia.

Contraindications

- Acute myocardial ischaemia (may increase oxygen demand)
- Disease of the atrioventricular (AV) node (may cause heart block)
- Renal impairment (especially digoxin)
- Before electrical cardioversion (may precipitate heart block).

Drug interactions

- Diuretics may cause hypokalaemia and worsen digoxin toxicity

- Verapamil, amiodarone and quinidine all increase plasma digoxin levels by reducing its clearance.

Treatment of digoxin toxicity

Treatment depends on severity: in very severe overdose, hyperkalaemia and hyponatraemia can occur because of the cellular effects.

1. Withdraw drug
2. Correct low serum K^+ by i.v. administration
3. Treat ventricular arrhythmias with phenytoin or lidocaine
4. Digoxin-specific antibodies will bind to and inactivate digoxin and can be used in life-threatening cases (very expensive).

4.3 Cardiac arrhythmias

Learning objectives

You should:

- be able to describe the phases of the action potential
- be able to list the major groups of antiarrhythmic drugs
- be able to name one drug from each group and describe the drugs you have named

Many minor cardiac arrhythmias often do not require treatment; for example, atrial or ventricular ectopics. Others are more serious and require treatment for termination or prevention. This may include correction of the underlying cause where possible; non-drug treatment, such as carotid sinus massage for supraventricular tachycardias; electrical cardioversion or pacemaking for serious supraventricular or ventricular arrhythmias; and drugs.

Antiarrhythmic drugs are usually classified according to the Vaughan Williams system, which is based on the changes in the action potential produced by drugs in isolated cardiac cells. Many drugs have mixed properties and do not fit neatly into any one class. The classification is of limited clinical value.

The action potential

The gradient of electrical charge across the membrane of a resting cardiac cell is −80 to −90 mV. This is maintained by movement of ions through specific ion channels in the membrane. Depolarisation and repolarisation of cardiac cells occurs in the following stages (Fig. 28):

Phase 0: rapid depolarisation caused by entry of Na^+ through the 'fast' sodium channel

Phase 1: early repolarisation, caused by closing of the sodium channel and opening of potassium channels

Phase 2: a plateau where there is a balance between K^+ exit and Ca^{2+} entry; the Ca^{2+} entry is through the opening of 'slow' channels

Phase 3: the late repolarisation phase caused by further K^+ exit and closing of the calcium channels

Phase 4: the slow depolarisation phase; the resting potential is restored and Na^+ and K^+ concentrations are restored by exchange pumps. There is a slow entry of Na^+ into the cell, decreasing the potential difference until the threshold potential is reached and a new action potential is triggered.

Classes of antiarrhythmic drug

Class I

Class I drugs block the rapid Na^+ current and slow phase 0. There are three subgroups: Ia, which delays repolarisation and lengthens the action potential; Ib, which accelerates repolarisation and shortens the action potential; and Ic, which has no effect on action potential duration but affects Purkinje tissue to slow conduction and prolong the QRS complex.

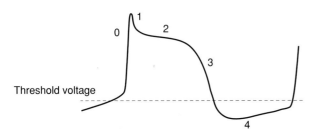

Fig. 28 The action potential in a Purkinje fibre. Cells from the atrioventricular node and other fibres show different patterns.

Class Ia. Disopyramide is the most commonly used in Europe. Disopyramide is used to treat atrial and ventricular arrhythmias. It may be given orally (as prophylaxis) or i.v. (for treatment). Its adverse effects include anticholinergic effects (urinary retention, blurred vision, dry mouth) and a negative inotropic effect, leading to hypotension or heart failure. It may precipitate cardiac arrhythmias in some patients.

Class Ib. Lidocaine (also used as a local anaesthetic, see Ch. 8) is given i.v. (poorly absorbed orally and subject to first-pass metabolism) to treat acute ventricular arrhythmias such as ventricular tachycardia, especially after myocardial infarction as it is particularly effective in ischaemic tissue. It is rapidly metabolised by the liver with a half-life of 2 hours during prolonged infusion. Single bolus doses have a much shorter duration of action (5–10 minutes) because of redistribution. Its toxic effects include drowsiness, paraesthesia and convulsions. It has little negative inotropic or proarrhythmic effect. *Mexiletine* is similar but is active after oral administration.

Class Ic. Flecainide is used orally or i.v. for atrial or ventricular arrhythmias. It is proarrhythmic and negatively inotropic, and it is usually reserved for very serious arrhythmias. It may also cause dizziness, headache and rashes.

Class II

The class II drugs are the beta-blockers, which have little effect on intracellular electrical activity except to slow phase 4. They may be given i.v. or orally, especially for atrial or exercise-induced arrhythmias. See above for adverse effects and other uses. *Sotalol* is the most widely used as an antiarrhythmic.

Class III

The class III drugs prolong the action potential by inhibiting repolarisation (phase 3). *Amiodarone* is used to treat atrial and ventricular arrhythmias. It also has Na^+-blocking effects (class I). It has little negative inotropic effect but it lengthens the QT interval. It is

---

Clinical sketch

A patient with recurrent ventricular tachycardia is treated with *disopyramide*. This controls his arrhythmia, but he complains of progressive shortness of breath.

Comment: Many antidysrhythmic drugs are negatively inotropic and this patient may have developed cardiac failure as a result of disopyramide therapy. Alternatively, the pathology underlying the arrhythmia (e.g. ischaemic heart disease) may have given rise to heart failure. It can be difficult to sort out which is responsible in a patient like this. Such dilemmas are not unusual in patients with multiple problems.

difficult to use because it has an exceedingly long half-life of 25–110 days, and because of its adverse effects: These include:

- proarrhythmia
- pneumonitis and pulmonary fibrosis
- hypo- or hyperthyroidism
- peripheral neuropathy
- hepatitis.

Minor effects include:

- corneal microdeposits of the drug (may cause halos around lights)
- photosensitivity of the skin and skin pigmentation.
- drug interactions, with decreased metabolism of warfarin, increased digoxin concentration.

Class IV

The calcium antagonists (verapamil mainly, but not dihydropyridines) are effective in AV nodal arrhythmias, where the action potential largely results from Ca^{2+} entry rather than Na^+ entry. Verapamil is used i.v. or orally to treat supraventricular arrhythmias.

Other drugs used in cardiac arrhythmias

The following three drugs do not fit into the classification given above.

Atropine. The anticholinergic drug atropine is used acutely in severe symptomatic bradycardias, as it blocks vagal tone. If long-term treatment is required, an electronic pacemaker is used.

Digoxin. Used for atrial fibrillation (see above).

Adenosine. This purine nucleoside acts on specific adenosine receptors in the sinoatrial node and causes bradycardia. It is used i.v. to treat supraventricular arrhythmias. It has no negative inotropic effects (unlike verapamil) and a very short half-life (less than 2 seconds) and so adverse effects are likely to be only transient; they include wheezing (asthma is contraindication), flushing and hypotension.

Drug of choice in arrhythmias

The antiarrhythmic drug of choice depends on speed of response required, presence of other conditions, including heart failure etc. Remember non-pharmacological methods (vagal stimulation manouevres, electrical cardioversion) may be more appropriate, depending on the circumstances:

- supraventricular tachycardia (not caused by Wolff–Parkinson–White): adenosine or verapamil for treatment, sotalol or verapamil for prophylaxis
- arrhythmias caused by Wolff–Parkinson–White: amiodarone, disopyramide, flecainide
- atrial flutter: drugs generally unsatisfactory; could use digoxin or disopyramide or amiodarone
- atrial fibrillation: digoxin to control the rate; disopyramide or amiodarone to cardiovert back to sinus rhythm (remember anticoagulation; Ch. 5)
- ventricular tachycardia: lidocaine, amiodarone.

Self-assessment: questions

Multiple choice questions

1. Drug combinations used in the treatment of angina include:
   a. Glyceryl trinitrate and salbutamol
   b. Digoxin and verapamil
   c. Nifedipine and isosorbide dinitrate
   d. Diazepam and atenolol
   e. Metoprolol and nifedipine

2. The following drugs are safe to use in patients with congestive cardiac failure:
   a. Propranolol
   b. Carbenoxolone
   c. Enalapril
   d. Amoxicillin
   e. Morphine

3. A patient with an acute myocardial infarction should usually be given:
   a. Thrombolytic therapy
   b. Paracetamol
   c. Diamorphine
   d. Nitrates
   e. Diazepam

4. With regard to the use of nitrates:
   a. Tolerance occurs only to the adverse effects and not to the antianginal effect
   b. Nitrates may have a diuretic effect
   c. Glyceryl trinitrate is given to relieve angina rapidly
   d. The major adverse effects of nitrates are predictable from their pharmacological action
   e. Liver metabolism rapidly terminates the action of all nitrates

5. Beta-blockers:
   a. May be used to treat tachycardia in patients with hypovolaemic shock or congestive cardiac failure
   b. Atenolol does not precipitate asthma
   c. Downregulation of adrenoceptors may occur in patients who take propranolol long term
   d. Lipophilic beta-blockers are more likely to cause CNS adverse effects
   e. Plasma concentrations are closely related to clinical activity

7. Drugs that may worsen cardiac failure include:
   a. Corticosteroids
   b. Calcium-channel blockers
   c. Nitrates
   d. Indometacin
   e. Daunorubicin

8. In congestive heart failure:
   a. Secondary hyperaldosteronism is a feature
   b. Fluid retention is a physiological response to a fall in cardiac output
   c. Positive inotropic drugs are the major treatment
   d. Diuretics prevent activation of the renin–angiotensin–aldosterone system
   e. Thiazides and loop diuretics may have vasodilator effects

9. In diuretic treatment:
   a. Thiazides may cause hypercholesterolaemia
   b. Hyperkalaemia is a common adverse effect of thiazides and loop diuretics
   c. High-dose thiazides are appropriate in severe hypertension
   d. Furosemide (frusemide) acts mainly in the distal convoluted tubule
   e. Potassium-sparing diuretics are the first choice in treating congestive cardiac failure

10. Digoxin:
    a. May be safely used in standard doses in patients with a glomerular filtration rate of 10 ml/min
    b. May cause tachyarrhythmias or bradyarrhythmias
    c. May cause hyponatraemia and hyperkalaemia in overdose
    d. May cause ST elevation on an ECG
    e. If given with diuretics, the serum K^+ should be monitored

11. ACE inhibitors:
    a. Are specific and only block breakdown of angiotensin
    b. Are effective vasodilators
    c. Improve life expectancy of patients with congestive cardiac failure
    d. May increase intrarenal blood flow
    e. Cough is the most common adverse effect

12. The following statements are correct:
    a. Many antiarrhythmics span several classes of the Vaughan Williams classification
    b. Lidocaine is excreted unchanged by the kidney
    c. Many antiarrhythmics have negative inotropic effects
    d. Amiodarone reaches a steady plasma concentration after about 25 days
    e. Adenosine is used to treat supraventricular tachycardias

Case history questions

Case history 1

A 65-year-old man presents to an A&E department with a history of severe central chest pain for 2 hours and typical ECG changes of an acute inferior myocardial infarction.

1. What drugs should he be given in the absence of any contraindication?
2. What contraindications would make you hesitate about giving each of these?

The patient suddenly develops an acute bradycardia.

3. What drug might you give to correct this?

The patient subsequently has an uncomplicated course.

4. What drug therapy would be appropriate for him to continue taking at home after discharge?
5. What advice might you give him?

Case history 2

A 60-year-old man who smokes and who has a history of chronic obstructive pulmonary disease (COPD) is diagnosed as having angina on exertion.

1. What drug therapy might he be given?
2. What advice might he be given?
3. What is nitrate tolerance and how can it be avoided?

He is also found to be hypercholesterolaemic, with a cholesterol of 8.6. mmol/l

4. How would you treat this initially?

His serum cholesterol fails to respond to your first treatment.

5. What would you consider next?

He uses nebulised high-dose salbutamol for his COPD but notices that this tends to bring on an attack of angina.

6. Why might this be?

Case history 3

A 45-year-old woman develops recurrent supraventricular tachycardias. She is treated with several drugs over a period unsuccessfully, and then given amiodarone, which seems to control the arrhythmias.

1. What blood tests should be considered before she starts on amiodarone?
2. If she starts taking it at the usual maintenance dose, how long will it be before the plasma concentrations of the drug reach steady state?
3. She is also taking warfarin because of a previous pulmonary embolism: does starting amiodarone pose any problems, and if so, how can the problems be managed?
4. Why was amiodarone not the first choice of antiarrhythmic drug?

Case history 4

A 70-year-old man develops dyspnoea and oedema and is found to have mild congestive cardiac failure.

1. What drug or drugs might he be started on?

He is also found to be in atrial fibrillation and this is assumed to be chronic.

2. How should this be treated?
3. If he does not respond adequately to your first choice of treatment for his heart failure, what drug or drugs might be added in later?
4. If he develops acute pulmonary oedema, how should this be treated?

He complains of knee pain and is prescribed indometacin.

5. Why might this be unwise?

Short note questions

Write short notes on the following:

1. The drug therapy that a patient might take for secondary prevention after a myocardial infarction.
2. The use of ACE inhibitors in cardiovascular disease.

Extended matching items question

Theme: treatment of cardiovascular disease
Options

A. Atenolol, aspirin, simvastatin
B. Amiodarone
C. Streptokinase
D. Isosorbide mononitrate, enalapril, glyceryl trinitrate
E. Verapamil
F. Isosorbide mononitrate, glyceryl trinitrate
G. Atenolol
H. Dipyridamole

For each of the questions 1–6, choose the most appropriate answer from options A–H. Each option may be used once, more than once or not at all.

1. Which therapy would be appropriate to reduce the rate of contraction of the left ventricle?
2. Which therapy would be appropriate to decrease oxygen demand on the heart?
3. Which therapy would be appropriate to facilitate secondary prevention of further episodes after myocardial infarction?
4. Which therapy would be appropriate to increase oxygen supply to the heart?
5. Which therapy would be appropriate for angina pectoris?
6. Which therapy would be appropriate when there is a requrement for sulphydryl groups for drug function?

Self-assessment: answers

Multiple choice answers

1. a. **False**. Glyceryl trinitrate is appropriate, but salbutamol is a β_2-agonist.
   b. **False**. Digoxin may increase oxygen demand and worsen ischaemic heart disease. It has no role in angina unless there is also atrial fibrillation. Verapamil is useful in angina and is sometimes combined with digoxin to control difficult cases of atrial fibrillation (because of its effects at the AV node).
   c. **True**. Both of these drugs are used in angina and act by different mechanisms and so can be usefully combined.
   d. **False**. The use of diazepam, a sedative, is inappropriate: it will have no effect on myocardial oxygen balance. Atenolol is valuable in angina. Beta-blockers are sometimes used in anxiety states because they reduce the somatic manifestations (tachycardia, tremor, etc.).
   e. **True**. Both drugs are used in angina and can be combined in more severe cases.

2. a. **False**. Beta-blockers have a negative inotropic effect that may worsen cardiac failure.
   b. **False**. Carbenoxolone is structurally related to aldosterone and may cause fluid retention.
   c. **True**. Enalapril should be used with diuretics as standard therapy in most cases of cardiac failure.
   d. **True**. But some penicillins have a large Na^+ load, e.g. carbenicillin, and should be avoided in cardiac failure.
   e. **True**. Morphine is used for its vasodilatating and sedative effects in addition to diuretics and vasodilators in acute left ventricular failure.

3. a. **True**. Standard treatment unless there is a clear contraindication. A patient who has recently had streptokinase could be given altepase.
   b. **False**. This would be inadequate as analgesia and has no antiplatelet action. Aspirin in contrast has been proven to improve mortality.
   c. **True**. Pain relief is very important, and strong opiates are the drugs of choice.
   d. **True**. Usually in the form of a GTN spray, but some would give them i.v.
   e. **False**. The patient may understandably be anxious, but this is better treated by pain relief and reassurance.

4. a. **False**. Tolerance occurs to both, although often more to the adverse effects; hence the need for a nitrate-free period when prescribing nitrates.
   b. **False**. Nitrates are effective in heart failure by reducing preload (venous vasodilatation).
   c. **True**. Standard treatment.
   d. **True**. Since nitrates are vasodilators, and the adverse effects are vasodilatatory in nature, this is a definition of a type A adverse effect (see Ch. 21).
   e. **False**. Although true for GTN, this is not true for isosorbide mononitrate.

5. a. **False**. This is likely to kill a patient.
   b. **False**. Even the β_1-specific blockers such as atenolol block β_2-adrenoceptors to some extent.
   c. **False**. Upregulation, i.e. increased number and sensitivity of receptors, occurs.
   d. **True**. Because they cross the blood–brain barrier more readily.
   e. **False**. The clinical activity often lasts longer than might be anticipated from the plasma half-life. The relevant factor is the duration of receptor binding, which is difficult to measure; plasma concentration is only a surrogate for this, which works reasonably well for some drugs but not for beta-blockers.

7. a. **True**. May cause Na^+ retention.
   b. **True**. Negative inotropes.
   c. **False**. Frequently used to treat cardiac failure.
   d. **True**. Along with most non-steroidal anti-inflammatory drugs, it may reduce prostaglandin production in the kidney and hence cause fluid retention and reduce the effects of diuretics.
   e. **True**. May cause a cardiomyopathy.

8. a. **True.** May cause Na^+ and fluid retention. Secondary hyperaldosteronism may be worsened by diuretic therapy.
   b. **True**. Ultimately it becomes harmful in cardiac failure.
   c. **False**. A very minor part of therapy for heart failure.
   d. **False**. Diuretics may increase activation of the renin–angiotensin–aldosterone system.
   e. **True**. This accounts for some of the action of furosemide (frusemide) in acute pulmonary oedema and for the action of thiazides in hypertension.

9. a. **True**. Probably not a long-term effect.
   b. **False**. Hypokalaemia is common.
   c. **False**. More likely to cause adverse effects with little increase in hypotensive effects.
   d. **False**. Furosemide is a loop diuretic that works mainly in the ascending limb of the loop of Henle.

e. **False**. Potassium-sparing diuretics are weak and loop diuretics are the first choice.

10. a. **False**. Digoxin is likely to have a very long half-life in a patient with such poor renal function, and the patient would be at risk of digoxin toxicity if usual doses were used.
    b. **True**. Almost any arrhythmia can result from digoxin: heart block or ventricular bigeminy are the most common.
    c. **True**. Because K^+ can no longer enter the cell nor Na^+ leave the cell as a result of the poisoning of the Na^+/K^+-ATPase.
    d. **False**. ST depression is the common change seen on ECG in a reverse tick pattern.
    e. **True**. Since diuretics may cause hypokalaemia, and hypokalaemia makes digoxin toxicity more likely.

11. a. **False**. Other peptides such as bradykinin are also affected.
    b. **True**. Hence their value in hypertension and cardiac failure.
    c. **True**. Hence should be widely used in these patients.
    d. **False**. May decrease intrarenal blood flow and cause renal impairment.
    e. **True**. Especially in women.

12. a. **True**. For instance amiodarone, which is mainly type III but also partially type I.
    b. **False**. Lidocaine is metabolised by the liver.
    c. **True**. This poses problems in managing many patients with cardiac disease.
    d. **False**. Steady state will occur after five half-lives—anything up to 500 days for amiodarone.
    e. **True**. Verapamil was in the past the most common first choice but adenosine is more widely used now.

Case history answers

Case history 1

1. Aspirin, glyceryl trinitrate (GTN), an opiate for pain relief, streptokinase. Other drugs proved to be of benefit but less often used include beta-blockers, i.v. nitrates.
2. A history of active peptic ulceration, surgery or cerebrovascular accident within the previous 6 months, allergy to aspirin or streptokinase.
3. Atropine (not isoprenaline which would increase myocardial oxygen demands and might worsen his myocardial infarction).
4. GTN to be used as required, aspirin and a beta-blocker or an ACE inhibitor. (The use of aspirin and a beta-blocker together has not been adequately tested yet, although individually they reduce the risk of reinfarction).
5. Life-style modification, graded exercise (perhaps as part of a rehabilitation programme), stopping smoking, management of acute angina, what to do in the event of further severe pain and what follow-up arrangements are made.

Case history 2

1. GTN to be used as required; prophylactic therapy: normally a beta-blocker would be the first choice in a patient with exercise-induced asthma. However, in this patient this might not be appropriate because of the COPD. Alternatives are, therefore, calcium-channel blockers and oral nitrates.
2. Stop smoking, life-style modification, how to cope with attacks of chest pain.
3. Loss of efficacy of nitrates in treating angina, probably the result of depletion of sulfhydryl groups. Avoid by building a nitrate-free period into the drug regimen, e.g. overnight.
4. Diet, management of other risk factors for ischaemic heart disease, exclude liver and thyroid disease and perhaps screen his family.
5. Drug therapy with diet, e.g. colestyramine or simvastatin.
6. Salbutamol stimulates β_1- and β_2-adrenoceptors in the heart and may cause tachycardia, increasing myocardial oxygen demand and possibly precipitating angina.

Case history 3

1. Thyroid function tests (hyperthyroidism may cause arrhythmias and the tests may be affected by amiodarone therapy), electrolytes, liver function tests.
2. A long time! Usually quoted as five half-lives: in the case of amiodarone, this could be between 125 and 500 days. Hence a loading dose is usually given.
3. Amiodarone may prolong the duration of warfarin activity and increase INR (international normalised ratio). This is best managed by careful regular measurement of INR when amiodarone is introduced and adjustment of the dose of warfarin accordingly.
4. Amiodarone has too many serious long-term effects to be first choice.

Case history 4

1. A diuretic, e.g. furosemide (frusemide), in a low dose, possibly but not necessarily with a K^+-sparing

diuretic. An ACE inhibitor would be useful in addition.

2. Digoxin and possibly warfarin (patients on diuretics taking digoxin will need careful monitoring of K^+ levels).

3. An ACE inhibitor if not already used (but stop a K^+-sparing diuretic if he has been on one), and possibly digoxin.

4. Intravenous opiate, furosemide and possibly nitrates, oxygen.

5. Indometacin may cause fluid retention and interfere with the effects of the diuretic. It may also not be necessary; why not use a simple analgesic?

Short note answers

1. These drugs include aspirin (for its antiplatelet effects), beta-blockers (proven to reduce mortality in the long term after myocardial infarction), an ACE inhibitor (proven also to reduce mortality after myocardial infarction, possibly by preventing morphological changes in the left ventricle), a lipid-lowering agent such as simvastatin (again proven to reduce mortality after myocardial infarction).

2. This should cover the use of ACE inhibitors in heart failure, hypertension and after myocardial infarction. A particularly good answer would also include their use in high-risk patients without such conditions such as patients with diabetes and ischaemic heart disease.

Extended matching items answer

1. E. This drug lowers the rate of contraction of the left ventricle and relaxes smooth muscle.

2. G. This (single) drug acts in stable angina by decreasing oxygen demand in the heart.

3. A. May all be used in secondary prevention after myocardial infarction (possibly in addition to other drugs).

4. G. This (single) drug acts in stable angina by increasing oxygen supply to the heart.

5. F. These drugs may all be used to treat angina pectoris.

6. F. These drugs all require the presence of sulphhydryl (-SH) groups to function.

5 Drugs and the blood

Overview

Thrombosis and embolism are important in the pathology of a range of diseases (e.g. myocardial infarction, venous thromboembolic disease). Drugs such as heparin and warfarin are used to treat and to prevent such conditions by preventing extension of the embolism or thrombosis, but carry a risk of causing bleeding. Antiplatelet agents have a weaker antithrombotic effect but may be particularly effective in conditions involving risk of arterial thrombosis (e.g. cerebrovascular disease or coronary heart disease). They are associated with less risk of bleeding. Formed thromboses can also be dissolved by thrombolytic drugs, for instance in myocardial infarction.

Anaemia is caused by failure of formation of blood or blood loss. Iron, vitamin B_{12} and folic acid are all essential in blood formation and are used therapeutically in deficiency states.

5.1 Coagulation and thrombosis

Learning objectives

You should:

- be able to list conditions where thrombosis and embolism may be important
- be able to explain how heparin and warfarin work and are used
- be able to explain how they are monitored
- be able to describe the common antiplatelet drugs
- be able to describe thrombolytic drugs.

Thrombosis or clotting of the blood occurs as a result of the interaction of several clotting proteins in the blood. Many of these are produced by the liver and act as a cas-

cade, amplifying their effect (Fig. 29). This is a vital mechanism in preventing blood loss after injury but it can also happen in other circumstances where it is less desirable. For instance, a myocardial infarction is usually caused by a thrombus developing on a damaged atheromatous plaque and blocking the coronary artery. A thrombotic stroke is similar. Thrombosis may form in one site and then move to block a blood vessel elsewhere: for instance patients with atrial fibrillation may develop thrombi in the non-contracting left atrium and are at high risk of a stroke—this can be reduced by anticoagulation.

Conditions where thrombi or emboli are harmful to patients are treated with anticoagulants, which are drugs that inhibit normal clotting.

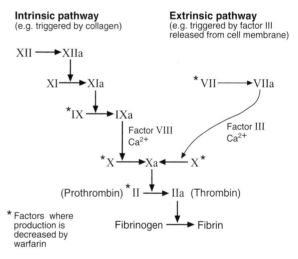

Fig. 29 The coagulation cascade. The intrinsic and extrinsic pathways amplify the response of blood damaged tissue. They converge in the formation of thrombin and interact in other ways also. Clotting factors are activated sequentially, increasing the response. Heparin enhances interaction between thrombin and antithrombin III, and between antithrombin III and many of the factors in the intrinsic pathway. The proteins are given roman numbers and the activated form is the 'a' form.

Indications for anticoagulation

The main indications for anticoagulant therapy are:

- treatment or prophylaxis of venous thromboembolic disease: deep venous thrombosis of the leg or pulmonary embolism

- atrial fibrillation, especially if the patient is very elderly, has poor left ventricular function or mitral stenosis
- mechanical prosthetic heart valve
- Unstable angina (use low-molecular-weight heparin (LMWH) only).

Risk Factors

Risk factors for venous thromboembolic disorders include:

- immobility (e.g. after surgery or illness)
- tissue damage (e.g. after surgery or myocardial infarction)
- genetic predisposition (e.g. factor V or prothrombin mutations)
- pregnancy or oestrogen therapy (see Ch. 12).

Contraindications to anticoagulation

None of these contraindications are absolute; the risks must be weighed against the benefits:

- renal or liver disease
- peptic ulcer disease
- recent surgery or trauma.

Heparin

Heparin is a naturally occurring mucopolysaccharide. It binds to antithrombin III and enhances its anticoagulant effect, inhibiting the formation of thrombin, factor Xa and other clotting factors. It is active in vitro as well as in vivo.

Heparin given parenterally, either subcutaneous (s.c.) or i.v. (usually as an infusion). It has a short half-life and is metabolised by the liver.

Low-molecular-weight heparins (e.g. dalteparin)

The low-molecular-weight heparins (LMWH, e.g. **dalteparin**) are purified derivatives that have more consistent activity than common unfractionated heparin. Consequently, they require less monitoring. They have a longer duration of action than unfractionated heparin and, therefore, are more convenient (for instance in the treatment of deep vein thrombosis, LMWH can be given s.c. once or twice a day compared with a continuous i.v. infusion of unfractionated heparin). However, they are more expensive.

Therapeutic uses of heparin

Heparin is indicated:

- where short-term or immediate anticoagulation is required
- in unstable angina.

Clinical sketch

A 25-year-old woman presents with a swollen left leg while taking an oral contraceptive pill. She has also experienced some chest pain and shortness of breath. Her mother died of a pulmonary embolus following an operation 4 years earlier.

Comment: This patient requires immediate investigation. The history is strongly suggestive of a deep vein thrombosis in the deep veins of the leg, associated with a pulmonary embolus. The combined oral contraceptive pill can increase the risks of such events. There may be a familial predisposition, which will need further investigation suggested by the history of her mother. Treatment will involve withdrawing the oral contraceptive pill (and providing alternative suitable contraception); immediate treatment will be i.v. heparin or subcutaneous low-molecular-weight heparin followed by warfarin for a period, usually of 6 months in this instance.

Two years on, the same patient is now off an oral contraceptive but presents with chest pain and shortness of breath. Ventilation profusion scanning confirms the presence of a pulmonary embolus.

Comment: This patient has now had two thromboembolic episodes and the usual advice would be that she should be treated with anticoagulation for life. This will require careful and regular monitoring and carries risks of bleeding, but in this case the benefits outweigh the risks.

Three years later the same patient has been taking warfarin with no problems. However, she develops a respiratory tract infection and is prescribed erythromycin.

Comment: Warfarin is the drug most commonly involved in serious drug interactions. It is metabolised by liver enzymes and if this metabolism is inhibited (for instance, by drugs such as erythromycin) its effects will be greatly intensified and this may lead to serious bleeding.

The duration of heparin therapy is determined by the indication. If it is to be followed by long-term oral anticoagulation, warfarin may be started immediately and heparin discontinued, usually within 72 hours.

Monitoring heparin

The degree of anticoagulation achieved is monitored by measuring the **APTT** (**activated partial thromboplastin time**), and the dose is adjusted, usually until the APTT is two to three times longer than a normal control.

There is no need to monitor the degree of anticoagulation when s.c. heparin is used as prophylaxis, nor when LMWHs are used.

Adverse effects

- Bleeding, locally at the site of injection or more distantly
- Hypersensitivity may occur rarely
- Thrombocytopenia may occur (regular platelet counts necessary if used for more than 5 days)
- Osteoporosis or hair loss in long-term use.

Reversal. In the event of bleeding caused by heparin, it may be sufficient to stop the heparin. If a faster reversal is needed, *protamine* can be given i.v.; it binds to heparin and reverses its effects. If given in excessive dose, however, protamine may itself have anticoagulant effects.

Oral anticoagulants: warfarin

Warfarin competitively inhibits the formation of the vitamin K-dependent clotting factors (II, VII, IX, X). Its onset of action is determined by the time required to clear those factors which are already formed, usually 48–72 hours to achieve its full effect. It is only active in vivo.

Warfarin is given orally. It is heavily protein bound (99%) and is metabolised by cytochrome P450 enzymes of the liver. Drug interactions may occur either by protein displacement or especially by effects of other drugs on liver enzymes (see below).

Therapeutic uses

Warfarin is used for long-term anticoagulation. It is given initially as a loading dose and later as a maintenance dose.

Monitoring oral anticoagulants

Warfarin dose is adjusted according to its anticoagulant effect, measured by the prothrombin time, often expressed as the **INR (International Normalised Ratio** in which internationally standardised reagents are used) and the dose adjusted to achieve the desired ratio to control values. For the treatment of thromboembolic disease this is usually 2–3, and for arterial disease, it is 3–4.5. The INR should be measured daily when therapy is initiated but monthly in long-term use when the patient is stable.

Adverse effects

- Bleeding: spontaneous or after minor trauma
- Teratogenetic: should not be given in the first trimester of pregnancy.

Drug interactions

Warfarin is probably the drug most commonly involved in serious drug interactions. Great caution is required when other drugs are coprescribed (see the clinical sketch on p. 60). Patients must be fully aware of the risks of drug interaction, with both prescribed drugs and with those that may be bought without prescription, and patients should carry an anticoagulant card.

- Drugs that inhibit cytochrome P450 enzymes will increase the effects of warfarin: cimetidine, erythromycin, ciprofloxacin, co-trimoxazole, metronidazole, fluconazole.

- Drugs which induce P450 enzymes will decrease the effects of warfarin: rifampicin, many antiepileptics. These lists are not exhaustive. If a patient has been stabilised on warfarin while taking one of these drugs, its withdrawal may have serious consequences.
- Drugs that have an antiplatelet effect, such as aspirin, may enhance the anticoagulant effect of warfarin and should generally be avoided.

Reversal of warfarin effects

The effects of warfarin can be reversed by administration of vitamin K_1. This can be given i.v., the dose determining whether the reversal is short term or long term. This will take several hours to act, and in urgent cases it may be necessary to replace the deficient clotting factors (usually by giving fresh frozen plasma or factor concentrate i.v.).

Antiplatelet drugs

Platelets are important in the initiation of thrombosis. Platelets are activated by tissue damage and release thromboxane A_2, a prostaglandin derivative that activates further platelets and promotes platelet aggregation, as well as causing vasoconstriction. The platelets block and narrow blood vessels and may precipitate the clotting cascade. Platelets are also activated by ADP (adenosine diphosphate) and by a glycoprotein acting at a specialised receptor, the glycoprotein IIb/IIIa receptor. Drugs can block several of these steps so as to reduce platelet activity and reduce the risk of thrombosis.

Aspirin. Even in low doses, aspirin inhibits cyclooxygenase, which is essential for the formation of thromboxane A_2. Aspirin also inhibits the formation of the antiaggregatory prostaglandin prostacyclin, to a lesser extent, but the balance is to prevent thrombosis.

Dipyridamole and clopidogrel. These drugs block adenosine receptors. Adenosine is one of the factors that initiate platelet aggregation.

Glycoprotein IIa/IIIb receptor antagonists. This new class of drug (e.g. *tirofiban*) is also an effective antiplatelet agent and is used in unstable angina (see Ch. 4). The drugs block the receptor essential for the final activation of platelet aggregation. They are most effective when used with aspirin and with LMWHs.

Therapeutic uses

The antiplatelet agents are particularly effective in conditions involving arterial thrombosis where platelets are more important, such as myocardial infarction or angina, and cerebrovascular accident or transient ischaemic attacks.

Aspirin as an antiplatelet agent

Aspirin is useful in a wide variety of rheumatological conditions and as an analgesic. (These effects are discussed in Ch. 7.) Aspirin is a highly effective and inexpensive antiplatelet drug. There is some controversy over the most appropriate dose of aspirin as an antiplatelet drug, since higher doses may cause more adverse effects and may increase the degree of inhibition of prostacyclin.

In ischaemic heart disease, aspirin reduces the risk of infarction in unstable angina, reduces the number of severe exacerbations in patients with stable angina and possibly slows disease progression. When given to patients with an acute myocardial infarction, it reduces mortality to a similar extent as thrombolytic therapy (see below). The combination of aspirin and thrombolytic drugs is more effective than either alone. When given to patients after myocardial infarction, aspirin reduces the risks of further ischaemic events.

In patients at high risk of cardiovascular or cerebrovascular events, aspirin should be considered in addition to lipid-lowering therapy.

In cerebrovascular disease, aspirin is also used to treat transient ischaemic attacks and as secondary prophylaxis to prevent further thrombotic cerebrovascular accidents.

After cardiovascular surgical procedures, aspirin also reduces the rate of closure of coronary artery grafts or of restenosis after coronary angioplasty.

Adverse effects of aspirin. Most important are gastric irritation and bleeding, and hypersensitivity.

Other antiplatelet drugs

Dipyridamole is used to prevent further cerebrovascular events, often in combination with aspirin. *Clopidogrel* is used in high-risk patients to prevent cardiovascular events; it is usually reserved for patients who are intolerant of aspirin. *Tirofiban* is used to treat acute unstable angina and is under study in a range of other cardiovascular conditions.

Thrombolytic drugs

Thromboses are dynamic—they are breaking down (thrombolysis) at the same time they are forming, with a variable balance between the two processes. Thrombolysis occurs when a blood protein plasminogen is converted to plasmin, which breaks down fibrin. Thrombolytic drugs activate plasmin and push the balance towards thrombolysis (Fig. 30).

Therapeutic uses

Thrombolytic drugs are most commonly used in the treatment of myocardial infarction. If given early, they

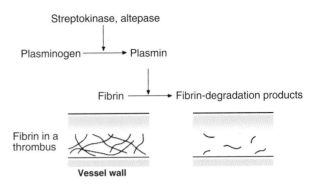

Fig. 30 The action of thrombolytic drugs.

can break down the thrombus that has caused the infarct, unblocking the artery, allowing reperfusion and limiting the extent of the damage. This has been proven to reduce mortality from myocardial infarction substantially.

Thrombolytic drugs are also used in the treatment of acute thrombotic stroke (must be given within 3 hours of the onset of the stroke—altepase only)

Contraindications to thrombolytic therapy

- Active peptic ulcer
- Bleeding condition of any sort
- Severe hypertension
- Recent surgery or trauma.

Adverse effects

- Bleeding
- Allergy (streptokinase only).

Streptokinase

Streptokinase is produced from β-haemolytic streptococci. It may react with antibodies in patients previously exposed either to streptokinase or a recent streptococcal

> **Clinical sketch**
>
> A patient presents with acute myocardial infarction. The pain started 4 hours before and there is marked ST elevation on the ECG. The patient had a previous myocardial infarction treated with streptokinase 2 years before.
>
> *Comment: This is an indication for urgent thrombolysis and antiplatelet therapy. The patient should be given aspirin. Patients given streptokinase may develop antibodies to the enzyme, which can render its antithrombotic effect erratic and undependable. For this reason, patients who have previously received streptokinase should generally receive altepase for subsequent infarction. Altepase is commonly given in combination with heparin.*

infection, leading to allergic reaction (1–2% of patients) or to unpredictable effectiveness. Streptokinase is given i.v. as a short infusion and its effects last about 3–4 hours.

Alteplase

Alteplase is a naturally occurring activator of plasminogen in humans produced by genetic recombinant techniques. Since it is not 'foreign', it does not cause allergic reactions. Alteplase is as effective, or possibly more effective, as streptokinase but may be associated with more haemorrhagic complications and is more expensive.

Antifibrinolytic drugs

Antifibrinolytic drugs might be useful in conditions where there is excessive bleeding. *Tranexamic acid* inhibits activation of plasminogen. It is used occasionally to try to stop uncontrolled bleeding, e.g. after dental extraction in haemophiliacs (in addition to clotting factors), after streptokinase overdose or in the treatment of severe menorrhagia.

5.2 Formation of blood

Learning objectives

You should:

- be able to describe the role of iron and haematinic vitamins
- be able to describe their replacement therapy in patients with deficiency.

Anaemia is defined as a deficiency of haemoglobin, below the normal for the patient's age and sex. There are many causes, and each case needs careful investigation; anaemia itself is not an adequate diagnosis. This discussion is limited to those anaemias caused by deficiencies that can be corrected pharmacologically.

Bear in mind that drugs can cause anaemia:

- drugs that cause bleeding, e.g. nonsteroidal anti-inflammatory drugs
- drugs that suppress the marrow, e.g. cytotoxic drugs or occasionally a severe adverse reaction to other drugs
- drugs that promote red cell breakdown, e.g. methyldopa or high-dose penicillin.

Iron-deficient anaemia

In iron-deficient anaemia there is either an inadequate intake of iron to meet physiological needs (e.g. in menstruation, in pregnancy or in elderly patients with a poor diet), or there is loss of iron (e.g. in patients with chronic bleeding).

Diagnosis

- Anaemia is hypochromic microcytic
- serum iron and iron stores are low.

Treatment

Iron is well absorbed from the small intestine when there is an iron-deficient state. Oral iron salts are usually used, often for 3–4 months to ensure that the anaemia is corrected and stores replenished. Failure to respond to oral iron is usually because of poor compliance (see Ch. 19) but may occasionally be the result of malabsorption or of continued blood loss.

Ferrous sulfate. Adverse effects include constipation, epigastric pain and nausea. If these are intolerable, a reduced dose or an alternative preparation should be used. The stools usually darken in patients taking oral iron.

Iron dextran. Occasionally oral forms cannot be tolerated, and iron (iron dextran) can be given by i.v. infusion or by deep intramuscular (i.m.) injection. The major risk of the infusion is anaphylaxis.

Vitamin B$_{12}$ deficiency

Vitamin B$_{12}$ is necessary for the adequate formation of nucleic acids. Deficiency usually arises from an autoimmune disease affecting the gastric mucosa so that a cofactor necessary for the absorption of the vitamin is not produced. The body usually has extensive stores and the anaemia will not arise for some months or years. Diagnosis is by finding out if the:

- anaemia is hypochromic but macrocytic
- bone marrow contains megaloblasts.

In severe cases (sometimes even without severe anaemia), the spinal cord may also be damaged.

Treatment

Treatment is by i.m. vitamin B$_{12}$ (*hydroxocobalamin*), avoiding the need for absorption from the gastrointestinal tract.

Clinical sketch

A 65-year-old woman presents with weight loss and a microcytic anaemia. The general practitioner prescribes ferrous sulfate, but the anaemia fails to respond.

Comment: Anaemia alone is not a sufficient diagnosis. This patient may well have a malignancy that has caused the weight loss and probably blood loss leading to the microcytic anaemia. Replacing iron stores is not going to stop further bleeding. This patient needs full investigation on first presentation.

Life-long treatment will be required, usually with 3-monthly injections.

Folic acid deficiency

Folic acid is also a cofactor for nucleic acid production, and deficiency also causes a hypochromic macrocytic anaemia. Body stores of folic acid are very limited, and deficiency is usually quickly apparent. Deficiency arises from malabsorption, from inadequate diet or from excessive demand, e.g. in pregnancy or in patients with rapid cell turnover (severe psoriasis or haemolytic anaemia). Folic acid replacement is by mouth, with very high doses being used if malabsorption is the underlying problem.

    Folic acid in pregnancy. See Chapter 19.

Other causes of anaemia

Erythropoietin, a glycoprotein released by the kidney, stimulates the bone marrow to produce red blood cells. In renal disease and especially in patients on dialysis, it is deficient and the patient may become anaemic. Erythropoietin can now be synthesised (*epoetin*) and given parenterally as a replacement to treat such patients. Adverse effects are usually the result of its overuse, when an attempt is made to restore haemoglobin levels fully to normal. This may result in severe hypertension with encephalopathy and thrombosis. Most patients are asymptomatic with a haemoglobin of around 10 g/dl (100 g/l) and experience no adverse effects.

    Colony-stimulating factors (CSF) encourage white cell proliferation in the marrow and are increasingly used in patients with neutropenia, especially after anticancer chemotherapy: they may also be used after anticancer chemotherapy (see Ch. 15).

Self-assessment: questions

Multiple choice questions

1. Heparin:
   a. Can be taken orally
   b. Activity may be enhanced by drugs that are heavily protein bound
   c. By the subcutaneous route reduces the risk of thromboembolic disease in hospitalised patients
   d. Is antagonised by proteamine
   e. Dosage is monitored by the international normalised ratio (INR)

2. Drugs that may interact with warfarin include:
   a. Phenytoin
   b. Metronidazole
   c. Dextropropoxyphene
   d. Trimethoprim
   e. Gemfibrozil

3. Warfarin:
   a. Is active in vitro
   b. Can be antagonised by vitamin K
   c. Hypersensitivity is a common adverse effect
   d. Should not be given to pregnant women in the first trimester
   e. Is used to treat pulmonary embolism

4. Aspirin:
   a. Inhibits the production of both aggregatory and antiaggregatory mediators
   b. Improves the prognosis in acute myocardial infarction
   c. Increases bleeding time
   d. Low doses may be safely given to patients with allergy to aspirin
   e. Is contraindicated in cerebrovascular disease

5. Thrombolytics:
   a. Depend on the presence of plasminogen
   b. Are contraindicated in patients with active peptic ulcer disease
   c. Dosage is adjusted according to bleeding time
   d. Activity of streptokinase may be decreased in patients with a recent streptococcal infection
   e. Bleeding is a potentially serious complication

6. In treating anaemia:
   a. Oral iron is often poorly absorbed by iron-deficient anaemics
   b. Patients with B_{12} deficiency may present with weakness of the legs
   c. Folate deficiency may occur because of gastrointestinal bleeding
   d. Erythropoietin is deficient in chronic renal disease
   e. Anaemia should always be treated in the first instance by blood transfusion

7. Drugs that may cause anaemia include:
   a. Indometacin (indomethacin)
   b. Carbimazole
   c. Methotrexate
   d. Penicillin
   e. Morphine

Case history questions

Case history 1

A 57-year-old man develops an extensive deep venous thrombosis after discharge from hospital, where he has recently had a cholecystectomy.

1. Should he be admitted to hospital?
2. What drug or drugs should he receive initially?
3. What drug should he receive for long-term management?
4. How is the dose determined?
5. What interactions must he be warned of?

Case history 2

A 25-year-old woman with menorrhagia and a poor diet presents with an iron-deficient anaemia.

1. How should the anaemia be treated?
2. What likely adverse effects of treatment should the patient be warned of?
3. If the patient fails to respond to treatment, what possible explanations should be considered?
4. When would i.v. therapy be considered?

Short note question

Compare and contrast warfarin and heparin as drugs.

Extended matching items question

Theme: blood/coagulation
Options

A. Heparin
B. International normalised ratio (INR)
C. Full blood count
D. Aspirin
E. Dipyridamole
F. Activated partial thromboplastin time (APTT)
G. Warfarin
H. Dalteparin
I. Vitamin K
J. Fresh frozen plasma
K. Proteamine
L. Cimetidine
M. Ranitidine
N. Altepase

A 30-year-old woman develops a deep vein thrombosis. She presents to the A/E department.

1. Select the most appropriate drug to use for anticoagulion immediately. How will it be administered?
2. Select the most appropriate means of monitoring her anticoagulation.
3. She is now treated with another drug, intended to be used for 3–6 months. How will this drug be monitored?
4. Identify two drugs from the list which might cause dangerous interactions with this drug.
5. Some weeks later, the patient is found to be dangerously overanticoagulated and requires an antidote. Which drug or drugs will you administer?
6. Later, she develops dyspepsia for which she requires gastric acid suppression: which drug should be used?

Self-assessment: answers

Multiple choice answers

1. a. **False**. Heparin must be used parenterally.
   b. **False**. Heparin is not itself protein bound and so is unaffected by other drugs in this way.
   c. **True**. Patients who are immobilised in hospital should be considered for subcutaneous heparin.
   d. **True**. Used in overdoses of heparin.
   e. **False**. The INR is used to monitor warfarin. The APTT is the correct test to monitor heparin. Clotting time is an alternative.

2. a. **True**. Liver enzyme induction.
   b. **True**. Liver enzyme inhibition.
   c. **True**. A liver enzyme inhibitor although this is often forgotten.
   d. **False**. No plasma protein binding or enzyme inhibition.
   e. **True**. Plasma protein displacement.

3. a. **False**. It is only active as a result of the inhibition of protein metabolism and so can only act in vivo and only after 1–2 days.
   b. **True**. Warfarin is a competitive antagonist for vitamin K.
   c. **False**. Bleeding is by far the most common adverse effect: hypersensitivity is rare.
   d. **True**. May be teratogenic.
   e. **True**. Although there are many other indications also.

4. a. **True**. Both prostacyclin (antiaggregatory from the endothelium) and thromboxane A$_2$ (proaggregatory, from the platelets) are affected. In theory, low-dose aspirin inhibits thromboxane more, since platelets have no nuclei and cannot secrete new thromboxane-manufacturing enzymes.
   b. **True**. By as much as streptokinase in some trials.
   c. **True**. Prevents formation of platelet plugs.
   d. **False**. In hypersensitivity, the dosage is usually unimportant in triggering a reaction.
   e. **False**. It is widely used for this indication.

5. a. **True**. Thrombolytics activate plasminogen to plasmin, which then breaks down established clots.
   b. **True**. The risks would seem to outweigh the benefits.
   c. **False**. There is at present no way of adjusting the dose according to need, and all patients receive the same dose.
   d. **True**. Antistreptococcal antibodies may be present and inhibit streptokinase.
   e. **True**. The most common and serious adverse effect.

6. a. **False**. In the absence of a specific malabsorption syndrome, iron is very avidly absorbed by iron-deficient patients.
   b. **True**. Lack of vitamin B$_{12}$ can cause damage to the spinal cord.
   c. **False**. Folate deficiency is the result of either an inadequate diet or excessive utilisation, e.g. in psoriasis, pregnancy, etc.
   d. **True**. Can now be given to such patients to correct their anaemia.
   e. **False**. Anaemia is a sign, not a diagnosis. Transfusion may interfere with investigations of the underlying cause as well as being potentially hazardous.

7. a. **True**. By gastrointestinal blood loss.
   b. **True**. By marrow suppression.
   c. **True**. By marrow suppression (folate antagonism).
   d. **True**. High-dose penicillins may cause haemolytic anaemia.
   e. **False**. This has never been recorded.

Case history answers

Case history 1

1. Yes. There is a risk of life-threatening pulmonary embolism.
2. Heparin should be given immediately, usually i.v.
3. Warfarin will usually be given for 6 weeks to 3 months after a deep venous thrombosis to reduce the risks of recurrence or extension of the clot.
4. Dose of warfarin is determined by its effects on clotting, as measured by the INR (international normalised ratio).
5. Warfarin is commonly involved in serious drug interactions; there are many examples, including those with liver enzyme inducers and inhibitors (see Ch. 20).

Case History 2

1. Oral iron, usually ferrous sulfate, for several months both to treat the anaemia and restore iron stores.
2. Constipation, darkening of the faeces and other gastrointestinal symptoms are the most common adverse effects of oral iron preparations.
3. The diagnosis should be reconsidered: if the patient genuinely has an iron-deficient anaemia, then could she be malabsorbing? However, the most likely explanations for failure to respond is either

continued heavy blood loss or poor compliance with the medication.

4. Intravenous iron is rarely necessary: perhaps if there was severe malabsorption or if the patient was unable to tolerate a variety of oral iron preparations.

Short note answer

The answer should consider:

1. Routes of administration (oral warfarin versus parenteral heparin)
2. Mechanisms of action (immediate versus more slowly developing effects on different clotting factors)
3. Potential adverse effects (most commonly bleeding for both)
4. Risks of interactions (greater for warfarin)
5. Clinical circumstances in which each are used (short-term anticoagulation for heparin, longer term for warfarin, and some examples of each would be appropriate).

Extending matching items answers

1. A or H. She should be given i.v. heparin or s.c. dalteparin. Dalteparin is a purified low-molecular-weight heparin, which is effective when given subcutaneously once per day. It is, therefore, more convenient (but more expensive) than unfractionated heparin.

2. F or none at all! A trick question. Your answer here depends on your answer to question 1. If given i.v. heparin, then the correct answer is the APTT, which should be twice as long as a normal control. If using dalteparin, then no monitoring is generally required.

3. B. The drug is, of course, warfarin, monitored by the INR (the ratio of the time taken for a patient's blood to clot when exposed to standardised reagents compared with that of a normal control). The desired range is usually 2–3.

4. D, I or L. Aspirin may case a pharmacodynamic interaction: by interfering with platelet aggregation it may increase the tendency to bleed. It might also cause gastric erosions or peptic ulcer disease, leading to bleeding. There might be a possible kinetic interaction also if aspirin displaces warfarin from plasma proteins, but this is not usually very significant (See Ch. 1). Cimetidine is a liver enzyme inhibitor and might cause an enhancement of the action of warfarin. Vitamin K would decrease the effect of warfarin; warfarin acts as a competitive Vitamin K antagonist.

5. I definitely and possibly J. Vitamin K is the antidote which works by increasing production of clotting factors. However, this may take hours and if an immediate effect is required (e.g. if the patient were actively bleeding) then replacing the clotting factors directly in the form of fresh frozen plasma might be necessary. In most cases of overanticoagulation, withdrawing warfarin for a few days is adequate.

6. M. Ranitidine would be the drug of choice here; cimetidine is similar in this action on gastric acid production but may interact with warfarin.

6 Drugs used in CNS disease

Overview

The observation that certain substances could alter consciousness was probably the start of primitive pharmacology, and alcohol, nicotine, caffeine and illicit recreational drugs remain in common use. Over the last 200 years, the empirical approach of isolating active molecules from naturally occurring materials has continued and doses have been formalised. It is only very recently that we have started to understand the molecular mechanisms by which drugs work in the central nervous system (CNS). Nearly all CNS drugs modify chemical synaptic transmission by changing the synthesis, storage, catabolism, release or receptor interactions of transmitter substances, or by perturbing transmitter-regulated ion conductance. One of the key factors in neurological disease is using knowledge of these processes to identify the problem area and to decide on the correct drug. This understanding of molecular mechanisms is also likely to see advances both in our understanding of disease mechanisms and in new drug design.

6.1 Anxiety and insomnia

Learning objectives

You should:

- be able to distinguish the terms 'sedation' and 'hypnosis'
- be able to describe the therapeutic use of sedative/hypnotics and appreciate the risks of their prolonged use
- be able to list some commonly used benzodiazepines
- be able to describe the mode of action, clinical pharmacokinetics and adverse effects of the benzodiazepines.

Clinical sketch

A middle-aged man has recently been bereaved and has insomnia as a result. His GP prescribes temazepam for 2 weeks.

Comment: this is an appropriate use of the drug to treat an acute problem with a clearly defined cause.

Clinical sketch

A middle-aged man has always suffered from anxiety and insomnia. He has been taking diazepam during the day and temazepam at night for many years. The doses of both drugs have gradually been increased (on the patient's request) over the years because of diminishing effectiveness.

Comment: this inappropriate long-term use of sedatives can sometimes be hard to avoid. However, the drugs have probably become part of the problem instead of offering any therapeutic benefit. The diminishing effectiveness of the drug is termed 'tolerance'.

Clinical sketch

A 20-year-old i.v. drug abuser is admitted deeply unconscious following an overdose of benzodiazepines and other substances. The benzodiazepine antagonist flumazenil improves his level of consciousness.

Comment: flumazenil 'reverses' benzodiazepines but has no effect on sedation from opiates. Unlike most benzodiazepines, flumazenil is eliminated very quickly and several doses may be needed.

The benzodiazepines

Gamma-aminobutyric acid (GABA) is a major inhibitory neurotransmitter that works by opening postsynaptic chloride channels. The benzodiazepines potentiate GABA and receptors for these drugs are found in close proximity to GABA receptors and chloride channels (Fig. 31). The dose–response curve (see Fig. 2) of benzodiazepines is shallow, and overdoses tend not to cause life-threatening toxicity other than in patients with respiratory impairment.

Examples

Diazepam is well absorbed when given orally, but absorption is slowed when it is taken with food. The parenteral formulations of diazepam should only be given i.v., as i.m. absorption is slow and erratic. Diazepam is converted (in the liver) to *active* metabolites many of which have very long half-lives: these may accumulate in elderly patients.

Temazepam is itself a metabolite of diazepam. It is well absorbed from the gut. It is cleared by conjugation to an inactive metabolite and has a short half-life.

Clonazepam too is well absorbed from the gut. A parenteral form is available for i.v. use.

Midazolam is usually given i.v. It is extensively protein bound and changes in plasma protein concentration can greatly affect the clinical response. Midazolam is cleared by metabolism to inactive derivatives and has a very short half-life.

Therapeutic uses

- Anxiety: diazepam is an appropriate choice for abolition of anxiety ('sedative' or 'anxiolytic' use).
- Insomnia: temazepam is an appropriate hypnotic because of its relatively short duration of action and lack of 'hangover'.
- Alcohol withdrawal: in chronic alcoholics withdrawal can induce confusion (delirium tremens) and seizures. Benzodiazepines exhibit **cross-**

tolerance with alcohol and are given to prevent withdrawal phenomena. The sedative drug is then gradually withdrawn over several days.
- Seizures: diazepam i.v. is the treatment of choice for status epilepticus; oral clonazepam is used for the prevention of several seizure types (see below).
- Medical procedures: i.v. midazolam is commonly used because of its short half-life.

Adverse effects

- Benzodiazepines impair intellectual function and motor skills: care is needed with machinery and patients should be advised not to drive after taking benzodiazepines.
- Psychological or physical dependence occurs (Ch. 18).
- Natural sleep is distinguished by two patterns: non-rapid eye movement (NREM), which accounts for about 75% of sleep time, and rapid eye movement (REM), during which most recallable dreams occur. Hypnotics reduce the time spent in REM and deep NREM. Patients may complain that their sleep is not fully satisfactory.
- Patients with respiratory impairment may be worsened by sedative drugs.

Contraindications

- Respiratory impairment
- Severe liver impairment.

Drug interactions

- Other sedative drugs (including alcohol, non-benzodiazepine sedatives (below), opiates, barbiturates, neuroleptics (see section 6.4) and antihistamines): cause additive CNS depression.
- Cimetidine: inhibits the metabolism of midazolam.
- Antimicrobials: some inhibit the metabolism of midazolam.
- The specific benzodiazepine antagonist *flumazenil* can be used in life-threatening overdoses.

Non-benzodiazepine sedative/hypnotics

These drugs are not structurally related, but all are thought to enhance the effects of GABA. All are indicated for short-term use and can cause dependence.

Examples

Zopiclone is given orally for insomnia. It is cleared by metabolism to less active derivatives and has a short half-life.

Chloral hydrate is well absorbed and subject to extensive first-pass metabolism. The drug's effects are mainly via its active metabolite, trichloroethanol. The parent drug has a very short half-life, but that of trichloroethanol is longer.

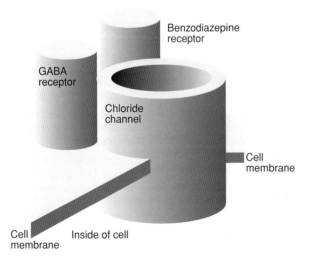

Fig. 31 Schematic representation of the benzodiazepine receptors.

Therapeutic uses

In the elderly, clomethiazole and chloral hydrate are sometimes used rather than benzodiazepines as hypnotics. Zopiclone can be used in all age groups.

Adverse effects

- Respiratory depression
- Dependence (particularly clomethiazole)
- Nasal irritation (clomethiazole)
- Gastric upset (chloral hydrate).

Contraindications

- Respiratory impairment
- Hepatic dysfunction.

Drug interactions

Cimetidine prolongs the half-life of clomethiazole.

6.2 Epilepsy

Learning objectives

You should:

- be able to define and classify epilepsy
- know the emergency management of status epilepticus
- be able to summarise the clinical pharmacology of the main antiepileptic drugs
- be capable of formulating a treatment plan for patients with common seizure types.

Definitions in epilepsy

- Epilepsy comprises recurrent episodes of abnormal cerebral neuronal discharge. The resulting seizures are usually clinically obvious and vary in pattern according to which parts of the brain are affected.
- Epilepsy can be caused by many neurological diseases, including infection, trauma, infarction and neoplasia.
- Heredity has an important role (especially in the idiopathic generalised epilepsies).

Common seizure types

The clinical manifestations of seizures are related to the part of the brain thought to be affected; classification based on these clinical features is of practical value since the response to drugs can often be predicted.

1. Generalised seizures

Clinical sketch

A patient with long-standing epilepsy is admitted because of recurrent tonic-clonic seizures for the preceding 12 hours. She is unconscious, stiff and is having repeated episodes of clonic limb movements. Management comprised protection of the airway, oxygen, i.v. diazepam or lorazepam and perhaps i.v. phenytoin (together with treatment of the pneumonia).

Comment: status epilepticus is a medical emergency. Diazepam is the first-choice drug but if it fails, then phenytoin is often effective. If neither is effective, the patient may require sedation and ventilation in an intensive care unit.

a. Absence (petit mal). These seizures have abrupt onset and cessation, with impaired consciousness, but with normal posture often retained. The EEG shows a typical 'spike and wave' pattern. First choice drugs: *valproate, ethosuximide*.

b. Tonic/clonic (grand mal). Consciousness is impaired and the patient usually falls to the floor. A phase of muscle contraction ('tonic') is followed by irregular muscle clonus and then by sleep. Injury may occur. First choice drugs: *valproate* or *carbamazepine*,

2. Partial seizures

a. Simple partial seizures. Features depend on the part of the brain affected, e.g. motor seizures (Jacksonian) result from discharge in the precentral gyrus. Consciousness is unimpaired. First choice drugs: *carbamazepine* or *valproate*.

b. Complex partial seizures (temporal lobe epilepsy). Consciousness is impaired with complex, often repetitive, actions. First choice drugs: *carbamazepine* or *valproate*.

Management of epilepsy

Patients require supportive care during a seizure: the airway should be protected and the patient laid in a semiprone (in case of vomiting) safe position. Most seizures stop spontaneously within 5 minutes; however major seizures occurring in sequence without remission, **status epilepticus**, require emergency management (Box 4).

Drugs used in epilepsy

Benzodiazepines

Diazepam is the first-choice drug in status epilepticus. Clomazepam is used in maintenance. They are described in more detail in section 6.1.

Box 4 Emergency management of status epilepticus

Status epilepticus, when seizures follow one another without recovery of consciousness, is a medical emergency and has a high mortality rate. Death is from cardiorespiratory failure.

- A loading dose of diazepam should be given i.v.
- This can be followed by a maintenance infusion of diazepam
- *Alternatively*, clomethiazole may be given as an i.v. infusion
- In resistant cases, phenytoin may be given as a *slow* i.v. infusion, following BNF guidelines.

Clinical sketch

An 18-month-old toddler is brought to A&E by his distraught parents. He has been unwell for 2 days with a viral illness and they have been 'wrapping him up warm'. He is having generalised clonic movements and his rectal temperature is 40°C. Treatment comprised rectal paracetamol and tepid sponging to reduce temperature, rectal diazepam and reassurance of the parents.

Comment: febrile convulsions are common in young children and have a good prognosis. Temperature needs to be lowered and the fit terminated with diazepam.

Clinical sketch

A 30-year-old woman has had epilepsy since a head injury 10 years ago. The fits were frequent, but she now takes carbamazepine, and has been fit-free for 4 years. She now holds a driving license that is renewed every 3 years. She is pregnant and wants advice.

Comments: There are a number of issues raised here. (a) it is usually possible to control fits with only one drug, as here. (b) Doctors have a duty to advise patients to behave sensibly: this often means immediate advice 'you should not drive'. They also have the responsibility to advise patients to report seizures to the Driver and Vehicle Licensing Agency and their insurance company. Patients may be allowed to drive again if they are fit-free for 12 months. (c) The risk of fetal malformation is increased by antiepileptic drugs and the patient needs to know this. If the woman decides to have the baby, the risks of the drug (to the fetus) need to be weighed against its benefits (to both mother and fetus); in most cases the drug is continued.

Carbamazepine

Carbamazepine blocks sodium channels postsynaptically, thereby reducing the response to excitatory neurotransmitter binding. Giving carbamazepine with food slows its absorption, and this can allow patients to tolerate higher doses. Carbamazepine is mainly cleared by hepatic metabolism. One of its metabolites (oxcarbamazepine) is also used as an antiepileptic. The half-life is about 36 hours after the first dose but, because it is a potent inducer of hepatic enzymes, half-life can fall by up to 50% with long-term use: this translates clinically into a need for dose adjustment. Carbamazepine plasma concentration is routinely measured but is not often a useful guide to management.

Therapeutic uses

- Drug of choice for partial seizures
- Extensively used for tonic/clonic seizures but is not effective against other generalised seizure types
- Chronic pain: including trigeminal neuralgia
- Manic-depressive disorders.

Adverse effects

- Concentration-related diplopia, ataxia and sedation
- Hyponatraemia leading to water intoxication
- Idiosyncratic reactions include aplastic anaemia, agranulocytosis, rashes and hepatic dysfunction
- Teratogenicity: spina bifida.

Contraindications and warnings

- Previous adverse drug reaction
- Porphyria can be exacerbated
- Women of child-bearing age should be advised of the teratogenic effects.

Drug interactions

- Carbamazepine is a potent inducer of liver enzymes and very prone to drug interactions. Notable examples include reduced effect of both oral contraceptive steroids and warfarin.
- Carbamazepine levels can rise when it is combined with dextropropoxyphene or sodium valproate.

Sodium valproate

The mode of action of sodium valproate is not completely understood, but its effects include increased CNS levels of GABA with potentiation of this transmitter and changes in both Na^+ and K^+ conductance. Giving valproate with food slows its absorption, and this may reduce symptomatic adverse effects. It is cleared by hepatic metabolism with a half-life of 10–20 hours. At high concentration, the clearance of valproate becomes 'zero order' (in clinical terms, blood levels rise disproportionately to dose increments). Plasma concentration monitoring is not a good guide to dose changes; concentrations do not correlate well with effect (perhaps in part because of variability in protein binding).

Therapeutic uses

Valproate has useful effects in most commonly seen seizure types.

Adverse effects

- Symptomatic toxicity includes gastrointestinal upset, weight gain, fine tremor (at high levels) and alopecia
- Idiosyncratic effects are uncommon but can be life-threatening; these include hepatotoxicity (particularly in children) and thrombocytopenia
- Teratogenicity: spina bifida and skeletal anomalies.

Contraindications and warnings

- Liver disease
- Women of child-bearing age should be advised of the teratogenic effects.

Drug interactions

Valproate can inhibit the metabolism of other anticonvulsants including carbamazepine.

Phenytoin

Phenytoin is an old compound, prone to symptomatic adverse effects; it is rarely the first choice agent for newly diagnosed epilepsy. Phenytoin has many effects within the CNS but probably works by maintaining the deactivation of voltage-sensitive sodium channels, thereby blocking the repetitive firing of neurones. It is usually well absorbed from the gut but this is very dependent on formulation; phenytoin absorption is unpredictable when given i.m. and this route should not be used. Phenytoin is extensively bound to plasma proteins but can be displaced by other drugs (see below). It is cleared by hepatic metabolism, but this can be saturated at concentrations readily reached in clinical practice (a 'zero-order' process): in clinical terms, blood levels rise disproportionately to dose increments (Fig. 32). The half-life of phenytoin, at therapeutic concentrations, is around 20 hours but it is prolonged at high concentration. Phenytoin clearance is reduced in patients

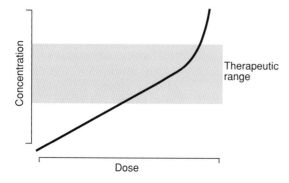

Fig. 32 Relationship between phenytoin dose and steady-state plasma concentration.

with liver disease and is enhanced in pregnancy. The therapeutic range is relatively narrow (40–80 µmol/l), and therapeutic drug monitoring is considered *essential*.

Therapeutic uses

- In status epilepticus i.v. phenytoin is a second-choice drug after a benzodiazapine. Phenytoin i.v. is dangerous and it *must* be given slowly (*read instructions in the BNF*) while monitoring the ECG and vital signs. Phenytoin readily precipitates if diluted in i.v. fluids; it is usually given by syringe-driver.
- Phenytoin can be used for partial seizures and tonic/clonic seizures, but not for other generalised seizure types.

Adverse effects

- Acute, concentration-dependent effects include diplopia, nystagmus, ataxia, nausea and sedation (usually only at very high concentration)
- Chronic effects are common and include gingival hyperplasia, hirsutism and coarsening of facial features, peripheral neuropathy, enhanced vitamin D metabolism (causing osteomalacia) and folate malabsorption
- Idiosyncratic effects include fever, rashes, lymphadenopathy
- Teratogenicity: cleft palate/lip and congenital heart disease.

Contraindications and warnings

- Porphyria can be exacerbated
- Women of child-bearing age should be advised of the teratogenic effects.

Drug interactions

- Phenytoin is an inducer of hepatic enzymes, reducing the effect of many drugs including warfarin, carbamazepine, oral contraceptive steroids and theophylline
- Plasma concentrations of phenytoin may be increased by hepatic enzyme inhibitors including sulphonamides (which also displace from protein binding), sulphonylureas, ketoconazole and cimetidine
- Plasma concentrations of phenytoin may be reduced by carbamazepine and antacids.

Phenobarbital

Phenobarbital potentiates the effects of GABA and antagonises the effects of the excitatory transmitter glutamate. It may be given orally, i.m. or by slow i.v. injection. The therapeutic range is 40–120 µmol/l in the short term; patients on long-term treatment develop tolerance and often maintain concentrations above 120 µmol/l. Most of a dose of phenobarbital is eliminated as inactive metabolites, but about 40% is excreted unchanged; this becomes relevant after overdosage, where raising urinary pH increases clearance (Ch. 1). Phenobarbital is used for partial and tonic-clonic seizures but is not the first-choice drug in industrialised nations; because of low cost it is commonly used in developing countries. Adverse effects include sedation and respiratory depression (especially in overdose). Phenobarbital is contraindicated in porphyria. Like carbamazepine and phenytoin, phenobarbital is an inducer of liver enzymes and increases the clearance of many drugs; in addition the sedative effects of phenobarbital are additive with other sedative/hypnotic drugs.

Vigabatrin

Vigabatrin works by inhibiting enzymatic breakdown of GABA and thereby increasing CNS concentrations of this inhibitory neurotransmitter. The drug is currently used in combination with other antiepileptic drugs as supplementary therapy for refractory seizures—particularly complex partial seizures. Vigabatrin is mainly eliminated unchanged by the kidneys; there is no correlation between drug concentrations and effect, and therapeutic drug monitoring is not routine. The main adverse effects are sedation, weight gain, confusion and (uncommonly) psychosis.

Lamotrigine

Lamotrigine inhibits the release of excitatory amino acid neurotransmitters (principally glutamate), which may be involved in the generation of seizure activity, and is mainly eliminated by glucuronidation in the liver. The therapeutic range is yet to be established and concentration monitoring is not routine. Lamotrigine can be used for the monotherapy of partial seizures but is also given in combination with other antiepileptic drugs for cases refractory to a single agent. Skin rashes are quite common (around 3%) but resolve when the drug is stopped. Rarely, lamotrigine has caused severe skin reactions, angioedema and multiorgan failure.

Gabapentin

Gabapentin is an amino acid analogue of GABA, but its mode of action does not seem to involve binding to GABA receptors; it may perturb GABA metabolism. Gabapentin is eliminated by the kidneys as the unchanged drug; drug concentrations are not routinely measured. Gabapentin is used in addition to other drugs in the treatment of refractory partial seizures and tonic-clonic seizures. The most common adverse effects are sedation and ataxia.

Topiramate

The mode of action of topiramate may involve effects on both sodium channels and GABA. Most of a dose is eliminated by the kidneys as the unchanged drug; there is no established concentration therapeutic range. Topiramate is used as an 'add-on' drug for patients with refractory partial or tonic-clonic seizures. Dizziness, cognitive slowing and fatigue are commonly reported.

Ethosuximide

Ethosuximide is used for generalised seizures (mainly absence) in children, but it is less frequently used than valproate because gastrointestinal adverse effects are common.

6.3 Depression and hypomania

Learning objectives

You should:

- be able to describe bipolar affective disorder
- be able to summarise the 'amine hypothesis'
- know the clinical pharmacology of tricyclic antidepressants, selective serotonin reuptake inhibitors and monoamine oxidase inhibitors
- be aware that antidepressant drugs can take several weeks to work
- be aware of the toxicity of antidepressant drugs, especially in overdose.

Clinical sketch

A 40-year-old woman has been depressed since the death of her husband 6 months ago. She has lost about a stone in weight and is unable to work. The doctor starts her on amitryptiline but there is no improvement for several weeks.

Comment: Sadness is a normal reaction to many life events. Usually this abates with time; but the term depression is used for abnormally protracted or severe sadness. It is common and, if ignored, may result in anorexia, 'retardation' (slow mental processes), somatic symptoms and disruption of normal life. Suicide may be attempted, and suicidal ideas should be asked about when assessing such patients. Choice of antidepressant drug can be difficult and is usually empirical: trials show them to be equipotent, and improvement in mood can take several weeks with all agents. The newer SSRIs (like fluoxetine) are safer than the tricyclic antidepressants after overdose.

lism. Amitriptyline's principal metabolite, nortriptyline, is active. Like all tricyclic antidepressants, amitriptyline has a large volume of distribution. The elimination half-life is slow.

Therapeutic uses

- Depression: there is a delay of about 2 weeks before benefit is seen. Amitriptyline is sedative, and this can be a useful property. Other tricyclics can be chosen that lack this sedative effect.
- Chronic pain: tricyclic antidepressants are also used for the treatment of neuralgia.

Adverse effects

As well as their therapeutic effect via uptake I, tricyclic drugs are antagonists of muscarinic and histamine H_1 receptors and α_1-adrenoceptors.

- Anticholinergic effects include urinary retention, constipation and tachyarrhythmias (especially problematic in overdose; see Ch. 17)
- Cardiac arrhythmia may also occur because of effects on intracardiac conduction
- Sedation is particularly a problem with amitriptyline
- Weight gain can occur
- Exacerbation of epilepsy
- Idiosyncratic adverse reactions include hepatotoxicity and blood dyscrasias.

Contraindications

- Glaucoma: pupil dilatation from antimuscarinic effects causes intraocular pressure to rise
- Prostatic hypertrophy: acute retention of urine is a risk
- Immediately after a myocardial infarction: risk of arrhythmias
- Epilepsy: reduced seizure threshold.

Drug interactions

Additive sedation is seen when amitriptyline is combined with alcohol or other sedatives. Tricyclic drugs should not be combined with non-selective monoamine oxidase inhibitors (MAOIs) because of a rare, but potentially fatal, hyperthermia syndrome.

Selective serotonin-reuptake inhibitors (SSRI)

SSRI drugs cause selective inhibition of 5-HT reuptake by postsynaptic nerve terminals.

Examples

Fluoxetine is well absorbed from the gut and is metabolised to an equipotent metabolite. Both parent drug and active metabolite are very slowly eliminated and may accumulate in severe liver or kidney disease.

The term depression is used for abnormally protracted or severe sadness. Hypomania is prolonged inappropriate elevation of mood; it may alternate with depression in so-called 'bipolar affective disorder'.

The amine hypothesis

The amine hypothesis that depression results from a 'depletion' of monoamine neurotransmitters (5-hydroxytryptamine (or serotonin; 5-HT) and noradrenaline) is at the centre of antidepressant development.

Drugs that interfere with monoamine release or storage, such as reserpine (a disused antihypertensive), can cause depression.

Drugs that potentiate monoamines (such as tricyclic antidepressants and selective serotonin-reuptake inhibitors (SSRIs)) can relieve it.

Drugs in depression and hypomania

Tricyclic antidepressants

Tricyclic antidepressants block the reuptake into the presynaptic neurone of noradrenaline and 5-HT, thereby increasing their availability to the postsynaptic membrane (so-called uptake 1; Fig. 33). *Amitriptyline*, an example of this drug group, is completely absorbed from the gut; however, it slows gut motility and its absorption is consequently slow. There is extensive first-pass metabo-

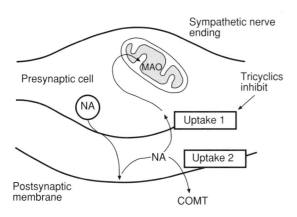

Fig. 33 Mode of action of tricyclic antidepressants. NA, noradrenaline; MAO, monoamine oxidase; COMT, catechol-*O*-methyltransferase.

Sertraline in contrast, has a shorter elimination half-life and is metabolised to inactive derivatives.

Therapeutic use

As with the tricyclic antidepressants, there is considerable delay between starting treatment and the onset of benefit. Unlike the tricyclic drugs, SSRIs do not have marked sedative, hypotensive or anticholinergic effects and have less effect on cardiac conduction. In overdose, the SSRIs are better tolerated than tricyclic antidepressants.

Adverse effects

- Vasculitic rash: a rare but serious reaction to fluoxetine
- Seizures: SSRIs can exacerbate seizures
- Symptomatic adverse effects include anorexia and sexual dysfunction
- Anorexia and weight loss
- Fluoxetine can cause hyponatraemia.

Drug interactions

The combination of lithium with fluoxetine may increase the risk of seizure.

Non-selective monoamine oxidase inhibitors (MAOIs)

The non-selective MAOIs are a long established group of drugs that inhibit the metabolism of noradrenaline and 5-HT by monoamine oxidase (of both subtypes; see below). *Tranylcypromine* is an example of the group. The non-selective MAOIs are used far less frequently than SSRIs or tricyclic antidepressants because of the risk of drug interactions. Foods containing tyramine and dopamine are contraindicated when taking the non-selective MAOIs because of the risk of severe hypertension. These foods include ripe cheese and pickled herring. Likewise nasal decongestants, which contain sympathomimetics, pethidine and levodopa should be avoided. The non-selective MAOIs should not be combined with tricyclic drugs or SSRIs (causes a rare, but often fatal, hyperthermia syndrome).

Reversible inhibitors of monoamine oxidase A (RIMA)

There are two subtypes of monoamine oxidase: MAO-A metabolises noradrenaline and 5-HT and is, therefore, relevant to depression, while MAO-B metabolises dopamine (see Section 6.5). *Moclobemide* is a reversible inhibitor of MAO-A. It is well absorbed from the gut and cleared by hepatic metabolism; its half-life is very short and it is given twice daily. Unlike the non-selective MAOIs, moclobemide does not carry a high risk of hypertensive

crises with sympathomimetics. Moclobemate does potentiate opiates but may be prescribed in combination with tricyclic drugs or SSRIs.

Lithium

The mode of action of lithium, which is used for the prophylaxis and treatment of bipolar affective disorder, is unknown. It is well absorbed orally and is excreted by the kidney; its clearance is reduced in patients with renal impairment. There is an established therapeutic range for lithium and monitoring is *mandatory*. Exceeding the upper limit of the therapeutic range is dangerous and a serum lithium concentration, 12 hours postdose, greater than 3.5 mmol/l is life threatening. Common adverse effects include renal damage (nephrogenic diabetes insipidus), hypothyroidism, rashes and oedema. Lithium may be teratogenic and women of child-bearing age must be made aware of this and offered contraception. Lithium should be avoided in patients with renal impairment because of the risk of accumulation. Psoriasis may be worsened by lithium, making this a relative contraindication. Diuretics and non-steroidal anti-inflammatory drugs can cause accumulation of lithium.

6.4 Schizophrenia

> **Learning objectives**
>
> You should:
>
> - be able to describe schizophrenia
> - be able to outline the 'dopamine hypothesis' of schizophrenia and appreciate the limitations of this hypothesis
> - know the clinical pharmacology of the 'standard' neuroleptic drugs and their main adverse effects
> - understand that clozapine, an 'atypical' neuroleptic drug, is reserved for resistant cases because of its adverse effect profile.

Schizophrenia is a common, severe 'functional' mental disorder that mainly affects young adults. The disease is characterised by:

- delusions (unshakable beliefs at variance with observed reality; these are commonly 'paranoid' or 'grandiose')
- hallucinations (most commonly auditory)
- disordered thinking (the patient is oriented in person, place and time, but logical connections between ideas are perturbed)

- lack of motivation or emotion (in chronic schizophrenia, this 'negative' symptom may become more prominent.

The aetiology is not fully understood. There is a large genetic element. In addition, abnormalities of the temporal lobes are detectable, and abnormality of dopaminergic transmission may have a role.

Established neuroleptic drugs

Neuroleptics (otherwise known as 'major tranquilizers') are structurally heterogeneous drugs that reduce the thought disorder that characterizes schizophrenia. All act by blocking dopamine D_2 receptors, primarily in the mesolimbic system. Antagonism of D_1 receptors does not contribute therapeutically but may cause dystonic reactions. Neuroleptics may also block receptors to 5-HT, histamine (H_1) acetylcholine (muscarinic receptors) and noradrenaline (α_1-adrenoceptors), and these actions contribute to their adverse effect profile. Examples include *chlorpromazine*, *haloperidol* and *flupentixol*.

Therapeutic uses

- Schizophrenia and related disorders
- Severe organic psychosis.

Clinical sketch

An 18-year-old student is seen in the A&E department after a determined suicide attempt. His parents are distraught. Over the previous year, his work has been deteriorating and he has lost touch with his family. He has few friends in college. Detailed assessment by a psychiatrist reveals paranoid delusions and auditory hallucinations. A diagnosis of schizophrenia is made and he is started on depot injections of a neuroleptic drug. He improves on this treatment, but not enough to resume his studies.

Comment: schizophrenia most commonly presents in young adulthood. Disruption of social contacts and work are major features. Most people respond to neuroleptics, but complete control of symptoms is unusual.

Clinical sketch

A 30-year-old woman has been schizophrenic since she was 20. Psychiatrists have tried many different drugs without much success. Eventually, clozapine is started, and improvement is noted.

Comment: clozapine is one of several 'atypical' neuroleptic drugs that are reserved for difficult cases. Serious adverse effects are common and monitoring of white cell counts is mandatory.

Adverse effects

- Exacerbation of depression.
- Blockade of D_1 receptors may result in parkinsonism and other extrapyramidal reactions including akathisia (severe restlessness) and acute dystonia (including torticollis). All these syndromes may respond to anticholinergic drugs. Tardive dyskinesia, the late onset of choreoathetoid movements, may occur in up to 40% of patients; it is probably caused by dopamine receptor upregulation and can be very difficult to treat.
- Autonomic effects include postural hypotension, premature ejaculation, visual disturbance, dry mouth, retention of urine and constipation (more common with chlorpromazine).
- Jaundice, rashes and agranulocytosis are rare but serious adverse effects.
- Hyperprolactinaemia can result from chronic dopamine antagonism and may cause gynaecomastia.
- Neuroleptic malignant syndrome is a rare but serious reaction to all these drugs, comprising hyperpyrexia and muscle rigidity.

Contraindications

- Hypersensitivity
- Glaucoma
- Parkinson's disease
- Impaired consciousness.

Drug interactions

Most of the interactions are pharmacodynamic and predictable from a knowledge of the receptor groups blocked by the drugs. Additive effects are seen between neuroleptics and other antidopaminergic, antimuscarinic, antihistaminergic and antiadrenergic drugs.

'Atypical' neuroleptic drugs

The atypical neuroleptics differ chemically from any of the established (older) compounds described above. All are thought to work by their effects on D_2 receptors and all tend to cause fewer extrapyramidal adverse effects: hence their attraction. The 'atypical' drugs are gradually becoming more commonly used by psychiatrists. Three examples are briefly described below.

Risperidone

The most common symptomatic adverse effects with risperidone include sleep disturbance, anxiety and rhinitis. Sudden death has occurred in a small number of patients with pre-existing cardiac disease, and this is a relative contraindication to the use of risperidone.

Olanzapine

Olanzapine was introduced in the late 1990s and its adverse effect profile is incompletely documented. Life-threatening adverse effects have included agranulocytosis and cardiac arrhythmias.

Clozapine

Clozapine is often effective in resistant cases of psychosis. However, because of the high prevalence of associated agranulocytosis, it was withdrawn in the 1970s. It was reintroduced in the 1990s but is reserved for resistant schizophrenia under close hospital monitoring. Other adverse effects include weight gain and convulsions.

6.5 Parkinsonism

Learning objectives

You should:

- be able to summarise the accepted neurotransmitter problem that underlies parkinsonism
- know the clinical features of parkinsonism
- appreciate that parkinsonism can be idiopathic (Parkinson's disease) or have identified causes
- be able to describe the clinical pharmacology of dopaminergic and anticholinergic antiparkinsonism drugs
- appreciate that the natural history of idiopathic Parkinson's disease is one of steady deterioration and that none of the existing drugs reduces mortality.

Clinical sketch

A 65-year-old man notices difficulty turning in bed and rising from a chair. This symptom worsens and is accompanied by shaking and a tendency to fall. His doctor diagnoses Parkinson's disease and starts a levodopa preparation.

Comment: These symptoms are typical of parkinsonism. Levodopa (L-dopa) preparations, and other dopaminergic drugs, are the preferred options.

Clinical sketch

A 50-year-old schizophrenic has been on neuroleptic drugs for many years. The features of parkinsonism are noted, and an anticholinergic preparation is started.

Comment: neuroleptic-induced parkinsonism is common. Dopaminergic therapy is illogical: the problem has resulted from the dopamine antagonism of the neuroleptic drug. Furthermore, dopaminergic drugs may worsen psychosis. Treatment aims to oppose the effects of cholinergic fibres, by using antimuscarinic drugs.

Parkinsonism comprises bradykinesia (or difficulty initiating movement), coarse tremor, rigidity and disordered posture. The patient shuffles ('festinating gait') and has a tendency to fall. The cause is degeneration of the substantia nigra in idiopathic disease, with marked reduction in local dopamine concentrations; this reduces the inhibition of excitatory cholinergic fibres.

Neuroleptic drugs can cause parkinsonism by blocking dopamine receptors. The aim of therapy is to restore the balance between dopamine and acetylcholine either by increasing the concentration of dopamine (dopaminergic drugs) or by blocking acetylcholine production (anticholinergic drugs).

Parkinson's disease

This is a disease of unknown cause that mainly afflicts the elderly. The commonest symptoms are tremor and slowness of movement. The patient's writing may become small and spidery ('micrographia').
The main physical signs are:

- coarse 'pill rolling' tremor; this settles during sleep but worsens during emotion. It is often symmetric
- rigidity
- bradykinesia: movements are slow and there is difficulty initiating movement
- postural changes: the patient is characteristically stooped, and the gait shuffles (so called 'festination')
- Speech is characteristically monotonous.

The natural history is one of gradual deterioration. The rate of progress is very variable.

Dopaminergic drugs

The dopaminergic drugs act by (a) providing the precursor of dopamine, (b) acting as dopamine agonists, (c) reducing dopamine metabolism or (d) causing local release of dopamine.

Levodopa

Levodopa (dihydroxyphenyl-L-alanine; L-dopa) is the precursor of dopamine and, unlike the latter, can cross the blood–brain barrier. Both within the CNS, and elsewhere in the body, levodopa is metabolised (by decarboxylation) to dopamine; it is the 'peripheral' synthesis of dopamine that results in many of the adverse effects of levodopa. To offset this, levodopa is combined with a decarboxylase inhibitor (either *carbidopa* or *benserazide*) that does not cross the blood–brain barrier. Consequently, peripheral decarboxylation is reduced but the CNS is unaffected. Levodopa is the drug of first choice; clinical response is usually good initially but declines with time.

Levodopa is absorbed by a facilitated carrier mechanism and, since certain other amino acids compete for transport, its absorption is reduced after meals. The drug is subject to extensive first-pass metabolism. Even when combined with a decarboxylase inhibitor, only about 10% of the levodopa dose enters the brain.

Adverse effects

- Nausea and vomiting: dopamine is the principal neurotransmitter of the vomiting centre in the brainstem, and dopamine agonists can cause nausea; this is reduced by the combination of levodopa with a decarboxylase inhibitor
- Dyskinesias (caused by overactivity in some dopaminergic pathways): seen in 80% of patients with prolonged use, including facial choreoathetosis, hemiballismus, dystonia, tics and myoclonus
- Cardiovascular: postural hypotension is common but some patients develop hypertension; tachyarrhythmias may occur
- Erratic response: marked variation in drug response occurs in a high proportion of patients after several years of treatment; in some, severe bradykinesia is seen several hours after dosing (end of dose phenomenon) while in others the fluctuation in response seems unrelated to drug doses and periods of severe bradykinesia alternate with periods of dyskinesia (on–off phenomenon). This is partly a pharmacokinetic phenomenon and may be limited by either frequent small doses or the use of a long-acting formulation.

Contraindications

- Glaucoma: intraocular pressure is increased
- Psychosis.

Drug interactions

Levodopa should not be given to patients taking a non-selective MAOI because of the risk of severe hypertension.

Direct dopamine agonists

Bromocriptine, *pergolide* and *ropinirole* are direct agonists at dopamine receptors. All are subject to extensive presystemic metabolism and are cleared mainly by hepatic metabolism. These drugs may be used as adjuvants to levodopa therapy, particularly where responses to levodopa are diminishing. They are also used as monotherapy in early Parkinson's disease, especially in younger patients.

Adverse effects

All dopamine agonists may cause nausea, dizziness, visual disturbance, vivid dreams and postural hypotension. Idiosyncratic reactions are rare.

Selegiline and entacapone

Dopamine is metabolised in the CNS by two pathways. MAO-B is inhibited by selegiline. Catechol-*O*-methyltransferase (COMT) is inhibited by entacapone.

Entacapone is given as an adjunct to levodopa.

Selegiline may be used in combination with levodopa either to restore the clinical response to the latter where this has been lost or in patients with 'on–off' symptoms. In one large study, patients on selegiline had increased mortality, and this is a cause of concern.

Adverse effects

Both entacapone and selegiline cause gastrointestinal upset and may induce confusion. The adverse effect profile of entacapone is not entirely known, since it has only recently been used widely.

Amantidine

Amantidine, an antiviral drug, probably increases dopamine release in the CNS. Its antiparkinsonian effects are weak, and it is not frequently used for this indication.

Anticholinergic drugs

Depletion of striatal dopamine, as in idiopathic parkinsonism, or blockade of dopamine receptors, as seen with neuroleptics, reduces inhibition of excitatory cholinergic neurones. This balance may be restored using antimuscarinic drugs. Examples include *trihexyphenidyl* (*benzhexol*) and *procyclidine* (which has an i.v. formulation that can be useful in acute dystonic reactions to neuroleptics). Anticholinergic drugs are most often given to patients with drug-induced parkinsonism. Their use in idiopathic Parkinson's disease is less common because the dopaminergic drugs are more effective. The adverse effects are those of systemic antimuscarinic drugs (Ch. 8), and contraindications include glaucoma and prostatic hypertrophy.

6.6 Migraine

Learning objectives

You should:

- be able to describe the features of classical migraine
- be able to summarise the pathophysiology of migraine and the role of 5-HT
- be able to formulate a management plan for acute migraine, and the prophylaxis of migraine
- be aware of the main adverse effects of antimigraine drugs.

5-hydroxytryptamine (5-HT) is a vasoactive amine that is released from platelets. The main organ-specific effects of 5-HT are:

- vasoconstriction (except in skeletal muscles and heart where it is vasodilator)
- venoconstriction, causing cutaneous flush
- increased peristalsis
- platelet aggregation.

Migraine is probably caused by the abnormal release of 5-HT within intracranial blood vessels, resulting in vasoconstriction; it is this that causes the typical 'aura', which may involve visual disturbance, speech abnormalities or even temporary hemiparesis.

Vasodilatation, possibly caused by 5-HT depletion, then follows and it is this that is associated with the headache, which is severe, classically unilateral and often causes prostration and nausea.

Migraine is common, particularly in adolescents, is often familial and tends to decrease in frequency as age advances. Most attacks show some response to simple analgesics, which should be tried first.

Drugs for the acute attack

Simple analgesics

Paracetamol (often combined with an antiemetic) is the drug of choice for most attacks.

Sumatriptan

Sumatriptan is a specific 5-HT agonist that opposes the vasodilatation responsible for the headache. It is formulated for oral and s.c. administration. Sumatriptan is well absorbed from both sites but is subject to presystemic metabolism when taken orally. It is used, early in an attack, to abort acute migraine. Adverse effects include:

- ECG changes and chest pain (especially after s.c. injection); it is contraindicated in ischaemic heart disease and severe hypertension
- drowsiness, nausea and vomiting.

Ergotamine

Ergotamine is an α-adrenoceptor antagonist, and a partial 5-HT agonist. The therapeutic benefit of ergotamine in migraine probably results from vasoconstriction, which opposes the vasodilatation responsible for the headache. It may be given by inhalation, sublingually, orally, s.c. or i.m. The bioavailability of the non-parenteral routes is very low, probably because of presystemic metabolism. Like sumatriptan, ergotamine should be taken during the prodromal illness, before the onset of headache. Although the drug's plasma half-life is short, its vasoconstricting effects are long lasting; consequently, once the maximum daily dose (about 6 mg) has been taken, no further ergotamine should be taken for 4 days. Parenteral administration should be reserved for use in hospital. Adverse effects include:

- arterial vasoconstriction: occasionally causing gangrene, myocardial infarction and renal failure; severe vasoconstriction can be seen in patients taking a beta-blocker
- retroperitoneal fibrosis: this is rare, and complicates long-term use
- headache: if used frequently.

Contraindication
Ergotamine is contraindicated in vascular disease.

Prophylaxis of migraine

Beta-blockers and tricyclic drugs

Beta-blockers and tricyclic drugs can be used to reduce the frequency of attacks.

Pizotifen

Pizotifen is an antihistamine with anti-5-HT activity. It can reduce the frequency of migraine attacks but often causes mild sedation.

Methysergide

Methysergide is a potent 5-HT antagonist that is reserved for patients with very severe symptoms. It should be used with great caution under hospital supervision because of the high risk of serious adverse effects. Treatment should be gradually withdrawn and stopped, for at least 4 weeks, every 6 months. Adverse effects include:

- fibrotic reactions: most commonly retroperitoneal fibrosis causing ureteric obstruction
- vasoconstriction: may exacerbate angina.

6.7 Other disorders

Alzheimer's disease

Alzheimer's disease is a degenerative brain disease of unknown cause that leads to dementia. It is characterised by a relative lack of the neurotransmitter acetylcholine, and by the presence of plaques of amyloid proteins. The predominant early features are memory loss and personality change. The disease is progressive, leading to global impairment of higher cerebral function. *Donepezil* is a reversible inhibitor of acetylcholinesterase. It is indicated for patients with mild-to-moderate Alzheimer's disease and may improve around 40% of such patients.

Multiple sclerosis

Multiple sclerosis is a common disease of unknown cause in which episodes of inflammation of white matter (of brain or cord) cause progressive disability. The disease generally starts in young people and pursues a course of relapses and remissions over many years. Acute exacerbations are generally identified by the development of new symptoms (such as optic neuropathy, cranial nerve lesions or cerebellar dysfunction). Such exacerbations are managed with short courses of *corticotrophin* (adrenocorticotrophic hormone) or steroids, which shorten the duration of such episodes. Patients with relapsing-remitting multiple sclerosis can benefit from *interferon beta*; it is indicated for the reduction of frequency and severity of relapses. Interferon-beta should not be used in patients with severe depression or poorly controlled epilepsy. It is generally held that the use of interferon beta should be monitored by a neurologist.

Self-assessment: questions

Multiple choice questions

1. Diazepam:
   a. Causes sedation, which is abolished by the elimination of the drug
   b. Interacts adversely with amitryptiline
   c. Can prove useful in very anxious asthmatics during an attack
   d. Can be given orally, over prolonged periods, to prevent seizures
   e. Is a suitable choice for the sedation of outpatients undergoing endoscopy

2. Carbamazepine:
   a. Is an appropriate choice to treat a patient with absence seizures (petit mal)
   b. Can be considered to be a prodrug
   c. Induces its own metabolism
   d. May be eliminated from the body after overdose using haemodialysis
   e. Potentiates the effects of warfarin

3. Sodium valproate:
   a. Is the treatment of choice for atonic seizures
   b. Induces the metabolism of warfarin
   c. Should always be withdrawn if a woman is trying to become pregnant
   d. Is the anticonvulsant of choice in patients with cirrhosis
   e. Potentiates phenytoin

4. Amitriptyline:
   a. Enhances the uptake of catecholamines by the presynaptic neurone (uptake I)
   b. Can be expected to lift mood within 2 days
   c. Is contraindicated in patients with glaucoma
   d. Is free of sedative effects
   e. Is the treatment of choice for someone who has become depressed following a myocardial infarction

5. Monoamine oxidase A inhibitors:
   a. Reduce noradrenaline metabolism
   b. Reduce 5-HT metabolism
   c. Predispose to hypertensive crises
   d. Are safely combined with tricyclic antidepressants in the treatment of depression
   e. Are safely combined with levodopa

6. Chlorpromazine:
   a. Should always be combined with an anticholinergic antiparkinsonian drug
   b. Works by enhancing the effect of dopamine at D_2 receptors
   c. Often improves depressive symptoms in patients with psychosis
   d. Is the treatment of choice for confusion in the elderly
   e. Is potentiated in chronic liver disease

7. Levodopa:
   a. Has a high oral bioavailability
   b. Should be given at higher dosage in parkinsonism if facial tics develop
   c. Should be withdrawn without delay if the 'on–off' phenomenon develops
   d. May be combined with MAO-B inhibitors
   e. Is converted to dopamine by MAO-B

8. In the management of migraine:
   a. During an acute attack, as much ergotamine should be used as needed to abolish headache
   b. Methysergide is an alternative to ergotamine for the treatment of an attack
   c. Sumatriptan may be used in patients with ischaemic heart disease
   d. Beta-blockers can give effective prophylaxis
   e. Most patients can be managed with simple analgesics like paracetamol

Case history questions

Case history 1

An 80-year-old woman is given diazepam to help her sleep at night. After 2 weeks, neighbours discover her in a state of self-neglect. She is taken to hospital where she is found to be somnolent and confused.

1. Why was diazepam a bad choice of drug in this case?
2. How should she be treated in hospital?

Case history 2

A woman with epilepsy, taking 200 mg phenytoin per day, continues to have seizures at an unacceptable rate. The drug level is measured and found to be 30 mmol/l (therapeutic range 40–80 mmol/l), so the dose is increased to 400 mg daily. After 1 week, the patient has nystagmus and cannot walk because of ataxia.

1. What has happened?

Case history 3

A 19-year-old man has gastroenteritis and is given metoclopramide. He develops acute torticollis (involuntary spasm of the neck muscles) 2 days later, which is very painful.

1. What is the likeliest diagnosis and what should be done?

Case history 4

A 60-year-old woman with schizophrenia has been taking haloperidol for many years and has been well controlled. However, her doctor thinks that her control is 'slipping' as she has recently started to move very strangely: when doing nothing, her arms writhe continuously in a rather jerky but semi-purposeful way.

1. What is the likeliest diagnosis and what should be done?

Case history 5

A patient with long-standing idiopathic Parkinson's disease finds that she is no longer getting so much benefit from her levodopa/carbidopa combination. Specifically, she finds that she is unable to rise from a chair because of stiffness well before her next dose is due.

1. What is the problem, and what should be done?

The same patient had her dose of levodopa increased; her parkinsonism was improved marginally, but after a couple of months she complains that shortly after taking the drug she suffers an hour of uncontrollable facial grimacing.

2. What is the problem, and what should be done?

The same lady develops nausea and dizziness, from an intercurrent illness, and is started on prochlorperazine.

3. What is the principal risk?

Case history 6

A 40-year-old woman, who smokes cigarettes, suffers from frequent migraine headaches. She takes propranolol as prophylaxis for migraine and uses ergotamine for the treatment of acute attacks.

1. What adverse drug reactions and interactions are likely to occur?

Case history 7

A 65-year-old man is given amitriptyline because of prolonged grief following the death of his wife. He is a cigarette smoker and suffers from angina pectoris. He is admitted to hospital 2 weeks later with noisy confusion. He is dehydrated, his pulse is irregular at 140 beats/min and he is anuric.

1. Advance some possible causes of his problems.

Short note questions

Write short notes on the following:

1. The therapeutic use of drugs for status epilepticus.
2. The clinical pharmacology of the drugs used in status epilepticus: deal with mechanisms of action, relevant pharmacokinetics, adverse effects and drug interactions.
3. The therapeutic use of drugs for complex partial seizures.
4. The clinical pharmacology of the drugs used in complex partial seizures: deal with mechanisms of action, relevant pharmacokinetics, adverse effects and drug interactions.
5. The modes of action, disposition and adverse effects of the drugs used in the treatment of depression.
6. Predicting the possible effects of chronic renal disease on response to (a) phenytoin and (b) lithium.

Extended matching items question

Theme: the clinical pharmacology of antiparkinsonian drugs
Options

A. It stimulates dopamine receptors
B. It crosses the blood–brain barrier
C. It blocks the metabolism of dopamine
D. It inhibits conversion of dopa to dopamine in the CNS
E. It does not cross the blood–brain barrier

F. It blocks acetylcholine receptors, thereby restoring the dopamine/acetylcholine balance

G. Because drug-induced parkinsonism results from the blocking of dopamine receptors by neuroleptics (so-called 'major tranquilizers')

H. Because drug-induced parkinsonism results mainly from excess acetylcholinergic activity in the CNS.

For each of the brief questions 1–4, choose the most appropriate answer from options A–H. Each option may be used once, more than once or not at all.

1. Why is dopamine not used for idiopathic Parkinson's disease?

2. Carbidopa, with which levodopa is formulated, is a dopa decarboxylase inhibitor (it blocks the conversion of dopa to dopamine): so why does its use not abolish the therapeutic effect of levodopa?

3. Why is levodopa contraindicated in drug-induced parkinsonism?

4. How does selegiline work?

Self-assessment: answers

Multiple choice answers

1. a. **False**. Diazepam is converted to pharmacologically active metabolites that persist in the body after the parent drug has been eliminated.
   b. **True**. Amitriptyline has marked sedative effects; if diazepam was taken simultaneously, the two sedatives would produce additive sedation.
   c. **False**. Diazepam may well kill asthmatics during an attack by causing respiratory depression. Anxiety in an asthmatic is appropriate and should be treated by tackling the asthma.
   d. **False**. Though diazepam can be used to stop a seizure, it is not used in prevention.
   e. **False**. Diazepam's effects are too long lived; a more appropriate choice would be midazolam.

2. a. **False**. Carbamazepine is indicated for partial seizures; it is useful for tonic/clonic seizures, but for no other generalised seizure types.
   b. **False**. Though carbamazepine does have a pharmacologically active metabolite, the parent drug possesses anticonvulsant activity.
   c. **True**. Carbamazepine is a potent enzyme inducer and, with chronic therapy, this enhances the elimination of the drug.
   d. **True**. Though structurally similar to the tricyclic antidepressants, carbamazepine has a small volume of distribution and can be removed by dialysis (this topic is more fully covered in Ch. 6).
   e. **False**. Carbamazepine induces the metabolism of warfarin and, therefore, reduces its effects.

3. a. **True**. Atonic seizures are not common; they are characterised by sudden loss of muscle tone causing the patient to collapse. Consciousness is often retained. Valproate is the drug of first choice.
   b. **False**. Valproate is a selective enzyme inhibitor, but it does not interact with warfarin.
   c. **False**. Standard advice for women on antiepileptic drugs is that treatment should continue during pregnancy despite the relatively small risk to the fetus.
   d. **False**. Valproate is contraindicated in patients with chronic liver disease because of the increased risk of drug-induced hepatic dysfunction.
   e. **False**. Valproate probably does not have clinically relevant effects on phenytoin.

4. a. **False**. Tricyclic antidepressants block uptake I.
   b. **False**. No therapeutic response is usually seen within the first 2 weeks.
   c. **True**. The anticholinergic effects of tricyclic drugs raise the intraocular pressure.
   d. **False**. Amitriptyline is a potent sedative and is usually given at night for this reason.
   e. **False**. Tricyclic antidepressants are contraindicated immediately after a myocardial infarction because of their effects on intracardiac conduction, and their anticholinergic effects.

5. a. **True**. MAO-A metabolises noradrenaline; MAO-B metabolises dopamine.
   b. **True**. MAO-A metabolises 5-HT.
   c. **True**. Sympathomimetics, as occur naturally in some foods and are the active ingredients in some proprietary cough mixtures, can cause severe hypertension in patients taking MAO-A inhibitors.
   d. **False**. The combination of tricyclic drug plus a MAO-A inhibitor may cause 'malignant hyperthermia'.
   e. **False**. The combination of levodopa and an MAO-A inhibitor may cause severe hypertension.

6. a. **False**. Not all patients develop parkinsonism, and there is no benefit starting therapy until they do.
   b. **False**. Neuroleptics are dopamine antagonists.
   c. **False**. Neuroleptics frequently exacerbate depression.
   d. **False**. Although neuroleptics may be indicated in organic psychosis, confusion in elderly patients is often worsened by sedative drugs.
   e. **True**. Chlorpromazine is metabolised in the liver.

7. a. **False**. Levodopa is subject to extensive first-pass metabolism.
   b. **False**. Levodopa may cause dyskinesias like tics.
   c. **False**. Sudden withdrawal of antiparkinsonian drugs may cause life-threatening deterioration; drugs must be withdrawn slowly in hospital.
   d. **True**. Selegiline may be combined with levodopa to restore the clinical response to the latter where this has been lost.
   e. **False**. Levodopa is formed by dopa decarboxylase.

8. a. **False**. Ergotamine is a potent vasoconstrictor and may cause severe peripheral ischaemia if recommended doses are exceeded.
   b. **False**. Methysergide is used prophylactically.
   c. **False**. Sumatriptan is contraindicated in patients with ischaemic heart disease because it may exacerbate angina.
   d. **True**. But caution is needed if ergotamine is used for acute attacks.

e. **True**. The majority of patients gain relief from paracetamol.

Case history answers

Case history 1

1. Diazepam itself is slowly eliminated, as are its active metabolites, and impaired hepatic or renal function slow their rate of elimination further. The elderly often have subclinical renal or hepatic impairment, and benzodiazepines accumulate, causing a so-called 'hangover effect'. With continued use confusion may develop.
2. The benzodiazepine should be stopped even though confusion may initially become worse. A specific benzodiazepine antagonist such as flumazenil is indicated in respiratory failure after overdose but not in the present circumstances. Prescription of further sedative drugs (e.g. in the event of noisy confusion at night) should be avoided.

Case history 2

The relationship between the dose of phenytoin and its plasma concentration is not linear (as it is with most drugs): relatively small dose increases frequently lead to a large rise in blood level. Doubling the dose, as here, can cause major toxicity.

Case history 3

This is an involuntary movement disorder induced by the antidopaminergic actions of the drug. Acute reactions, as in this patient, are common with some neuroleptics and antiemetics (see Ch. 11) and may come in the form of akathisia (inability to sit still) or acute dystonias such as torticollis (as here) or retrocollis. The pharmacological basis of the reaction is not clear, but anticholinergic drugs such as benztropine or procyclidine are indicated; as the latter may be given i.v., it is probably indicated here because of the pain. After i.v. dosing, improvement should occur within about 5 minutes.

Case history 4

This patient's symptoms illustrate tardive dyskinesia. This complicates chronic neuroleptic use in about 40% of cases. Elderly women are the most common group affected, though it can occur in either sex and at any age. The movements described are typical: so-called choreoathetoid movements. Early recognition is advisable as neglected cases can be more difficult to treat. The current hypothesis is that there is increased sensitivity to dopamine, possibly receptor upregulation, resulting from the chronic use of an antagonist. Most doctors would reduce the neuroleptic dose (and stop the drug if possible), even though this may worsen the dyskinesia in the short term; diazepam is often helpful to control symptoms.

Case history 5

1. This unfortunate patient has developed a common problem in late Parkinson's disease referred to as 'end of dose akinesia'. She may be helped by increasing the frequency of her levodopa doses.
2. She has gone on to develop 'on–off' effects where the high concentration of levodopa shortly after dosing induces acute diskinesia; such patients 'see-saw' between akinesia and dyskinesia, with only brief spells of normal movement. This can be difficult to treat: the dose of levodopa should probably be reduced, and a supplementary drug such as bromocriptine or selegiline started. In the worst cases, the patient may need admission to hospital to allow gradual withdrawal of all drugs, a 'drug holiday'; when reintroduced, the benefit from levodopa is restored, but this is usually only temporary.
3. Prochlorperazine is a neuroleptic drug (though it is not used for schizophrenia) that works by blocking dopamine receptors: the patient's parkinsonism could be made much worse. This is very poor prescribing.

Case history 6

This woman is at risk from atherosclerosis caused by smoking. Both the beta-blocker propranolol (see Ch. 3) and ergotamine are vasoconstrictor and might exacerbate peripheral vascular disease. She would be at particular risk should she exceed the recommended dose of ergotamine during an attack, for its effects accumulate.

Case history 7

At this man's age, a degree of prostatic hypertrophy can be expected. Tricyclic antidepressants have anticholinergic effects, which tend to increase the tone of the sphincter while reducing the tone of the bladder wall: this can cause acute retention of urine. His bladder should be easily palpable. Acute retention is painful and causes tachycardia and confusion. He should be catheterised and the tricyclic drug should be stopped. However, it sounds as if this patient either has atrial fibrillation, which may have been precipitated by the anticholinergic effects of the drug, or else multiple ectopic beats. The possibilities of myocardial infarction and of tricyclic overdose should be considered.

Short note answers

1. Status epilepticus (multiple seizures without recovery of consciousness in between episodes) is life threatening because it causes hypoxia, and it may damage the brain independently of hypoxia. Diazepam (given slowly i.v.) or lorazepam are the drugs of first choice. If these fail to stop seizures, then phenytoin (given as a very slow i.v. injection) is the next choice.
2. Refer to sections above.
3. Complex partial seizures (temporal lobe seizures) respond to carbamazepine, sodium valproate and lamotrigine. Monotherapy is usually achievable. Doses of drug should start small, and dose increases should be judged by the patient's response to treatment, rather than 'drug levels'. Therapeutic drug monitoring of carbamazepine does have a role, especially in the assessment of (a) apparent lack of response to a large dose and (b) suspected drug toxicity.
4. Refer to sections above.
5. Deal with each of the following areas.

Modes of action

- For the tricyclic antidepressants, describe the fate of noradrenaline after release into the synaptic cleft, mention uptake 1 and uptake 2.
- For SSRIs, the role of blockage of the reuptake of 5-HT into the neurone is not fully understood, but 5-HT may modulate noradrenaline release.
- For MAOIs, describe the substrates of MAO-A (noradrenaline and 5-HT) and MAO-B (dopamine). Mention that MAOIs selective for MAO-A(RIMA) are now available.

Disposition

- Tricyclic drugs are mostly well absorbed from the gut. All have large volumes of distribution (this is relevant to the overdose situation, they are not dialysable). Most are metabolised to active metabolites.
- SSRIs. Fluoxetine is well absorbed, metabolised to an equipotent metabolite and eliminated slowly.
- Most MAOIs are well absorbed and metabolised to active derivatives.

Adverse effects

- Mention the antimuscarinic properties of tricyclic antidepressants, which may, therefore, exacerbate glaucoma, retention of urine, constipation and tachyarrhythmias. Mention weight gain, sedation (especially amitriptyline) and idiosyncratic reactions.
- For SSRIs, mention vasculitis, anorexia and exacerbation of seizures.
- Mention weight gain, anticholinergic effects and gastrointestinal upset with MAOIs. Mention the risk of hypertensive crisis with sympathomimetic compounds found in cough medicines, cheese and red wine; this is not a problem with RIMAs.

6. Chronic renal diseases may alter drug response either by changing their plasma protein binding (albumin concentrations may fall and waste products may compete for binding sites) or by reducing their clearance. (This subject is dealt with more fully in Ch. 20.)

Phenytoin is extensively bound to albumin but cleared by hepatic metabolism to inactive derivatives. Hypoalbuminaemia or uraemia cause the unbound drug fraction to rise: at a given total plasma concentration the drug, therefore, seems to be more effective and more toxic. Phenytoin doses should be reduced.

Lithium is a metallic ion that is distributed in body water and is not bound to plasma proteins. It undergoes no metabolism but is cleared unchanged by the kidney. Renal impairment causes drug accumulation.

Extended matching items answer

1. E. Levodopa crosses the blood–brain barrier, where it is metabolised to the neurotransmitter dopamine. Dopamine itself cannot easily cross the blood–brain barrier.
2. E. Carbidopa does not cross the blood–brain barrier easily, so its effects are confined to the extracerebral metabolism of levadopa (which is responsible for many of the drug's adverse effects).
3. G. It would be illogical to give levodopa in this setting. Instead, the acetylcholinergic system is antagonised using drugs like benztropine and benzhexol.
4. C. Selegiline is an inhibitor of the enzyme monoamine oxidase B (MAO-B), which metabolises dopamine. MAO-A metabolises noradrenaline and 5-HT.

7 Analgesics

Overview

Pain can arise from damage to somatic areas (e.g. skin, bone), the viscera (e.g. heart, gut) or the CNS (neurogenic pain). Analgesics are classified by their mode of action and include opioids, non-opioids and non-steroidal anti-inflammatory drugs. Analgesics vary widely in their potency and the right drug should be chosen for the type and level of pain.

7.1 Pain

Learning objectives

You should:

- be aware of the different sources of pain and the occurrence of referred pain
- be able to assess likely levels of pain and the therapeutic response needed.

Somatic pain can arise from damage of any kind, to skin, bone, fascia, meninges, peritoneum, pleura and teeth. Somatic pain is usually well localised; the sensory modality is conducted to the CNS along small myelinated *delta* fibres and non-myelinated *C-fibres*.

Visceral pain can arise from damage to heart, gut and bladder, but not brain, liver, lung and spleen. Visceral pain is often poorly localised and may be *referred* to a distant site. It is not transmitted to the CNS by specific fibres but rather by changes in the rate of discharge of afferent autonomic fibres.

Neurogenic pain can result from damage to the CNS itself: such neurogenic pain is felt in the periphery. Neuralgia is a classical example. Such pain tends not to respond to the drugs described below and it can be dif-

ficult to treat (see Ch. 6); tricyclic antidepressants or antiepileptic drugs may be useful.

Endorphins

The endorphins are endogenous compounds released in the CNS in response to pain. Many endorphins have been identified; they vary widely in structure but are all small peptides. The endorphins act by binding to opioid receptors in the CNS, of which there are three main subtypes: μ, κ and σ.

- μ-receptors cause analgesia at a supraspinal level and are also responsible for drug-induced euphoria, respiratory depression and drug dependence
- κ-receptors cause analgesia at a spinal level and also induce miosis and sedation
- σ-receptors seem to have no clinically useful properties but cause dysphoria and hallucination.

The morphine-like (opioid) drugs are the only class known to act by mimicking these peptides. Development work in new pain relief drugs is also looking at potential inhibitors of endorphin breakdown and other molecules that might interfere with nociception (sense of pain).

7.2 Analgesic drugs

Opioid analgesics

Learning objectives

You should:

- know the mode of action of the opioids and their major actions in the intact individual
- appreciate that opiates are mainly eliminated by hepatic metabolism
- be able to list the major adverse effects of opiates and know how naloxone reverses their effects
- be able to describe the appropriate clinical use of opiates and appreciate that they can be addictive
- be aware that strict law governs the storage of many opiates, and the records that must be kept by the doctor
- appreciate that the antipyretic effects of paracetamol are useful in lowering fever

- appreciate that paracetamol is useless against inflammatory diseases such as rheumatism

- appreciate that NSAIDs are also used as analgesics (at a lower dose than that used for anti-inflammatory effects)

- appreciate that compound analgesics, although in common use, rarely have much benefit over the use of paracetamol or low-dose NSAID.

Clinical sketch

A young man is involved in major trauma and sustains both pelvic and head injuries. He is given diamorphine for the pain from his fractures, but his level of consciousness gradually worsens in the next hour; arterial gases reveal carbon dioxide retention. A computed tomographic (CT) scan shows brain swelling.

Comment: opioid analgesics are contraindicated in patients with head injury. Respiratory depression causes retention of carbon dioxide and may worsen brain swelling.

Clinical sketch

A man with severe alcoholic liver disease is admitted with an exacerbation of chronic liver failure. He is given dihydrocodeine for headache, and becomes unrousably comatose.

Comment: all opiates are contraindicated in patients with decompensated liver disease, and even drugs like codeine can worsen the level of consciousness.

Clinical sketch

A woman with ischaemic heart disease presents with a myocardial infarction. She is in great pain, clammy and breathless. She is given i.v. diamorphine as a slow injection. This relieves the pain and dyspnoea but makes her vomit.

Comment: this is appropriate use of the drug, but the nausea could have been anticipated. The breathlessness may have been caused by pulmonary congestion, and the vasodilator effects of diamorphine are useful. Her blood pressure would be very likely to fall, and this is a common adverse consequence.

Analgesics are classified according to their mode of action, into opioids, non-opioids, and non-steroidal anti-inflammatory drugs (NSAIDs). As suggested by their name, this last group has the additional therapeutic property of reducing inflammation (Ch. 9). Analgesics vary in their potency and are used for a wide variety of pains ranging from mild, such as 'tension headache', to severe, such as terminal malignancy.

Mode of action

Opioid analgesics, which are structurally quite different from the endorphins, are agonists at endorphin receptors. The effects of opiates on specific organs are as follows:
- CNS
  —analgesia: the perception of both somatic and visceral is impaired, and the response to pain is altered; the patient may feel 'at ease' even though pain is still perceived
  —euphoria: a sensation of wellbeing; this is the main sensation sought by addicts
  —sedation: a dose-dependent effect that may lead to respiratory depression
  —other effects: cough suppression, nausea and miosis (small pupils)
- gastrointestinal tract
  —reduced gut motility leading to constipation
  —tone of biliary tree may be increased
  —sphincter of Oddi may contract.
- cardiovascular system
  —peripheral arteriodilatation and venodilatation,
  —possibly as a result of effects on the vasomotor centre in the CNS
  —blood pressure may fall in subjects with reduced blood volume.

Examples and clinical pharmacokinetics

The examples have certain features in common. All are well absorbed from i.m. and s.c. sites but are subject to extensive first-pass metabolism in the liver if given orally. All are widely distributed and cross the blood–brain barrier readily. All are metabolised in the liver.

Morphine is a potent analgesic with a duration of analgesia of about 4 to 6 hours.

Diamorphine (heroin) is more potent than morphine, possibly because it crosses the blood–brain barrier more readily. The duration of analgesic action is 4–6 hours.

Pethidine is a synthetic opioid with a shorter duration of action (2–4 hours) than morphine or diamorphine and a lower potency.

Codeine has a higher bioavailability than morphine but is less potent.

Buprenorphine is a synthetic opioid with both agonist and antagonist effect at opioid receptors. It may precipitate a withdrawal reaction in opiate addicts. Its oral bioavailability is low, and buprenorphine is given either sublingually or parenterally. Buprenorphine has a long duration of action (4–8 hours) but is less potent than morphine.

Fentanyl is a potent synthetic opioid mainly used in anaesthesia.

Dextropropoxyphene is approximately as potent as codeine and is used in compound analgesics. It inhibits liver enzymes and may give rise to drug interactions as a result.

Tramadol is a synthetic compound that, like buprenorphine, has mixed agonist and antagonist activity. It also has effects on other, non-opioid, receptors. There is no advantage over opioids.

Therapeutic uses
Somatic and visceral pain. Opiates are useful for both types of pain. They are, however, contraindicated in biliary colic (see above) and are useless against neurogenic pain. The severe visceral pain of myocardial infarction is treated with morphine or diamorphine, usually by slow i.v. injection accompanied by an antiemetic. In terminal disseminated cancer, s.c. infusions (often at a rate controlled by the patient) can be very useful, and oral slow-release preparations are available.

Pulmonary oedema. Morphine or diamorphine are commonly used to treat pulmonary oedema, in combination with loop diuretics. The opiate acts partly by relieving respiratory distress and partly by reducing venous return.

Diarrhoea. Oral opiates can be useful against diarrhoea, though the priority is maintenance of hydration, especially in children.

Cough suppression. This effect is particularly useful in terminal illness.

Adverse effects

- Addiction is a risk if opiates are used regularly for long periods: withdrawal then causes an unpleasant, but not clinically serious, reaction (Ch. 18). With continuous exposure larger doses are required to produce the same effects: this is called tolerance. These problems should not be used to deny patients necessary analgesia
- Respiratory depression is a problem after overdose and in patients with chronic respiratory disease
- Nausea
- Constipation.

Contraindications

- Acute or chronic respiratory disease: patients with chronic retention of carbon dioxide caused by type II respiratory failure are particularly at risk
- Hepatic failure (see the clinical sketches on p. 90)
- Head injury (see the clinical sketches on p. 90).

Drug interactions
Opiates produce additive sedation when given with other sedative drugs or alcohol.

Opiate antagonists

Naloxone is the main antagonist in widespread use for opiate overdose. Opiate effects, such as respiratory depression and coma, are dramatically reversed within 2 minutes of giving i.v. naloxone. However, naloxone has a short half-life and must sometimes be given repeatedly to those who have taken large overdoses.

Paracetamol (acetaminophen)

Mode of action
Paracetamol probably works by inhibiting the enzyme prostaglandin synthetase within the CNS. Furthermore, inhibition of prostaglandin E_2 synthesis in the hypothalamus accounts for the drug's antipyretic effects. (NB: paracetamol does not lower a normal body temperature.) Little inhibition of prostaglandin synthesis is seen peripherally and paracetamol has little or no anti-inflammatory properties.

Clinical pharmacokinetics
The clearance of paracetamol is described in Ch.17, where the effect of overdosage is covered.

Therapeutic uses

- Analgesia: paracetamol is effective, safe and causes little gastric irritation. In standard doses it is virtually free of adverse effects
- To correct fever: this can prevent febrile convulsions in young children.

Non-steroidal anti-inflammatory drugs as analgesics

NSAIDs inhibit cyclo-oxygenase and block production of prostaglandin E_2 both centrally and peripherally. They are effective as both anti-inflammatories and analgesics.

Aspirin and *ibuprofen* are available as simple analgesics without prescription in the UK.

Most other NSAIDs require a prescription. They are intended for use in inflammatory conditions (see also Ch. 9) but are often used, sometimes inappropriately, as simple analgesics.

Therapeutic uses

- Analgesia in common pain: aspirin and ibuprofen are widely used for common pain, such as headache and dysmenorrhoea
- Analgesia in bone metastases: NSAIDs can be a useful adjunct to opioids in the terminal care of patients with bone metastases
- Antipyretic: aspirin used to be a common remedy for childhood fevers, but fears about its role in Reye's syndrome have caused a switch to paracetamol for paediatric use.

Adverse effects

- Gastrointestinal upset (Ch. 9)

- Peptic ulcer disease
- Allergy
- Renal impairment.

Compound analgesics

Many analgesic drug combinations are marketed: they are often expensive, are rarely more potent than use of a single drug and can be dangerous in overdosage. Examples include:

co-proxamol: paracetamol plus dextropropoxyphene
co-codamol: paracetamol plus codeine
co-codaprin: aspirin plus codeine.

Self-assessment: questions

Multiple choice questions

1. The following are appropriate choices of drug:
   a. Diamorphine for pulmonary oedema
   b. Pethidine for biliary colic
   c. Paracetamol for arthritis
   d. Aspirin for dyspepsia
   e. Morphine for joint pain in haemophiliacs

2. Paracetamol plus dextropropoxyphene (co-proxamol):
   a. Is safe in patients with severe renal failure
   b. Is safe in patients with liver impairment
   c. Is as potent an analgesic as morphine
   d. Can induce addiction
   e. If taken in overdose, may cause both CNS and hepatic dysfunction

3. In patients with painful bony metastases:
   a. Oral morphine may be used
   b. The combination of an opioid with a non-steroidal anti-inflammatory drug (NSAID) is beneficial
   c. Opioids do not produce important adverse effects in such patients
   d. When using parenteral morphine (via an infusion pump) it is important that the rate of infusion is not controlled by the patient
   e. Carbamazepine or tricyclic antidepressants may have better analgesic effects than opioids

Case history questions

Case history 1

A registered i.v. drug abuser is admitted with a deep vein thrombosis and pleuritic chest pain. Ventilation-perfusion scanning reveals a pulmonary infarct. Blood cultures grow *Streptococcus pyogenes*. He is treated with dalteparin and antibiotics. He claims to be on methadone, but it is the weekend and you cannot check with the drug dependency centre. His pleuritic pain is severe, and he wants pain-killers.

1. What should you do?
2. What are the risks of stopping methadone abruptly?

Case history 2

A man is admitted with severe abdominal pain: you suspect acute appendicitis. The surgeon is scrubbed and will not be available for about half an hour.

1. What should you do?

Short note question

Contrast the modes of action, disposition, clinical use and adverse effects of aspirin and paracetamol.

Extended matching items questions

Theme: prescribing the best drug
Options

A. Paracetamol
B. Dihydrocodeine
C. Aspirin
D. Ibuprofen
E. Methysergide
F. Indometacin

For each of the case histories 1–3 prescribe the best drug for the patient from options A–F. Each option may be used once, more than once or not at all.

1. A 30-year-old man with unilateral headache, which was preceded by visual disturbance and is accompanied by nausea and prostration.
2. A 65-year-old woman with osteoarthrosis and reflux oesophagitis.
3. A young woman with tendonitis.

Theme: predicting adverse effects of analgesics
Options

A. Liver damage
B. Kidney damage
C. Gastro-intestinal bleeding
D. Coma
E. Respiratory arrest
F. Angioedema
G. Shock
H. Rash

For each of the case histories 1–3 predict the most likely adverse reaction to the named drug from options A–H. Each option may be used once, more than once, or not at all.

1. A 50-year-old man with alcoholic cirrhosis is admitted with mild confusion. He complains bitterly of severe back pain, and the doctor prescribes dihydrocodeine.
2. A woman with a past history of peptic ulcer disease is given diflunisal for dysmenorrhoea.
3. An 80-year-old man with severe chronic bronchitis suffers a nasty fall and is admitted 24 hours afterwards with pneumonia. The partial pressure of oxygen in his arterial blood is found to be very low, while that of carbon dioxide is markedly elevated. He is in a great deal of pain from two broken ribs, and this is making physiotherapy very difficult. The doctor gives him an injection of diamorphine.

Self-assessment: answers

Multiple choice answers

1. a. **True**. Diamorphine reduces anxiety and breathlessness and is vasodilator, thereby reducing venous return.
   b. **False**. Pethidine can cause smooth muscle contraction and may exacerbate biliary colic.
   c. **False**. Paracetamol has no anti-inflammatory properties.
   d. **False**. Aspirin may exacerbate peptic ulcers and, because of its effects on clotting, may cause gastrointestinal bleeding. However, proprietary effervescent antidyspeptics may contain aspirin.
   e. **False**. Haemophilia is a life-long problem that causes repeated painful intra-articular bleeds. Frequent use of opioids may lead to addiction.

2. a. **False**. The effects of dextropropoxyphene are enhanced in renal failure; paracetamol, however, is safe.
   b. **False**. Opioids undergo extensive liver metabolism and, in the presence of hepatic failure, may induce fatal coma. The role of paracetamol in severe liver disease is more contentious; in theory the patient may be more prone to toxicity, but in practice many physicians are forced to use the drug because alternatives are usually less safe.
   c. **False**. This drug combination is probably no more potent than paracetamol alone.
   d. **True**. Dextropropoxyphene does induce dependence.
   e. **True**. Co-proxamol is particularly dangerous when taken in large doses: the opioid effects are clinically obvious (depression of consciousness and respiration) but those of the paracetamol may be missed unless drug levels are assayed.

3. a. **True**. Although morphine has a low bioavailability, it is given in a slow-release formulation, which can easily be used in the community.
   b. **True**. The NSAID is often a very effective addition to the opiate.
   c. **False**. Constipation is the main problem encountered, and this is often very distressing to the dying patient. It needs to be tackled vigorously.
   d. **False**. Current practice is to give limited control of infusion rates to the patient: doses of drug are often found to be lower, and many patients find analgesia improved.

e. **False**. Terminally ill patients may need antidepressants, but these drugs have 'analgesic' properties only in neurogenic pain.

Case history answers

Case history 1

1. It is reasonable to give him *oral* methadone, in a moderate dose, until you can check with his usual doctor. Such patients are manipulative and will often request that the dose be increased. This should be resisted: it is not in the patient's best interests.
2. Stopping opiates abruptly does cause a somatic illness 'cold turkey': sweating, shivering, goose bumps and drug-craving. However this is not life threatening. A NSAID would be the best choice for relief of the pleuritic chest pain: parenteral opiates should be avoided.

Case history 2

Half an hour is not a very long time to wait for a surgical opinion: although, of course, it will seem longer to the unfortunate patient. Here, the risks of opiates outweigh their benefits: the surgeon will want to assess an alert patient and examine the abdomen in the absence of strong analgesia. This should be sympathetically explained to patient and family.

Short note answers

Modes of action. Both inhibit prostaglandin synthetase, paracetamol weakly and aspirin relatively more strongly. Aspirin has anti-inflammatory, analgesic and antipyretic effects; paracetamol is analgesic and antipyretic but has no significant anti-inflammatory properties.

Disposition. Both drugs are well absorbed from the gut. Aspirin is hydrolysed, by tissue esterases, into salicylic acid and acetate. Both drugs are extensively bound to plasma proteins. Paracetamol is eliminated by hepatic metabolism (conjugation reactions at therapeutic doses; in overdose, paracetamol is oxidised to a reactive, and toxic, metabolite; Ch. 17). Salicylate is mainly eliminated by conjugation in the liver, but a clinically relevant fraction is excreted unchanged by the kidney: renal clearance of salicylate is increased by alkalinisation of the urine.

Clinical use. Both drugs are available without prescription in the UK. Paracetamol is used to treat mild pain (including headache and dysmenorrhoea) and to lower temperature, especially in young children at risk of febrile seizures. Aspirin should not be given to young children because of the possible association with Reye's syndrome; otherwise, aspirin is used for mild pain. Few patients can tolerate the doses of aspirin required for anti-inflammatory effects, and alternative NSAIDs are usually employed. Recently, aspirin has become standard for the secondary prevention of myocardial infarction and is becoming increasingly used for the secondary prevention of non-haemorrhagic stroke.

Adverse effects. At therapeutic doses, it is unusual for paracetamol to cause adverse effects, but aspirin causes gastrointestinal bleeding even at therapeutic doses. Aspirin may exacerbate peptic ulcer. In patients with haemophilia or von Willebrand's disease, aspirin should be avoided because of its antiplatelet effects. In overdose, paracetamol causes concentration-dependent liver damage, which can develop into fulminant hepatic failure; aspirin overdose is characterised by metabolic acidosis.

Extending matching items answers

Theme: prescribing the best drug

1. A. The brief description is typical of migraine, which is usually relieved by simple analgesics such as paracetamol. Methysergide (Ch. 6) is used for the *prevention* of migraine as a drug of final resort (because of the frequency of severe adverse effects).

Indometacin (Ch. 9) can cause headache and is not indicated in migraine. Dihydrocodeine may exacerbate nausea, as may aspirin and (to a lesser extent) ibuprofen.

2. A or B. This is a difficult, but common, problem. The pain of osteoarthitis can be very disabling, but the various NSAIDs exacerbate oesophageal reflux or peptic ulcer. Some doctors might give NSAIDs while also giving either a histamine H_2 antagonist (e.g. ranitidine) or a proton pump inhibitor (e.g. omeprazole). However paracetamol and dihydrocodeine, either separately or in combination, may give adequate pain relief.

3. D. Ibuprofen will be better tolerated than aspirin by most patients. Indometacin may be used for severe cases, but adverse effects are much more common.

Theme: predicting adverse effects of analgesics

1. D. Opioids, even mild ones, are absolutely contraindicated in patients with liver failure.

2. C. Diflunisal (which you may have needed to look up in BNF) is one of the many commonly used NSAIDs. Gastrointestinal bleeding is a common adverse effect.

3. E. This man has type II respiratory failure (Ch. 10) in that he has carbon dioxide retention. All sedative drugs, including opioids, which cause marked sedation are contraindicated.

Drugs used in anaesthesia

Overview

Anaesthetics are used to prevent pain for a limited period during surgery or other procedures whereas analgesics are used to control pain. In this chapter, the use of local and general anaesthetics is described and the use of skeletal muscle relaxants, which facilitate surgery by reducing muscle tone.

8.1 Pain prevention

Learning objectives

You should:

- be aware of the indications for use of local or general anaesthetics

- understand the principles upon which drug use in surgery is based.

Broadly, surgery may cause two types of pain: *somatic*, which is produced by cutting skin, peritoneum or other ectodermal structures, and *visceral*, which is produced by traction on organs or omentum. While analgesics are used to *control* pain, anaesthetics are used to *prevent* it, for a limited period, during surgery. This has long been attempted with drugs, probably since prehistory: alcohol or opioids were the (unsatisfactory) mainstay until the discovery of ether, other inhaled drugs and cocaine.

Local anaesthetic agents are extensively used for both minor and major procedures: instilled locally they prevent somatic pain and abolish much tactile sensation; instilled epidurally, they allow abdominal surgery, though visceral pain may not be entirely prevented.

The state of general anaesthesia is complex but includes loss of consciousness, amnesia, analgesia and impairment of sensory and autonomic function. Depending on the drug, general anaesthetics may be given i.v.—most frequently for *induction*—or by inhalation— often for *maintenance* of anaesthesia.

Even with general anaesthetics, much surgery would be technically difficult because of the high tone of abdominal and other muscles. Skeletal muscle relaxants are widely used to facilitate major surgery and during mechanical ventilation; consequently, these drugs will also be dealt with in this chapter.

8.2 Local anaesthetic agents

Learning objectives

You should:

- be able to describe the mode of action of local anaesthetics at both the molecular and whole neurone levels

- appreciate that drug absorption, from injection site into the circulation, usually *terminates* the effects of local anaesthetics

- be aware of the relevance and dangers of formulation of local anaesthetic with epinephrine (adrenaline)

- appreciate that local anaesthetics are eliminated by hepatic metabolism

- be able to list the main adverse effects of local anaesthetics.

Mode of action

At the molecular level. When a neurone is stimulated, sodium channels open and Na^+ rapidly diffuses into the cell from the higher extracellular concentration; this depolarises the cell membrane and transmits the nerve impulse. Local anaesthetics reversibly block activated sodium channels (Fig. 34) by binding to receptors situated 'within' the channel. They have low affinity for the receptor when the channel is resting (Fig. 34A) and bind mainly to activated and inactivated channels (Fig. 34B,C). Local anaesthetics are mainly ionised at physiological pH, but only the unionised fraction is capable of crossing the cell membrane and gaining access to the receptor.

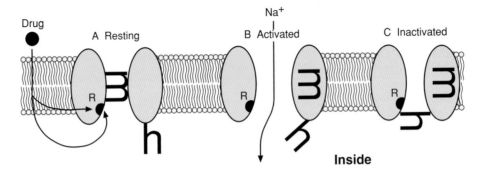

Fig. 34 Effect of local anaesthetic agents on sodium channels. **A.** When resting, the 'm' gate is shut and Na⁺ cannot diffuse. **B.** On activation, the 'm' gate opens and the 'h' gate begins to shut. **C.** When inactivated, the 'h' gate has interrupted the influx of Na⁺ and energy must be expended to return the channel to its resting configuration. Local anaesthetics must access their receptors (R) from within the cell or from within the membrane; they have no direct access from outside the cell. They have greater affinity for activated and inactivated channels than for resting channels.

At the neurone level. Local anaesthetics block the conduction of action potentials along axons (and other excitable membranes such as cardiac muscle; see Ch. 3). Their effects are more marked in rapidly firing neurones than in resting fibres because of the higher affinity of the drug for the receptor in the active state. Furthermore, the effects of local anaesthetics vary between differing neurones: Small diameter fibres (e.g. those carrying pain modalities) with little or no myelination are more susceptible than the larger more extensively myelinated fibres (e.g. motor neurones). See the clinical sketch below.

> **Clinical sketch**
>
> After dental anaesthesia, a patient is apprehensive because he can still feel the dentist's touch.
>
> *Comment: this is expected, and the patient should be reassured. Neurones for light touch are myelinated and hence less susceptible than those carrying pain awareness. The level of anaesthesia is likely to be acceptable.*

Examples and clinical pharmacokinetics

Lidocaine (lignocaine). This is the most commonly used local anaesthetic. The drug achieves local anaesthesia when applied to conjunctiva and mucous membranes. It is most often used as a local injection. Lidocaine is extensively metabolised to inactive derivatives (see also Ch. 3). It can be formulated with adrenaline (epinephrine), which causes local vasoconstriction and slows its absorption (this usually terminates local anaesthetic action). Gangrene can result if this preparation is used to 'ring block' a digit (see the following clinical sketches).

Cocaine. Cocaine is mainly used topically in ear, nose and throat (ENT) surgery. It need not be formulated with adrenaline because it prevents the uptake of cat-

> **Clinical sketch**
>
> A dentist chooses lidocaine plus epinephrine (adrenaline) for anaesthesia during routine work.
>
> *Comment: by causing vasoconstriction, epinephrine slows lidocaine absorption and, therefore, prolongs its activity.*

> **Clinical sketch**
>
> Lidocaine plus epinephrine (adrenaline) is drawn up by an A&E doctor for 'ring block' anaesthesia, to allow him to suture the finger of a young child. Just before injection, he checks the label on the ampoule and discovers his error.
>
> *Comment: the vasoconstriction can cause gangrene. You should always double check the content of a syringe before it is injected.*

echolamines and, therefore, produces vasoconstriction. It is extensively metabolised.

Bupivacaine. This drug, which is more lipophilic than lidocaine, has a longer duration of action than other local anaesthetics.

Adverse effects

- CNS: in the doses used for minor local procedures, serious CNS toxicity is rare; high plasma drug concentrations, resulting from incautious or accidental i.v. use, may result in seizures
- Cardiovascular system: the antiarrhythmic and proarrhythmic effects of local anaesthetics have been described in Chapter 3
- Allergy.

8.3 General anaesthetic agents

Learning objectives

You should:

- understand the clinical use of injected general anaesthetic agents (thiopental and propofol) as induction agents
- appreciate the clinically important aspects of the pharmacokinetics of thiopental and propofol
- be able to describe the clinical use of ketamine
- appreciate the diverse nature of the inhaled general anaesthetic drugs and our poor understanding of their modes of action
- know the role of inhaled agents in the maintenance of anaesthesia and appreciate why they are used less often for induction
- be able to describe the pharmacokinetic principles underpinning the use of anaesthetic gases and their use clinically in combination
- know the main adverse effects of the main inhaled anaesthesic agents.

Injected general anaesthetics

Intravenous anaesthetics act much more rapidly than inhaled agents, producing unconsciousness in about 30 seconds, and are less intimidating for the patient. Hence they are preferred for induction of anaesthesia.

Thiopental

Thiopental is a barbiturate that enhances the effect of the inhibitory transmitter gamma-aminobutyric acid (GABA). It readily crosses the blood–brain barrier, and, at standard doses, surgical anaesthesia is achieved after the lapse of one circulation time. Thiopental diffuses out of the brain rapidly (being distributed to other tissues): this distribution phase has a half-time of about 3 minutes and terminates the anaesthetic effect. The elimination half-life is about 9 hours, but this has little bearing on the clinical effects. Elimination is mainly by hepatic metabolism. Thiopental is used for induction of anaesthesia. It is a potent respiratory depressant, but in the setting of controlled ventilation this is not usually an issue. Thiopental does not increase intracranial pressure.

Propofol

The mode of action of propofol is unknown. Propofol rapidly crosses the blood–brain barrier and, like thiopental, its CNS effects are terminated by distribution (out of the brain) rather than elimination. It may cause pain on injection and may cause tremors. It may also cause a drop in blood pressure because of vasodilatation.

Ketamine

Ketamine is not used as an induction agent. Instead, it tends to be used to induce 'dissociative anaesthesia' in which the eyes remain open and spontaneous respiration is maintained, but pain is not appreciated and the patient is amnesic. This state can be maintained for around 15 minutes after a slow i.v. injection, which is sufficient to allow re-dressing of burns or similar short-duration procedures. Ketamine is not used much in adult medicine because there is a high incidence of unpleasant nightmares during emergence from anaesthesia; this is less of a problem with young children. The drug induces salivation, and the airway must be carefully protected. Heart rate, blood pressure and intracranial pressure are all increased.

Inhaled general anaesthetic agents

Pharmacokinetics

Rapid induction and recovery are important in inhaled anaesthesia allowing flexible control of the depth of anaesthesia. The main factors that determine the speed of these processes are the physical properties of the gas (its solubility in blood and lipid (membranes)) and physiological factors (lung and heart).

To achieve their effects, inhaled anaesthetics must pass from the alveolar air into the blood and thence into the CNS. This needs to happen rapidly but the extent and rate at which these happen depend upon:

- the partial pressure of the agent in the inspired air
- the solubility of the agent in blood: very blood-soluble drugs take longer to achieve high partial pressure in the blood and vice versa
- pulmonary physiology: the arterial tension of highly soluble drugs, such as halothane, is very dependent on ventilation; similarly, pulmonary blood flow changes the arterial tension of very soluble inhaled anaesthetics (e.g. in patients with low cardiac output, the reduced blood volume exposed to the drug steepens the rise in arterial tensions).

Elimination of the agent from the body is mainly by transfer from tissues to blood and from blood to alveolar air. Some hepatic metabolism also occurs (but this varies between drugs).

The rate at which consciousness returns after ceasing drug administration depends mainly on the relative solubility of the drug in the CNS and blood. For example, nitrous oxide, which is relatively insoluble, is 'washed out' rapidly, whereas halothane is more soluble and recovery takes longer.

The *duration* of the anaesthetic procedure is important for very soluble agents since, after long exposure, drug may accumulate in diverse tissues and clear from them slowly.

Mode of action

At the molecular level. The lack of structural similarity in the general anaesthetics has given rise to the concept that no specific receptor is involved in their mode of action. Rather, it is thought that these lipophilic drugs interact with the lipid of the cell membrane and thereby 'distort' membrane ion channels.

At the clinical level. If anaesthesia is *induced* using older inhalational agents, patients pass through four stages:

I. **Analgesia.** The patient has not lost consciousness but pain is reduced. This is exploited in the use of a mixture of nitrous oxide, N_2O, with air to achieve analgesia during the second stage of labour.
II. **Excitement.** The patient appears to be delirious, and there is amnesia thereafter.
III. **Surgical anaesthesia.** There is no blepharospasm upon brushing the eyelashes. Breathing is regular.
IV. **Respiratory depression.** This develops as stage III deepens, and eventually respiration ceases in stage IV. Mechanical ventilation is, of course, needed.

Nowadays anaesthesia is almost always induced with i.v. drugs and the stages are not recognisable. However, they do indicate an important point about the action of inhaled general anaesthetics, which is that different neurones manifest different sensitivity: the dorsal horn cells of the spinal cord are particularly sensitive to inhaled agents, whereas brainstem neurones are fairly resistant.

Examples and clinical pharmacokinetics

Nitrous oxide. This drug, which is a gas at room temperature, has a rapid onset of action and recovery because of its low solubility (see above). It is not metabolised.

Halothane. This is a volatile liquid at room temperature, is more soluble than nitrous oxide and, therefore, has slower onset and recovery rates; it is more potent than nitrous oxide. The drug is mainly eliminated via the lungs. However, the fraction metabolised in the liver may be important to the adverse effect profile—the processes involved are complicated, but involve production of free radicals within the liver.

Isoflurane and enflurane. These drugs are volatile liquids at room temperature; their solubility and potency is somewhere between those of nitrous oxide and halothane. Enflurane undergoes a degree of hepatic metabolism, but that of isoflurane is negligible.

Therapeutic use

Inhaled general anaesthetics are often used in combination to minimise the disadvantages of any one drug (e.g. the relatively low potency of nitrous oxide) while taking full advantage of their 'strengths'.

Adverse effects

- *Cardiovascular.* Halothane, enflurane and isoflurane all reduce the blood pressure, mainly by lowering cardiac output, though isoflurane also reduces systemic vascular resistance. Nitrous oxide has little effect on blood pressure.
- *CNS.* All inhaled general anaesthetics, with the exception of nitrous oxide, reduce tidal volume and depress responses to carbon dioxide. This is not usually a practical problem as ventilation is under careful control during general anaesthesia. More of a problem is the increase in intracranial pressure induced by all these agents (nitrous oxide the least), especially in the setting of head injury.
- *Liver.* Halothane frequently causes asymptomatic elevation of transaminases and may infrequently cause severe hepatitis.
- *Uterus.* Halothane, isoflurane and enflurane relax uterine muscle. This is a problem if vaginal delivery is in progress but can be used therapeutically if uterine contraction needs to be inhibited.
- *Malignant hyperthermia.* This is a rare, but potentially fatal adverse reaction to halothane, resulting from violent muscle fasciculation.

8.4 Relaxation of skeletal muscle and its reversal

Learning objectives

You should:

- appreciate that skeletal muscle relaxants allow adequate muscle relaxation to avoid potentially hazardous levels of general anaesthetic
- appreciate that, under the influence of muscle relaxants, breathing ceases and secure artificial ventilation is immediately essential
- be able to describe the basic physiology of the motor end plate and the modes of action of depolarising and non-depolarising agents
- be able to describe the mode of action of the anticholinesterases and their clinical use to reverse depolarising muscle relaxants
- Describe the use of anticholinesterases in myasthenia gravis
- know how the 'edrophonium test' is used in myasthenia gravis
- be able to list the major adverse effects of the different drug groups.

Skeletal muscle relaxants

The motor end plate

Somatic motor neurones terminate at specialised parts of the cell membrane of striated muscle fibres termed **motor end plates**. When the transmitter acetylcholine is released into the synaptic cleft, it binds to **nicotinic acetylcholine receptors** on the motor end plate. This causes the opening of cation channels in the cell membrane and depolarisation; if sufficient acetylcholine is released, then a wave of depolarisation spreads through the fibre, which goes on to contract.

Acetylcholine is removed from the motor end plate partly by acetylcholinesterase, an enzyme present in the cleft, and partly by diffusion.

Contraction of skeletal muscle can be prevented by *antagonists* of acetylcholine at the nicotinic receptor (**non-depolarising drugs**) and also, paradoxically, by *agonists* at the same receptor (**depolarising drugs**).

Non-depolarising drugs (acetylcholine antagonists)

These non-depolarising agents structurally resemble acetylcholine and are competitive antagonists at nicotinic acetylcholine receptors. All examples are given i.v. after the induction of anaesthesia but usually before endotracheal intubation. The effects of all examples may be reversed by anticholinesterases such as neostigmine.

Examples

Tubocurarine. This is eliminated unchanged via the kidneys and has a long terminal half-life; its gross effects last between 30 and 60 minutes.

Pancuronium. This is mainly excreted unchanged but has a shorter elimination half-life than that of tubocurarine.

Vecuronium and atracurium. These are shorter acting drugs preferred for brief procedures.

Adverse effects

Hypotension: many non-depolarising drugs cause histamine release with consequent vasodilatation; at higher doses they may block autonomic nicotinic receptors.

Contraindications

Non-depolarising drugs have more potent effects in patients with myasthenia gravis (Ch. 20).

Drug interactions

- General anaesthetics cause a degree of muscle relaxation. Therefore, the effects of muscle relaxants are superimposed on existing relaxation.
- Aminoglycosides have nicotinic antagonist properties and may enhance non-depolarising drugs.

Depolarising drugs

Like the non-depolarising drugs, these compounds also resemble acetylcholine structurally. Having bound to the nicotinic receptor, they stimulate it (i.e. they are *agonists*) and sodium channels open; this causes transient muscle contraction. Thereafter, though the end plate remains depolarised, the muscle fibre membrane is refractory, and the muscle becomes flaccid.

Suxamethonium

Suxamethonium (succinylcholine) is the only example of a depolarising drug in common use. It has an extremely short duration of action because it rapidly diffuses away from the end plate and is then metabolised by a plasma enzyme **butyrylcholinesterase** (also called pseudocholinesterase). It is given i.v. and has a half-life of about 5 minutes. Because its duration of action is short, it can be useful for brief procedures; it can be given in repeated doses for longer procedures.

Adverse effects

- Atypical butyrylcholinesterase: about 1 in 2800 patients inherits a butyrylcholinesterase with markedly reduced activity; the drug should be avoided in such patients because of its markedly prolonged duration of action
- Arrhythmias: suxamethonium can produce life-threatening bradyarrhythmias
- Malignant hyperthermia: this is a rare, but potentially fatal, adverse reaction resulting from muscle fasciculation
- Hyperkalaemia: can be a problem, particularly during the anaesthesia of trauma victims.

Anticholinesterases

The anticholinesterases act by inhibiting acetylcholinesterase in the synaptic cleft, thereby prolonging the duration of acetylcholine. They may therefore be used (a) to 'compensate' for autoimmune destruction of acetylcholine receptors (as in myasthenia gravis) or (b) to 'overcome' the presence of an antagonist (such as a non-depolarising muscle relaxant).

Examples

Neostigmine forms a complex with acetylcholinesterase. Its duration of action is mainly determined by the turnover of this drug–enzyme complex, rather than by pharmacokinetic processes. In myasthenia gravis, doses are needed every 2 to 4 hours. Neostigmine does not readily cross the blood–brain barrier.

Pyridostigmine is similar to neostigmine but longer lasting.

Physostigmine crosses the blood–brain barrier well. This gives it utility in anticholinergic poisoning (such as 'deadly nightshade' consumption by children).

Edrophonium (Tensilon) is a very short-acting anti-cholinesterase used in diagnostic tests: i.v. injection rapidly produces short-lived improvement of muscle weakness in myasthenia gravis (which can be a difficult diagnosis in its early stages).

Adverse effects

- *Heart*: the effects of both sympathetic and parasympathetic systems are potentiated, but the parasympathetic predominates and the heart rate and stroke volume fall.
- *Muscular weakness* can occur at high dosage (excessive acetylcholine causing depolarisation).

Self-assessment: questions

Multiple choice questions

1. Anticholinesterases:
   a. Markedly reduce peripheral vascular resistance
   b. Are negatively chronotropic
   c. Can cause muscle weakness in myasthenia gravis
   d. All cross the blood–brain barrier well
   e. Have their effects reversed by edrophonium

2. Local anaesthetic drugs:
   a. Diffuse across the cell membrane in their unionised (uncharged) form
   b. Bind to receptors on the external surface of the cell membrane
   c. Block sodium channels
   d. May be potentiated locally by combination with vasoconstrictor drugs
   e. Cause seizures at high plasma concentration

3. Nitrous oxide:
   a. Is very soluble in blood compared with other inhaled anaesthetics
   b. Is very soluble in brain tissue compared with other inhaled anaesthetics
   c. Works by binding to specific receptors on neurones

   d. Has potent analgesic properties
   e. Depresses respiration

4. Halothane:
   a. Is a liquid at room temperature
   b. Is eliminated from the body mainly by hepatic metabolism
   c. Lowers the cardiac output
   d. Increases the intracranial pressure
   e. Crosses the placenta

5. Suxamethonium:
   a. Is mainly metabolised in the liver
   b. Has a long duration of action
   c. Causes depolarisation of motor end plates
   d. Causes histamine release
   e. Is reversed by neostigmine

Short note questions

Write short notes covering the uses, mode of action and adverse effects of the following in general anaesthesia:

1. Thiopental
2. Nitrous oxide
3. Halothane
4. Pancuronium
5. Neostigmine.

Self-assessment: answers

Multiple choice answers

1. a. **False.** Modest vasodilatation may occur.
   b. **True.** By opposing the breakdown of acetylcholine, these drugs increase the effects of the vagus at the sinoatrial (SA) node.
   c. **True.** Paradoxically, if too much anticholinesterase is used, patients develop weakness.
   d. **False.** Only physostigmine crosses extensively into the brain.
   e. **False.** Edrophonium is a short-acting anticholinesterase used in myasthenia gravis to distinguish weakness caused by excessive anticholinesterase dosage from that caused by the disease.

2. a. **True.** In common with all drugs, the unionised fraction is lipid soluble.
   b. **False.** The receptors are internal.
   c. **True.**
   d. **True.** Cocaine needs no vasoconstrictor, since it stimulates release of catecholamines.
   e. **True.** Especially when used i.v. (e.g. to treat arrhythmias, see Ch. 4).

3. a. **False.** Nitrous oxide is relatively insoluble.
   b. **False.** Because nitrous oxide is relatively insoluble, it has a rapid onset of action and recovery.
   c. **False.** The inhaled anaesthetics are thought to act by induction of changes to neuronal membranes.
   d. **True.**
   e. **True.** In common with all general anaesthetics.

4. a. **True.**
   b. **False.** Although halothane is partly eliminated by hepatic metabolism, this is a minor pathway; most is exhaled.
   c. **True.** It, therefore, lowers blood pressure.
   d. **True.** A particular problem after head injury, where intracranial pressure is already raised.
   e. **True.** May cause apnoea in the neonate.

5. a. **False.** Suxamethonium (succinylcholine) is metabolised by a plasma enzyme.
   b. **False.** It acts for about half an hour in normal subjects.
   c. **True.**
   d. **False.** This is an adverse effect of the non-depolarising drugs.
   e. **False.**

Short note answers

1. Thiopental is an i.v general anaesthetic agent with a very rapid onset of action and a short duration of activity; it is used for the induction of anaesthesia.
   - Thiopental is a barbiturate.
   - Mention its effects on the GABA receptor, its steep dose–response curve and its depressant effect on respiration.
   - Mention that its effects are terminated by distribution rather than elimination.

2. Nitrous oxide is an inhaled anaesthetic, used for the maintenance of general anaesthesia.
   - Describe the solubility of inhaled agents such as nitrous oxide in lipid membrane, and mention the current hypothesis that it is this property which explains their activity.
   - Nitrous oxide has a rapid onset of action (though not enough for its pleasant use as an induction agent) and recovery.
   - It has relatively few adverse effects and is widely used with other anaesthetic gases; however, nitrous oxide is not very potent when used alone.

3. Halothane is a volatile liquid at room temperature
   - Halothane has a slower onset of action and recovery than nitrous oxide but is more potent.
   - It reduces blood pressure.
   - Halothane is metabolised in the liver and can be hepatotoxic if used repeatedly for the same patient.
   - It can cause a rare but potentially fatal syndrome known as malignant hyperthermia.

4. Pancuronium is a muscle relaxant, an essential class of drug for abdominal surgery.
   - Describe the mode of action of non-depolarising agents like pancuronium.
   - Pancuronium is excreted more rapidly than tubocurarine but even so is usually reversed using an anticholinesterase.

5. Neostigmine is used to terminate the effects of pancuronium.
   - Describe the metabolism of acetylcholine by acetylcholinesterase in the cleft between the motor end plate and the motor neurone.
   - Explain that this is not confined to nicotinic receptors on striated muscle but extends to nicotinic receptors of the autonomic nervous system too (parasympathetic effects predominate and the heart rate and stroke volume fall).

Drugs for arthritis

Overview

Arthritis means joint *inflammation* (redness, local heat and loss of function) and not simply joint pain (which is termed arthralgia). The most common causes of non-suppurative arthritis are rheumatoid disease, a result of disordered immune function, osteoarthritis, a result of 'wear and tear', and gout, caused by deposition of uric acid crystals in joints. The treatment of each differs, but the non-steroidal anti-inflammatory drugs (NSAIDs) are used in all three.

9.1 Causes of arthritis

Learning objectives

You should:

- be aware of the causes of joint inflammation

- understand that treatment differs with the underlying mechanism by which inflammation is provoked.

Osteoarthritis is very common, especially in the elderly. It often involves large, weight-bearing joints (vertebral column, hips and knees). It is caused by failure of normal repair of joint cartilage following minor injuries. Fractures that involve an articular surface and damage caused by other joint diseases predispose towards osteoarthritis. In some patients it is a familial trait. Treatment usually involves non-steroidal anti-inflammatory drugs (NSAIDs) and may require local steroid injections; joint replacement may become necessary.

Rheumatoid arthritis is the result of disordered immune function. It is a chronic inflammatory condition principally involving the joints but often also involving lung, heart, eye, blood vessels and spleen. It causes a symmetrical polyarthritis, usually of small peripheral joints (hands, wrists and feet) though any joint may be involved. The disease has a very long course of relapses and remissions and may cause gross deformity. Treatment of rheumatoid arthritis usually involves NSAIDs and may require disease-modifying drugs (*penicillamine* or *gold*), *corticosteroids* (locally as injections, and systemically) and/or other immunosuppressing agents.

Gout results from excess tissue levels of uric acid, which is the end product of purine metabolism. While the cause of hyperuricaemia is usually unidentifiable, it may result from metabolic diseases or occur during treatment of malignancy (where sudden necrosis of the malignant clone during chemotherapy increases purine turnover). Acute attacks of gout typically present as monoarthritis. The first metatarsophalangeal joints are commonly involved, but any joint (apart from the axial skeleton) may be affected.

9.2 Non-steroidal anti-inflammatory drugs (NSAIDs)

Learning objectives

You should:

- know how NSAIDs work and be able to distinguish cyclo-oxygenase II (COX-II) inhibitors from other NSAIDs in terms of adverse effects and cost

- be able to describe the therapeutic uses of NSAIDs both for inflammatory conditions and for pain

- be able to list the main adverse effects, contraindications and drug interactions of NSAIDs.

At the whole animal level, NSAIDs are anti-inflammatory, analgesic and antipyretic (they have no effect on temperature in the absence of fever). At a cellular level, the inflammatory response involves the release of mediator substances that attract further inflammatory cells to the locality and increase vascular permeability. Many of the mediator substances are synthesised from phospholipid in membranes of the endoplasmic reticulum, through the intermediate substance **arachidonic acid** (Fig. 35). NSAIDs inhibit **prostaglandin synthetase (cyclo-oxygenase (COX))**, which has two isoenzymes:

- COX-I has housekeeping functions, including gastric cytoprotection: inhibition can have harmful effects including mucosal damage
- COX-II is a gene product of inflammatory cells: inhibition has anti-inflammatory effects.

Most NSAIDs are non-selective (e.g. aspirin, ibuprofen, naproxen, indometacin), but specific 'COX-II inhibitors' have been developed recently (e.g. rofecoxib).

Examples

Aspirin (acetylsalicylic acid). Aspirin is converted to salicylate, its active metabolite, in the tissues. Salicylate is partly excreted unchanged and is partly conjugated; its half-life is about 4 hours. Aspirin overdose is covered in Chapter 17.

Ibuprofen is extensively metabolised in the liver. Its half-life is about 2 hours.

Naproxen has a longer half-life (about 12 hours) and is excreted as an inactive glucuronide.

Indometacin is partly excreted unchanged and partly as inactive metabolites.

Rofecoxib Antacids reduce extent of absorption to a small degree. Rofecoxib is mainly eliminated by hepatic metabolism.

Therapeutic uses

Anti-inflammatory. Although aspirin and ibuprofen are NSAIDs at high dose, at usual doses their effects are confined to analgesic and antipyretic actions; anti-inflammatory doses of aspirin are often poorly tolerated because of gastrointestinal effects. Naproxen is used as a NSAID in the treatment of rheumatoid arthritis, osteoarthritis, gout and other inflammatory conditions. Indometacin is the most potent NSAID generally available, though it is also prone to common adverse effects. Many other structurally heterogeneous NSAIDs are available. The COX-II inhibitors, such as rofecoxib, can be expected to have fewer serious gastrointestinal adverse effects than non-specific agents. However, they are much more expensive than the older drugs, and not required by every patient.

Antipyretic effects. All NSAIDs are antipyretic, but their use for this indication is limited by their toxicity relative to paracetamol. In children, fever can be complicated by 'febrile convulsions', and thus antipyretics are commonly used. The safest drug in this regard is paracetamol, and not an NSAID.

Clinical sketch

A 50-year-old woman has metastatic breast cancer. Her doctor has prescribed morphine, and to this is added naproxen.

Comment: NSAIDs are very useful additions in pain relief from bony secondaries.

Clinical sketch

A 75-year-old woman with heart failure has painful, swollen knees. She takes ramipril and big doses of furosemide (frusemide) for her heart failure. The doctor gives her indometacin for her knees. She is admitted to hospital with severe pulmonary oedema and renal failure 2 weeks later.

Comment: indometacin is a very potent NSAID. It causes salt and water retention, hence the worsened heart failure. The combination of ACE inhibitor (ramipril), loop diuretic (furosemide) and NSAID may have contributed to the renal failure.

Clinical sketch

A 60-year-old man is taking warfarin for atrial fibrillation; he has not read the 'drug interaction booklet' that the hospital gave him when the warfarin was started. Reading about the benefits of aspirin in heart disease, he starts himself on a regular dose. He is admitted with life-threatening gastrointestinal bleeding.

Comment: NSAIDs can cause gastric erosions. Furthermore, aspirin predisposes to bleeding (see text for the mechanism).

Clinical sketch

A 50-year-old man develops an acutely painful big toe; his foot is red and swollen and he cannot put on his shoe or walk. The doctor diagnoses gout and starts naproxen: the inflammation begins to settle within the next 48 hours.

Comment: gout can be extremely disabling. NSAIDs are the drug of choice for acute attacks, and steroids may also sometimes be needed.

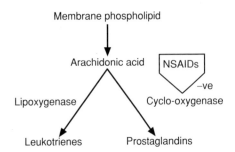

Fig. 35 The site of action of non-steroidal anti-inflammatory drugs (NSAIDs).

Analgesia. See Chapter 7.
Antiplatelet. See Chapter 5.

Adverse effects

- *Gastrointestinal effects:* all NSAIDs can cause dyspepsia and also peptic ulceration and bleeding. Peptic ulceration may be asymptomatic or may manifest as dyspepsia, iron-deficiency anaemia, haematemesis and melaena or ulcer perforation; the COX-II inhibitors are less prone to this adverse effect
- *Sodium and water retention:* a particular problem in heart failure and hypertension
- *Renal impairment:* chronic exposure to large doses of NSAIDs may cause papillary necrosis; acutely, all NSAIDs may reduce the glomerular filtration rate, particularly when combined with certain other drugs (see drug interactions below)
- *Asthma:* attacks may be precipitated by NSAIDs, most commonly aspirin
- *Indometacin:* rarely causes hepatitis and blood dyscrasias.

Contraindications

- Peptic ulcer
- Renal failure
- Haemophilia: aspirin worsens the bleeding diathesis, but ibuprofen and indometacin are usually safe
- Asthma (only in those sensitive to aspirin).

Drug interactions
Aspirin

- Warfarin is potentiated: the interaction is mainly pharmacodynamic—through inhibition of platelet aggregation—and partly pharmacokinetic because of displacement of warfarin from protein binding
- Probenecid and sulfinpyrazone: at low dose, aspirin opposes their uricosuric effects.

All NSAIDs, including aspirin

- Diuretics: NSAIDs cause salt retention and reduce the potency of diuretics. This may result in deterioration in blood pressure or control of heart failure. Less commonly the combination of potent diuretic (e.g. furosemide) and a NSAID may precipitate or worsen renal impairment
- Lithium: clearance of lithium is reduced
- Aminoglycosides, semisynthetic penicillins and cephalosporins. Acute renal failure may occasionally be precipitated (especially when multiple 'nephrotoxic drugs' are combined).

9.3 Disease-modifying antirheumatic drugs

> ### Learning objectives
>
> You should:
>
> - understand the role of 'disease-modifying drugs' in the management of rheumatoid disease
> - be aware that the decision to start such drugs is usually made with specialist advice
> - be able to list the main adverse effects of the commonly used drugs.

> ### Clinical sketch
>
> A 30-year-old woman presented to her GP a year ago with severe arthritis: this required a hospital admission. She was started on regular NSAID. However, her rheumatologist is unhappy with her progress: in particular radiographs show inexorable worsening of joint erosions. Oral penicillamine is started. After several months her clinical progress is improved, but she has many adverse effects from the drug.
>
> *Comment: penicillamine takes months for its therapeutic benefit to become evident, and adverse effects are common (and often serious).*

Although NSAIDs are the mainstay of treatment in rheumatoid arthritis, they do not alter the natural history of this crippling disease. The disease-modifying antirheumatoid drugs (DMARDs) improve symptoms (as do NSAIDs) but also slow disease progression. They include gold, penicillamine, sulfasalazine, some antimalarial drugs and immunosuppressive agents. Their effects take months to become apparent, and their use (which should be supervised by rheumatologists) is often limited by toxicity. Although formerly used as 'reserve' drugs, they are often now used early in the course of the disease.

Gold (sodium aurothiomalate)

The mode of action is unknown, though gold concentrates in synovial membranes and seems to inhibit lysosomal enzymes. Sodium aurothiomalate is given as i.m. injections; an oral dosage form is available but is incompletely absorbed. Gold is reserved for patients with active and progressive disease. About one third of patients develop adverse reactions.

Adverse reactions

- Skin reactions: dermatitis, and mucosal lesions
- Nephritis: proteinuria is common
- Blood dyscrasias.

Contraindications

- Hypersensitivity
- Pregnancy
- Pre-existing blood dyscrasias.

Penicillamine

The mode of action of penicillamine is unknown. It induces changes in white cells and alters immune function. Little is known about the drug's disposition because of difficulties in assay. The drug is given orally for prolonged periods. Severe adverse effects occur in about 40% of patients.

Adverse effects

- Nephropathy: proteinuria is common, and some patients develop immune-complex nephritis
- Blood dyscrasias
- Skin reactions: this common adverse effect may respond to dose reduction
- Loss of taste
- Autoimmune diseases: a variety of conditions including autoimmune haemolytic anaemia and thyroiditis may be seen.

Sulfasalazine

Sulfasalazine is mainly unabsorbed until it reaches the colon: microorganisms then split the molecule to produce 5-aminosalicylic acid (5-ASA) and sulfapyridine, both of which are absorbed. In rheumatoid arthritis, it is the sulfonamide component, not the 5-ASA, that has disease-modifying activity (see also Ch. 11). Adverse effects are common (see Ch. 11) and include severe skin reactions and blood dyscrasias.

Antimalarial drugs

Chloroquine and hydroxychloroquine have 'disease-modifying activity'. Both can cause retinopathy when given for many years.

Other drugs

Glucocorticoids. This group of drugs (see Ch. 12) is used for its anti-inflammatory properties in many diseases, including rheumatoid arthritis and gout (see below).

Methotrexate. This anticancer drug (Ch. 15) can be used as an immunosuppressant in diseases such as rheumatoid arthritis.

Azathioprine. This is a derivative of the anticancer drug 6-mercaptopurine. Azathioprine is used in severe rheumatoid arthritis and other inflammatory diseases (such as systemic lupus erythematosus). The chief toxicity, which is dose dependent, is bone marrow suppression.

Ciclosporin. This drug is the mainstay of treatment to prevent graft rejection. Its use in rheumatoid disease is restricted to severe and unresponsive disease. Its adverse effects include hair growth, liver dysfunction and nephrotoxicity. In common with all drugs that suppress immunity over long periods of time, ciclosporin increases the risk of malignancy (particularly lymphoma). Ciclosporin has little bone marrow suppressing effect.

Infliximab. This is a monoclonal antibody against tumour necrosis factor. It is used in both rheumatoid disease and Crohn's disease.

9.4 Drugs used in gout

Learning objectives

You should:

- know the therapeutic options in the management of acute gout
- be aware that allopurinol and uricosuric drugs may make acute gout worse, and know their therapeutic use
- be able to list the main adverse effects of colchicine, allopurinol and uricosuric drugs.

Clinical sketch

A 50-year-old man develops agonising inflammation of his first metatarsophalangeal joints on both feet. He is unable to walk and has a low-grade fever. The joints are red, exquisitely tender and the surface skin shows signs of desquamation. His plasma urate level is extremely high. His doctor starts the NSAID naproxen and gives a short course of prednisolone.

Comment: this treatment will probably improve the symptoms within a week, at which point the steroid would be stopped. Drugs like allopurinol or uricosuric agents are contraindicated at this stage: they will precipitate a further attack. Such prophylactic drugs should be delayed for several weeks and then started under 'cover' from an NSAID.

Clinical sketch

A 60-year-old man, who still suffers acute attacks of gout periodically, has tissue deposits of urate crystals (*tophi*). His doctor gives him sulfinpyrazone to lower his plasma urate levels. During an episode of severe viral gastroenteritis, when he is very dehydrated, he develops agonising loin pain, which radiates to his left testicle.

Comment: this is likely to be a ureteric uric acid stone. By raising the urine concentration of urate, drugs like sulfinpyrazone can cause stone formation, especially during dehydration.

Clinical sketch

A 12-year-old boy has acute leukaemia. His doctors start allopurinol before the first dose of chemotherapy.

Comment: the destruction of the malignant clone will release a great deal of purine, which will be metabolised into urate in the absence of allopurinol. This urinary urate load may threaten renal function.

Allopurinol

Allopurinol inhibits the enzyme xanthine oxidase (Fig. 36), thereby interrupting purine metabolism at hypoxanthine—a much more soluble compound than uric acid. Hypoxanthine does not cause arthritis and is readily excreted. Allopurinol is given orally but is incompletely absorbed. It is used for the prophylaxis of gout; it is also used during the chemotherapy of haematological malignancy (e.g. leukaemia) to prevent renal dysfunction from the massive uric acid excretion that results from the death of the malignant clone.

Adverse effects

- Gout may be precipitated or exacerbated because of the early rise in uric acid concentration and the drug should not be used until about 3 weeks after an acute attack; many physicians start allopurinol under 'cover' from a NSAID to minimise the chances of a new acute attack

- Gastrointestinal effects are common
- Allergic rashes.

Drug interactions

- 6-Mercaptopurine and azathioprine are both potentiated. They are structurally similar to allopurinol and are metabolised by xanthine oxidase
- Warfarin is potentiated.

Uricosuric agents

Uric acid is filtered by the glomerulus but, in common with other relatively strong acids and bases, it is subject to both reabsorption and secretion in the proximal tubule (Fig. 37). Uricosuric drugs inhibit reabsorption, increasing uric acid clearance. Examples include **probenecid** and **sulfinpyrazone**, which are used for the prophylaxis of acute gout and the treatment of patients with large accumulations of uric acid in their tissues ('chronic tophaceous gout'). Urinary levels of this relatively insoluble acid are increased, and precipitation may occur—especially when urine volumes are small and at low pH.

Adverse effects

- Exacerbation of acute attacks: when first given, uricosurics inhibit urate secretion rather than its reabsorption; this increases urate levels and may worsen gout and, consequently, uricosuric drugs are generally started about 3 weeks after an acute attack, and many physicians routinely start treatment under the 'cover' of a NSAID or colchicine
- Gastrointestinal upset
- Uric acid stones can form in the urinary tract
- Allergic rashes.

Contraindications

- Previous urinary tract stones
- Impaired renal function
- Recent acute gout.

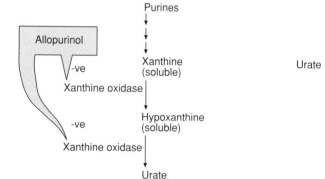

Fig. 36 The mode of action of allopurinol.

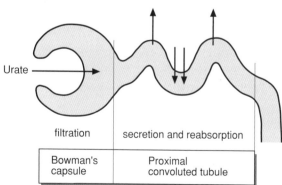

Fig. 37 Excretion of uric acid.

Self-assessment: questions

Multiple choice questions

1. Aspirin:
   a. Should be avoided in patients taking warfarin
   b. Commonly causes gastrointestinal bleeding
   c. Is the drug of first choice for rheumatoid arthritis
   d. Should be avoided in asthmatics
   e. Is excreted unchanged

2. Indometacin:
   a. May be used to treat headache
   b. Causes few gastrointestinal adverse effects
   c. Is less likely than aspirin to interact adversely with warfarin
   d. Reduces the clearance of lithium
   e. Is relatively contraindicated in heart failure

3. Penicillamine
   a. Is indicated for gout
   b. Is the first choice drug for rheumatoid arthritis
   c. Should not be combined with NSAIDs
   d. Can only be given by injection
   e. Is usually well tolerated

Case history questions

Case history 1

An 84-year-old woman takes a NSAID for osteoarthritis; she is also taking furosemide (frusemide) and captopril for heart failure. Following a fall, she breaks her hip and receives emergency surgery, where a prosthetic joint is implanted. The surgeons start her on ceftazidime as prophylaxis against infection. Post-operatively her renal function declines alarmingly.

1. What may account for her renal failure, and what should be done?

Case history 2

A 40-year-old man with mild hypertension presents with arthritis, which is diagnosed as acute gout. He takes bendroflumethiazide for his blood pressure.

1. Which of the following treatments would it be correct to start:
   a. Indometacin and allopurinol
   b. Indometacin and probenecid
   c. Indometacin alone, and allopurinol in due course
   d. Aspirin alone
   e. Allopurinol alone

The man gets better from the acute attack and remains on the thiazide for his hypertension, and allopurinol for gout prophylaxis. Over the next year he has six further bad attacks of gout.

2. In what way would you alter his drugs?

Short note questions

Write short notes on:

1. Drug treatment of acute and chronic gout.
2. Drug treatment of severe, progressive rheumatoid disease.

Self-assessment: answers

Multiple choice answers

1. a. **True**. Aspirin increases the bleeding time by its effects on platelet function; furthermore, by causing gastrointestinal bleeding diatheses, all NSAIDs may induce life-threatening bleeds in patients with prolonged prothrombin times.
   b. **True**.
   c. **False**. Aspirin needs to be given at high dose to induce an anti-inflammatory effect. Many patients cannot tolerate these high doses.
   d. **True**. Aspirin may precipitate asthma in some patients; this is thought to occur through its inhibition of prostaglandin synthetase.
   e. **False**. Aspirin (acetylsalicylic acid) is hydrolysed to salicylate (phase I metabolism) and thereafter conjugates (phase II).

2. a. **False**. Indometacin is a potent NSAID that is not used as a simple analgesic but for its anti-inflammatory properties; indometacin may cause headache.
   b. **False**. It is very prone to cause gastrointestinal effects.
   c. **True**. Although warfarin is displaced from plasma protein binding, this is not clinically important; indometacin has less potent antiplatelet effects and interacts little with warfarin.
   d. **True**. See Chapter 6.
   e. **True**. Indometacin may cause pronounced salt and water retention.

3. a. **False**. Penicillamine is not used for gout.
   b. **False**. NSAIDs are usually for first-choice agents. Penicillamine is used for aggressive disease (often for extra-articular manifestations, such as vasculitis). It is started and monitored by specialists.
   c. **False**. Penicillamine is often used with NSAIDs.
   d. **False**. It is given orally.
   e. **False**. It frequently causes adverse events.

Case history answers

Case history 1

It is possible that her blood pressure may have fallen as a result of the fracture or the anaesthetic causing acute tubular necrosis, but her drugs are probably responsible. NSAIDs, furosemide, captopril and ceftazidime are all nephrotoxic, and their effects are additive. The necessity for antibiotic prophylaxis needs to be reconsidered, the captopril should probably be stopped and the NSAID should certainly be stopped. The patient's state of hydration and the risk of withdrawal of furosemide (acute pulmonary oedema) need to be carefully considered. Specialist advice would certainly be required.

Case history 2

1. It would only be correct to start (c): indometacin alone with allopurinol in due course. Most physicians would start a NSAID alone for immediate therapy: this should begin to control symptoms within 2 days, but failure to improve may necessitate addition of glucocorticoid. Aspirin would not be a good choice because it causes retention of urate when first started. Any NSAID may worsen control of hypertension, but this can be compensated for by increasing antihypertensive dosage. When symptoms have resolved, a prophylactic drug may be started (under NSAID cover to begin with). Starting either allopurinol or a uricosuric alone immediately would worsen the gout.
2. Thiazide diuretics elevate plasma urate and should be changed to an alternative drug.

Short note answers

1. The urgent priority in *acute gout* is relief of symptoms using an anti-inflammatory drug:

   - the usual choices are indometacin, naproxen or ibuprofen, although any NSAID may be used
   - in the presence of peptic ulcer disease, or recent upper gastrointestinal haemorrhage, treatment becomes more difficult; colchicine may be used but generally causes severe diarrhoea
   - patients with severe gout may require systemic steroids as well as NSAID treatment.

   The NSAID should be continued until the arthritis has subsided; most physicians would continue to give a NSAID during the introduction of allopurinol or uricosuric therapy.

   The treatment of *chronic gout* aims to reduce the risk of further acute arthritis, to preserve renal function and to avoid formation of gouty tophi. Patients who have had more than one clinical attack of gout should probably be offered treatment with either:

- uricosuric drugs (probenecid or sulfinpyrazone) which increase the renal clearance of uric acid; they are contraindicated in patients with renal failure because there is the risk of uric acid stone formation, which may further worsen renal function, and the uricosurics work less well in the presence of renal impairment
- allopurinol (more commonly used) which inhibits the enzyme xanthine oxidase and reduces the formation of uric acid; it is preferable in patients with renal failure (although doses should be reduced, as the risk of adverse effects increases in renal failure).

A summary of the main adverse effects of NSAIDs, colchicine, uricosurics and allopurinol should be given.

2. The usefulness and limitations of NSAIDs should be covered:
   - NSAIDs reduce inflammation and help symptoms but do not change the rate of disease progression
   - the principal adverse effects of NSAIDs should be discussed: gastrointestinal bleeding, gastrointestinal ulceration, dyspepsia, antiplatelet effects, salt retention and exacerbation of heart failure, exacerbation of renal impairment.

The use of gold, penicillamine and sulfasalazine should be covered:

- indications
- route of administration
- course of therapy
- adverse effects.

10 Respiratory disorders and hypersensitivity

Overview

This chapter covers the use of drugs and oxygen in the treatment of asthma, chronic obstructive bronchitis and respiratory failure. Asthma is caused by inflammation of the small bronchi. Most attacks are mild. Acute severe attacks of asthma are potentially life threatening. Drugs are used in both acute asthma and to control chronic asthma. Chronic obstructive pulmonary disease results from damage to respiratory cilia and requires antibiotics for acute attacks as well as drugs to dilate airways as in asthma. Respiratory failure can complicate a number of conditions and requires oxygen therapy, drugs or mechanical ventilation, depending on the circumstances. Because the immune system plays a role in asthma, it is convenient to cover hypersensitivity in the same chapter.

Learning objectives

You should:

- be able to describe the basic pathophysiology of asthma and chronic obstructive pulmonary disease

- understand what is meant by 'acute severe asthma', and appreciate the severity of this condition

- be able to outline a management plan for a patient with acute severe asthma and discuss the indications for mechanical ventilation in this condition

- be able to outline a management plan for a patient with stable asthma, both to prevent attacks and treat acute episodes

- List the main classes of drug used for asthma and chronic obstructive pulmonary disease, their main adverse effects and the interactions of these drugs.

10.1 Drugs for asthma and chronic obstructive bronchitis

Asthma is caused by inflammation of small bronchi—usually resulting from type I hypersensitivity—resulting in recurrent, reversible episodes of airways obstruction. This causes three main features: dyspnoea, wheeze and cough. The antigen (commonly the excreta of the house dust mite or a pollen) is usually inhaled. However, asthmatics also have attacks in response to non-allergic stimuli including exercise, emotion and viral respiratory infection; in many cases (often where symptoms have come on in later life), no allergy can be demonstrated. Obstruction results from (a) mucous membrane oedema secondary to inflammation; (b) contraction of bronchial smooth muscle, under the influence of the autonomic nervous system and inflammatory mediators; and (c) thick mucus plugs, which may obstruct the lumen altogether in the most severe cases (Fig. 38). The principal clinical features are paroxysmal cough, wheeze and shortness of breath. Most attacks are mild, but asthma

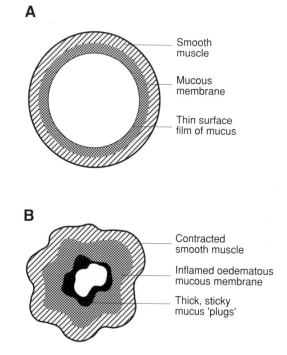

Fig. 38 Airways obstruction in asthma. **A.** Normal airway. **B.** Airway during an asthmatic attack.

still kills around 2000 people in the UK annually, despite available drugs.

Chronic obstructive pulmonary disease (COPD) is a very common complication of cigarette smoking and results from damage to respiratory cilia, which causes chronic colonisation of the lower airways by *Haemophilus influenzae* and *Streptococcus pneumoniae*. It includes emphysema and chronic bronchitis: most patients have elements of both. Chronic bronchitis is clinically defined as 'a cough productive of sputum for more than 3 months in 2 consecutive years' but, in addition, there is usually associated small airways obstruction, and so patients are often wheezy and breathless. The airway obstruction in COPD is often fixed rather than reversible, and inflammation is not such a prominent feature. The drugs used to treat COPD are the same as those used for asthma, but patients with COPD usually require antibiotics for exacerbations.

Acute severe asthma and its management

An attack of asthma in an adult should be considered *severe* if any of the following are present:

- the patient is unable to complete sentences in one breath
- respiratory rate is greater than 25 breaths/min

Clinical sketch

A 60-year-old cigarette smoker developed 'asthma' aged around 40. He is now on regular doses of inhaled salbutamol (he has a nebuliser at home) and cannot drop his dose of oral prednisolone below 7.5 mg daily (the doctor has tried him on inhaled high-dose beclometasone, but systemic steroids have always been found essential to avoid hospital admissions). He develops severe back pain suddenly. Radiographs confirm a collapsed thoracic vertebra and osteopenia.

Comment: Some patients do need long-term systemic steroids. As always the risks of such treatment need to be weighed against the benefits. Osteoporosis is a common hazard, which might be reduced by specific therapies.

Clinical sketch

A 70-year-old man has closed angle glaucoma. His ophthalmologist advises beta-blocker eye-drops. Unknown to the ophthalmologist, the patient has long-standing chronic obstructive pulmonary disease. Shortly after the start of the eye-drops, the gentleman requires an admission to intensive care for a life-threatening attack of airway obstruction.

Comment: although beta-blocker eye-drops are used topically, they are eventually swallowed and absorbed.

Clinical sketch

A 50-year-old smoker is admitted during the winter following a 'headcold'. She now has severe breathlessness, wheeze and a cough productive of copious green sputum. She is treated with β_2-agonist, systemic steroids and broad-spectrum antibiotics.

Comment: this is one of the commonest syndromes to be found in adult wards. Short courses of systemic steroids have been found beneficial in clinical trial. Antibiotics are tailored against Gram-positive organisms such as Haemophilus influenzae *and* Pneumococcus *sp.*

- heart rate is greater than 110 beats/min
- peak expiratory flow rate (PEFR) is less than 50% of the predicted value.

An attack should be considered to be *life threatening* if any of the following features develop:

- PEFR is less than 33% of predicted value
- the chest is silent on auscultation
- cyanosis
- feeble respiratory effort
- bradycardia
- hypotension
- exhaustion, confusion or coma.

Management

1. The patient must be admitted to hospital, and given a high concentration of oxygen
2. High doses of inhaled nebulised β_2-agonist should be given
3. High doses of systemic steroid should start at once (since onset will be delayed)
4. Clinical monitoring (including charting of PEFR, and repetition of arterial gases) should be intensive
5. If there is failure to improve (or deterioration) over

Clinical sketch

A 20-year-old woman is admitted with severe asthma and mild left-sided 'sharp' chest pain. She is hypoxic. Initial treatment is with inhaled 40% oxygen regular nebulised salbutamol and regular i.v. hydrocortisone. She fails to improve and becomes exhausted. The doctor is asked to give a night sedative 'to settle her down': this is declined. Auscultation reveals reduced breath sounds on the left and a chest radiograph shows a pneumothorax. She is moved to the intensive care unit; a chest drain is inserted and she is ventilated.

Comment: this sort of case is not unusual. You should remember that (a) not all asthmatics respond satisfactorily to first-line treatment, (b) pneumothorax must always be excluded and (c) sedative drugs are contraindicated.

the next few hours then nebulised *ipratropium* and/or i.v. *aminophylline* may be started

6. If there is further deterioration then mechanical ventilation should be considered.

At all times, sedative drugs are contraindicated, and respiratory stimulants are not usually helpful.

It is important to be aware that further deterioration can occur despite initial good response to treatment.

Severe asthma is a medical emergency, and patients need careful observation even though they seem to respond rapidly.

Chronic asthma and its management

Many patients with chronic asthma can be managed with occasional use of a bronchodilator such as a β₂-agonist. If this is required more than once daily, regular inhaled anti-inflammatory drugs are needed:

- in adults, inhaled steroids are most commonly used
- in children, *sodium cromoglicate* may be preferred (mainly because of the possible adverse effects of regular steroid exposure); its effectiveness is uncertain
- some patients need high doses of inhaled steroids and regular use of bronchodilators
- a very small minority of patients need regular oral steroid.

The roles of leukotriene receptor antagonists and other newer drugs are yet to be established. At the moment they are most commonly added to the treatment of patients with 'unstable' asthma, and those with relatively 'resistant' disease.

Patients need to understand:

- which of their drugs are indicated for acute attacks
- which of their drugs are indicated mainly for prevention of attacks
- how to take their drugs (particularly in the case of complicated inhaler devices)
- when to seek urgent medical help.

Increasingly, GPs hold 'asthma clinics' and 'nurse practitioners' specializing in asthma provide a link between hospital and community care.

Box 5 describes the topical use of drugs in asthma.

Anti-inflammatory drugs

Glucocorticoids

The preferred route of administration for glucocorticoids is by inhalation: high local concentrations of steroid can then be achieved with small doses, which minimises adverse effects. *Beclometasone* and *budesonide* are formulated for inhalation via several different devices. The mode of action, pharmacokinetics and adverse effects of steroids are dealt with in Chapter 21.

Box 5 Topical use of drugs in asthma

In acute severe asthma, which is a medical emergency, drugs are often used systemically: steroids may be given by injection or by mouth and beta-agonists may be given by i.v. infusion.

For the maintenance of patients with asthma, it is logical to use drugs topically when possible:

- if the drug is delivered directly to its site of action, high concentrations can be rapidly achieved
- total doses can be kept low, thereby reducing adverse effects; this is particularly important with the use of topical steroids

Drugs can be delivered topically in three main ways (although there is a wide range of commercially available delivery systems).

1. Nebulisation of drug solution: this is usually done in hospital (using a stream of oxygen or air) but can be achieved at home using electric pumps.

2. Hand-held metred-dose inhalers, using pressurised canisters: essentially the same technology as furniture polish!

3. Hand-held dry-powder devices: these usually rely on puncturing a plastic 'capsule', which contains the drug, and then dispersal of the drug by a 'turbine', which is powered by the patient's inspiration through the mouthpiece.

Inhaled glucocorticoids are useful for the *prevention* of attacks by the reduction of bronchial inflammation. Inhaled steroids are not indicated for acute attacks, but systemic steroids (particularly hydrocortisone) are life-saving drugs under such circumstances.

Sodium cromoglicate

Cromoglicate appears to inhibit the influx of Ca^{2+} that occurs in mast cell membrane after a specific antigen has reacted with surface IgE. The influx of Ca^{2+} seems to be necessary for degranulation and formation of leukotrienes and prostaglandins. Because cromoglicate is so insoluble in water it is not absorbed when given orally. Instead, the drug is formulated as an aerosol for inhalation to prevent asthma attacks. It is *useless* in the treatment of an attack. Cromoglicate reduces bronchial response to inhaled antigens and to non-specific triggers such as exercise; it is of most use in atopic asthmatics, though non-topic patients may also benefit. Used regularly, it seems to reduce inflammation and may abolish bronchial hyperreactivity. Different formulations of the drug are also used for seasonal rhinitis (hay fever). Cromoglicate is useless in COPD. Adverse effects are confined to laryngeal irritation.

Leukotriene pathway inhibitors

The leukotrienes (see below under type I hypersensitivity) are inflammatory mediators and potent bronchoconstrictors. Inhibitors of 5-lipoxygenase (such as *zileuton*) and leukotriene receptor antagonists (such as *montelukast*) both interfere with this 'leukotriene pathway', although by different mechanisms. Both may be taken orally. However, these groups of drug are relatively new, and their role in asthma therapy remains to be clarified.

Bronchodilators

Beta-agonists

Selective β_2-adrenoceptor agonists are used as bronchodilators in asthma. (See Ch. 2 for details of adrenoceptor classification and function.)

Salbutamol is well absorbed when given orally but is subjected to extensive first-pass metabolism. More usually, the drug is given as an inhaled powder or aerosol either for treatment of acute attacks or for maintenance. If salbutamol is given as a nebulised solution (driven either by pressurized oxygen or by electronic pump) then high concentrations are achieved in the lungs. Salbutamol may be given i.v. in an emergency.

Terbutaline is also given topically as a metered-dose inhaler or as nebulised solution. It has a longer duration of action than salbutamol.

Salmeterol is a longer-acting derivative of salbutamol. It is used for maintenance treatment by inhalation only, in patients not adequately controlled by inhaled steroids.

Therapeutic use

- Acute severe asthma: nebulised β_2-agonists, usually salbutamol, give rapid symptomatic improvement
- Maintenance of symptomatic asthma: most asthmatics take inhaled β_2-agonists as required for symptomatic relief; some patients need regular doses. Salmeterol can be useful for patients with bad asthma who need regular treatment with a β_2-agonist
- COPD: bronchodilators are used both in acute exacerbations of COPD and as maintenance treatment.

Adverse effects

- Tachycardia: sinus tachycardia is a common adverse effect but does not usually necessitate a change in therapy; a reduction in dose is sometimes required
- Fine tremor is a frequent finding but is rarely severe enough to warrant changing therapy

- Change in arterial oxygen: a transient fall can occur in acute–severe asthma treated with any bronchodilator.

Anticholinergics

Stimulation of the bronchi by the parasympathetic fibres of the vagus nerves causes bronchoconstriction and secretion of mucus. Muscarinic antagonists, such as *ipratropium*, oppose these effects. Ipratropium is used topically by inhalation or by nebuliser; very little is absorbed systemically. Because little of the drug is absorbed, systemic effects are few. Local absorption in the mouth may result in diminished salivary flow. Rarely, ipratropium may exacerbate glaucoma.

Aminophylline

Aminophylline is a soluble derivative of theophylline that is widely used. The mode of action is unknown (aminophylline blocks the metabolism of cyclic AMP, but it is doubtful whether this is the basis of the therapeutic benefit). Aminophylline may be given orally, rectally or i.v. Oral absorption is good, and the drug is not subject to first-pass metabolism. Aminophylline is mainly cleared by hepatic metabolism (to inactive derivatives); the elimination half-life is short but sustained-release formulations allow less frequent dosing (once or twice daily). The drug has a narrow therapeutic range (5–20 mg/l) and therapeutic drug monitoring is recommended, given the drug's adverse effects at high concentration.

Therapeutic uses

- Acute severe asthma. Aminophylline is *not* a first-choice agent but may usefully be combined with β_2-agonists. Aminophylline is usually given as a *slow* i.v. loading dose (given over about 10 minutes) followed by constant-rate infusion until improvement is seen. *Caution* is needed if the patient takes oral theophylline preparations, as toxicity is more likely.
- Control of asthma and COPD. Regular doses of oral theophylline may be needed in addition to other bronchodilators.

Adverse effects

- Seizures occur at high aminophylline concentrations and are most common when the drug is given rapidly i.v.
- Tachyarrhythmias may be life-threatening; like seizures, they are concentration related and common if the drug is given rapidly i.v.
- Tremor
- Nausea
- Insomnia.

Drug interactions

Because theophylline is mainly cleared by biotransformation, its effects are enhanced by enzyme inhibitors and opposed by enzyme inducers (see Ch. 21).

10.2 Respiratory failure: oxygen therapy and respiratory stimulants

Learning objectives

You should:

- know the classification of respiratory failure into types I and II
- be able to contrast the use of oxygen in types I and II failure
- be able to describe the roles of respiratory stimulants and mechanical ventilation.

Respiratory failure is defined as an arterial partial pressure of oxygen (Po_2) less than 8.0 kPa (when breathing atmospheric air at sea level). It may complicate asthma, COPD, pneumonia, pulmonary embolism and pulmonary fibrosis. 'Controlled oxygen therapy', respiratory stimulant drugs and mechanical ventilation may be needed, depending on circumstances.

Clinical sketch

A young woman on oral contraceptive steroids suddenly collapses with vague chest pain and severe dyspnoea. She is centrally cyanosed, has a pulse rate of 140 beats/min, a blood pressure of 60/20 mmHg, and marked jugular venous engorgement. Her arterial gases are Po_2 6.0 kPa, Pco_2 1.2 kPa and pH 7.52. The chest radiograph is normal, but spiral computed tomographic scans show massive pulmonary emboli in both main pulmonary arteries.

Comment: this patient probably needs urgent surgery. The inspired oxygen concentration should be as high as is needed to normalise the arterial partial pressure. Oxygen masks deliver up to 80%, depending on flow rate, while nasal cannulae will deliver up to 35%. In some cases even 80% oxygen will often be inadequate, in which case positive-pressure ventilation may be needed.

Clinical sketch

A 70-year-old cigarette smoker with severe COPD is admitted with an infective exacerbation. Her arterial gases are Po_2 5.0 kPa, Pco_2 9.2 kPa and pH 7.10. She is started on 35% oxygen, on which her gases are: Po_2 6.5 kPa, Pco_2 10.2 kPa and pH 6.98. She is changed to 28% oxygen and an infusion of doxapram is started. Her

gases improve to Po_2 6.0 kPa, Pco_2 8.8 kPa and pH 7.22.

Comment: In chronic type II failure, high inspired oxygen concentrations may worsen carbon dioxide retention, cause acidosis and may lead to death. In this circumstance, 24–28% inspired oxygen is usually recommended; if the patient remains unacceptably hypoxaemic, then respiratory stimulants may be considered.

Clinical sketch

A 20-year-old man is admitted after an overdose of several sedative drugs including opiates and barbiturates. He is deeply comatose, and naloxone fails to change this. His gases are Po_2 5.2 kPa, Pco_2 8.7 kPa and pH 7.00.

Comment: naloxone antagonizes the opiate but not the barbiturate. This man needs ventilation.

Clinical sketch

A 55-year-old smoker has chronic type II respiratory failure. He is provided with an oxygen concentrator at home.

Comment: the mortality rate for chronically hypoxaemic patients is lowered by long-term oxygen, which should be breathed for more than 15 hours of each day. Such 'domicillary oxygen' can be delivered as cylinders, or by using more cost-effective oxygen concentrators. There are strict criteria that determine when this should be started.

Classification of respiratory failure

Type I

Type I respiratory failure is caused by ventilation–perfusion mismatching; Po_2 is low and Pco_2 is normal or low. Common causes include:

- pulmonary embolism
- pneumonia
- asthma
- adult respiratory distress syndrome (ARDS).

Management involves:
- inhaled oxygen concentrations high enough to normalize arterial gases
- Mechanical ventilation if arterial oxygen cannot be maintained otherwise
- Treatment of the underlying cause.

Respiratory stimulants have no role (the patient is already hyperventilating).

Type II

Type II respiratory failure is caused by hypoventilation and the Pco_2 is high. Common causes include:

- sedative drug overdose (acute and self-limiting if supportive therapy is adequate)
- COPD (chronic).

It is crucially important to remember that, whereas normal respiration is mainly driven by changes in pH, in patients with chronic type II failure, respiration is driven by hypoxia. Too great a correction of hypoxia can be life threatening.

Management involves:

- carefully monitoring of inhaled oxygen concentrations
- respiratory stimulants may be useful
- mechanical ventilation is indicated for acute cases (such as drug overdose).

Doxapram

Doxapram is the only respiratory stimulant in regular use in type II respiratory failure. It produces a concentration-related increase in neuronal activity in the respiratory centre; this causes tidal volume to rise, PO_2 to rise and PCO_2 to fall. It is given by i.v. infusion. The benefit achieved by doxapram is short lived and the drug should be regarded as 'buying time' to allow more fundamental problems, such as infection, to be addressed. At high doses, doxapram may induce seizures.

10.3 Hypersensitivity

Learning objectives

You should:

- be able to describe briefly the mechanisms of the four types of hypersensitivity
- be able to describe the clinical syndromes of anaphylaxis and angioedema, and outline the emergency management of these syndromes
- appreciate that 'type B' adverse drug reactions are often caused by hypersensitivity.

The immune system, there for our protection against microorganisms, can cause disease when inappropriate responses lead to tissue damage: **hypersensitivity**. Hypersensitivity responses can be 'triggered' by drugs, causing such diverse clinical syndromes as asthma, anaphylaxis, vasculitis, glomerulonephritis and arthritis. Hypersensitivity can be classified into four groups, I–IV, based on the immune response.

Type I (immediate)

Drugs are often too small to function as antigens, but they may be capable of binding to protein forming an antigenic complex: the drug is then termed a **hapten**. Exposure stimulates production of antigen-specific IgE antibodies by plasma cells and these become attached to the membrane of mast cells and basophils (Fig. 39). Repeat exposure results in recognition of the antigenic drug–protein complex by IgE, and the release by the mast cells and basophils of preformed mediator substances (histamine, kinins and 5-HT) and the rapid synthesis of others (leukotrienes and prostaglandins). The net effects of the mediators are mucosal inflammation, increased capillary leakiness, secretion of mucus and contraction of smooth muscle. Drugs commonly pro-

---

Clinical sketch

A 40-year-old woman has had penicillin in the past without incident. During a hospital admission she is given high-dose benzylpenicillin i.v. for cellulitis of the leg. While the infusion is running, she becomes breathless and wheezy: the nurses stop the infusion and summon the doctor. Five minutes later, when the doctor arrives, she is cold and clammy and stridor is audible from the end of the bed. Her blood pressure is unrecordable. She is given epinephrine (adrenaline) i.m; i.v access is obtained and chlorphenamine, hydrocortisone and fluids are given i.v. The foot of her bed is raised.

Comment: this woman has developed anaphylaxis and angioedema in response to benzylpenicillin. The life-saving actions were immediate interruption of the suspect drug and i.m. epinephrine. Raising the foot of the bed may increase venous return, and hence increase cardiac output.

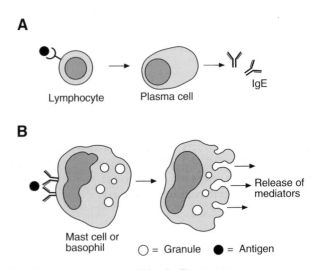

Fig. 39 Type I hypersensitivity. **A.** First exposure. **B.** Re-exposure.

ducing type I reactions are *penicillins* and *cephalosporins*. Common syndromes are asthma (above), rhinitis/conjunctivitis/eczema, angioedema and anaphylaxis.

Seasonal rhinitis

People prone to seasonal rhinitis/conjunctivitis, asthma and eczema are termed 'atopic'. Seasonal rhinitis is common and, though not life threatening, is a frequent cause of time off school and work. The classical pathogenesis is illustrated in Figure 39. Symptoms are maximal in the summer months when pollen counts are high and comprise rhinorhoea, sneezing and sore eyes.

Treatment

Treatment is with systemic antihistamines and topical sodium cromoglicate and topical steroids. **Histamine type I receptor antagonists** 'block' those histamine receptors found on mucus-secreting cells and capillaries in the mucous membranes of the upper airways. Examples include chlorphenamine, which causes sedation, and loratidine, which causes less sedation. If a sedative effect is required (e.g. in the management of a child with sleep disturbance because of urticaria), then a drug like chlorphenamine is preferred. More usually sedation is an undesirable effect, because it impairs skills such as driving and the use of machinery; under these circumstances a drug like loratidine, which produces less sedation, is indicated.

Anaphylaxis/angioedema

Mediator-induced venodilatation may be marked enough to lower cardiac output, causing life-threatening shock: this is termed **anaphylaxis**. Capillary leakiness in the larynx can cause life-threatening upper airways obstruction, termed **angioedema**. Anaphylaxis and angioedema may be present simultaneously.

Management

The suspected drug should be stopped (mainly relevant to i.v. infusions), and the airway maintained. **Intramuscular adrenaline (epinephrine)** is life-saving and may need to be repeated every 10 minutes (judged by response of blood pressure). Histamine H_1 antagonists (see above) should be given parenterally. A glucocorticoid should be given but is of secondary importance because of the delay in its onset of action. If the blood pressure is low, then the feet should be elevated to increase venous return. Intravenous fluid may also be necessary.

Type II (autoimmunity)

Drugs may induce immune responses to 'self'. The mechanisms are incompletely understood but include: (a) covalent binding of the drug to a cell surface so that

the cell becomes haptenated; (b) binding to a circulating protein, producing a hapten that resembles a cell antigen; and (c) alteration of cell metabolism so that cellular antigens change and become recognised by the immune system as foreign. In all cases the immune system is activated, and cell damage occurs. Clinical features can include systemic lupus erythematosus (SLE)-like syndromes and blood dyscrasias.

SLE-like syndromes

SLE is a common autoimmune disease with features that include arthritis, vasculitis, nephritis and rashes. *Hydralazine* (Ch. 3) and *isoniazid* (Ch. 13) can induce an SLE-like syndrome; this is usually reversible when the drug is stopped.

Blood dyscrasias

Methyldopa can induce autoantibodies towards erythrocytes, causing haemolytic anaemia. Some drugs may induce autoimmunity towards bone marrow precursor cells, causing pancytopenia (in which all cell series are affected) or agranulocytosis (in which the granulocyte series is affected): these syndromes may prove irreversible when the drug is stopped and can be fatal.

Clinical sketch

A woman is given sulfadoxine–pyrimethamine for the treatment of uncomplicated falciparum malaria acquired in west Africa. Within 24 hours she is extremely ill with fever, severe rash and ulcerating mouth lesions. She has proteinuria and goes on to die from renal failure.

Comment: this is 'Stevens–Johnson syndrome' resulting from a type III hypersensitivity to the sulphonamide. Sulfadoxine is particularly dangerous in this regard, because it is eliminated very slowly.

Type III (immune-complex)

Type III hypersensitivity is characterised by circulating antigen–antibody complexes (immune complexes), and their subsequent deposition on basement membranes. Attraction of cells of the immune system and local activation of complement cause tissue damage. Drugs commonly producing the type of reaction are *penicillins* and *sulphonamides*.

Serum sickness. Commonly seen with incompatible blood transfusions, this comprises urticaria (hives), fever and arthralgia.

A young man is found to be hyperthyroid and is started on carbimazole. One month later he presents with a febrile illness, conjunctivitis and a sore throat. His granulocyte count is extremely low.

Comment: this is agranulocytosis, a rare but potentially fatal adverse reaction to carbimazole. It is an immune mediated 'type B' adverse reaction.

Vasculitis. This may cause severe, occasionally life-threatening, skin reactions (e.g. erythema multiforme, Stevens–Johnson syndrome) and impaired renal function.

Type IV (delayed)

Whereas type I responses are seen within minutes of exposure, and those of type II and III usually within hours, type IV responses can take days to evolve. Antigens are phagocytosed by macrophages, transported to local lymph nodes and presented to lymphocytes. The lymphocyte clone then proliferates and travels to the site of antigen delivery. The classical example of a class IV reaction is that towards tuberculin injected into the skin as a Mantoux test, where inflammation takes 72 hours to develop. Contact dermatitis is the only common adverse drug reaction of this class; it may result from many skin preparations and from nickel salts.

Self-assessment: questions

Multiple choice questions

1. Salbutamol:
   a. Takes about 1 hour to produce bronchodilatation
   b. Is a selective agonist at β_1-adrenoceptors
   c. Should be stopped if it causes tremor
   d. Must be taken regularly
   e. May be valuable for acute left ventricular failure

2. Ipratropium:
   a. Is a nicotinic antagonist
   b. May cause intraocular pressure to rise
   c. Is of no value in the treatment of acute severe asthma
   d. Causes a dry mouth
   e. Encourages oral candidiasis

3. The following statements are true:
   a. Doxapram is preferable to mechanical ventilation for young asthmatics with severe respiratory failure
   b. In acute severe asthma, the inhaled oxygen concentration should be low (24–28%)
   c. Ciprofloxacin has no effect on the disposition of theophylline
   d. Glucocorticoids potentiate the effects of salbutamol
   e. Antihistamines have no place in the treatment of acute severe asthma

4. Inhaled sodium cromoglicate:
   a. Is beneficial in chronic bronchitis
   b. Is beneficial in acute severe asthma
   c. May cause hoarseness
   d. Is beneficial in allergic conjunctivitis
   e. Is anti-inflammatory

5. Drug hypersensitivity reactions:
   a. May involve more than one hypersensitivity mechanism
   b. May cause renal failure
   c. Should always be treated with systemic steroids
   d. May cause joint pain
   e. Usually occur upon first drug exposure

6. Histamine H_1 antagonists:
   a. Have a major role in the treatment of asthma
   b. Have a major role in the prevention of asthma
   c. Should not be combined with alcohol
   d. Have a major role in the treatment of anaphylaxis
   e. May cause dyskinesia

Case history questions

Case history 1

> A 20-year-old non-smoker with severe asthma presents as an emergency. She is given nebulised salbutamol, i.v. hydrocortisone and i.v. ampicillin. Later that night her breathing is no better and she is exhausted and sweaty but cannot sleep because of breathlessness. The doctor gives her temazepam because of her obvious agitation and insomnia.

1. What is likely to happen next and what comments do you have on her management?

Case history 2

> A 50-year-old smoker with chronic obstructive pulmonary disease takes salbutamol, ipratropium and aminophylline. He presents to his doctor with an infective exacerbation of his bronchitis; as he is allergic to penicillin the doctor starts erythromycin.

1. What is the potential risk?

Case history 3

> A woman takes co-amoxiclav (amoxicillin plus clavulanic acid) for a urinary tract infection. On the third day she feels unwell and shivery and complains of joint pains; subsequently she loses consciousness briefly. In hospital she is found to have a temperature of 38°C and lymph node enlargement. A diagnosis of bacteraemia is made and the co-amoxiclav is continued.

1. What alternative diagnosis should have been considered?

> During the night after admission, she is very unwell and develops a generalised rash plus ulceration of her buccal mucosa.

2. What should be done?

Short note questions

Write short notes on:
1. The modes of action, adverse effects and clinical use of drugs employed in the management of chronic asthma.
2. The emergency management of anaphylaxis and angioedema.

Self-assessment: answers

Multiple choice answers

1. a. **False**. The effect is almost immediate.
   b. **True**. Although salbutamol has greater affinity for β_2-adrenoceptors, β_1-adrenoceptors are stimulated, especially at high drug concentration. This may lead to tachycardia.
   c. **False**. Tremor is common but rarely bad enough for drug withdrawal.
   d. **False**. Salbutamol is usually taken when needed for wheeze and dyspnoea.
   e. **True**. Given i.v., salbutamol induces marked vasodilatation (β_2) as well as bronchodilatation. It is not a first-choice drug for left ventricular failure but can be useful.

2. a. **False**. It is a muscarinic antagonist.
   b. **True**. This may result from systemically absorbed drug, but it is more likely that part of the aerosol reaches the conjunctiva and is absorbed locally. Antimuscarinics cause the pupil to dilate (mydriasis) and this may occlude entry to the canal of Schlemm; this is only relevant if the patient has closed-angle glaucoma.
   c. **False**. See the management of acute severe asthma at the start of this chapter.
   d. **True**. Like atropine.
   e. **False**. Inhaled steroids do this.

3. a. **False**. Doxapram is occasionally useful in patients with type II respiratory failure and allows inhaled oxygen concentrations to be kept high without worsening hypercapnia. Young asthmatics with severe respiratory failure will rarely benefit from doxapram, and its use will waste valuable time: such patients need to be ventilated.
   b. **False**. Oxygen concentrations should be high (40%) to try to correct hypoxia; caution is only needed in patients with chronic type II respiratory failure. Blood gases should be measured in all cases of severe respiratory distress to help to resolve this issue.
   c. **False**. Ciprofloxacin (Ch. 13) is an enzyme inhibitor and reduces the clearance of theophylline.
   d. **True**. Glucocorticoids interact with β_2-agonists pharmacodynamically, by upregulating the expression of receptors.
   e. **True**. Their use confers no additional benefit.

4. a. **False**. Chronic bronchitis is secondary to mucosal damage, usually from smoking, and exacerbations are caused by infection.
   b. **False**. Cromoglicate is only of prophylactic value.
   c. **True**.
   d. **True**.
   e. **True**. Though the exact mode of action is unclear.

5. a. **True**. The division into types I, II, III and IV hypersensitivity is convenient, but adverse reactions can involve more than one mechanism.
   b. **True**. Drug allergy may cause renal damage by inducing vasculitis or 'interstitial nephritis'.
   c. **False**. Systemic steroids may be needed for life-threatening disease, but most drug reactions settle quickly upon withdrawal of the drug.
   d. **True**. Arthralgia and arthritis may both be a consequence of types II or III hypersensitivity.
   e. **False**. Previous exposure is usually required.

6. a. **False**.
   b. **False**. Antihistamines are of little use in either setting.
   c. **True**. Antihistamines are sedative.
   d. **True**. After epinephrine (adrenaline) has been given subcutaneously, an antihistamine, such as chlorphenamine, should be given i.v.
   e. **True**. This is not a common adverse reaction but is well documented.

Case history answers

Case history 1

This patient has been badly managed and may die because of the sedative. She was correctly given a β_2-agonist and early systemic steroid. She needs to be closely observed. Antibiotics were not required. Exhaustion and sweating are features of life-threatening disease, and sedatives are absolutely contraindicated.

Case history 2

Erythromycin is an inhibitor of drug-metabolising enzymes and potentiates theophylline: drug levels will rise. Commonly this induces nausea, headache and insomnia; arrhythmias and seizures are less common but more serious.

Case history 3

1. Although this woman did not initially have a rash, hypersensitivity should have been considered—particularly in view of the arthralgia. Her loss of

consciousness was probably simple syncope. Continuation of the drug worsened her condition, and it sounds as if she developed a severe skin reaction (like erythema multiforme) during the night.

2. Co-amoxiclav should be stopped, systemic steroids are indicated and specialist help is needed from a dermatologist.

Short note answers

1. a. In very mild asthma, occasional doses of inhaled β_2-agonist may be sufficient.
   b. If this is needed more than once daily, then an anti-inflammatory drug should be given regularly. In adults, inhaled steroid is probably the drug of first choice, but sodium cromoglicate is preferred as the drug of first choice in children.
   c. If asthma is not adequately controlled by low-dose inhaled steroid, then doses should be increased (high-dose aerosols and other delivery systems are available).
   d. Regular oral steroids are reserved for the most severely compromised patient: they will contribute to osteoporosis and other medical problems if they are needed for many years.
   e. Aminophylline (oral) and ipratropium bromide (inhaler) may be needed in addition by some patients to control symptoms.

This question, therefore, calls for the above overview, plus a summary of the clinical pharmacology of inhaled β_2-agonists, ipratropium, inhaled and oral steroids and aminophylline.

2. Describe what you mean by the terms:
   a. the main problem with anaphylaxis is shock (caused by vasodilatation)
   b. angioedema causes acute laryngeal narrowing
   c. the two often co-exist
   d. they are both medical emergencies.

Once you have clarified what you are treating, list the management steps:

   a. if a drug infusion (or blood transfusion) is in progress it should be stopped (it may be the cause of the problem)
   b. epinephrine (adrenaline) should be given i.m. and may be repeated at intervals: this drug may be life-saving
   c. high concentrations of inhaled oxygen are required
   d. The feet should be raised: this may raise the blood pressure by increasing venous return; use your judgement though as this may be difficult to achieve outside hospital and, if the patient arrests, the posture may make CPR difficult
   e. severe cases of laryngeal oedema may call for a tracheostomy.

Drugs and the gastrointestinal system

Overview

Conditions related to excessive secretion of gastric acid are extremely common, and include peptic ulcer, gastro-oesophageal reflux and non-specific dyspepsia. Acid-suppressing drugs are very important and widely used in treating these conditions. *Helicobacter pylori* is associated with peptic ulcer disease but not with simple dyspepsia or with reflux oesophagitis. Eradication of *H. pylori* drastically reduces the relapse rate in peptic ulcer disease.

The causes and treatment of nausea and vomiting are considered. Constipation and diarrhoea are very common symptoms and some causes and symptomatic treatment are considered. Irritable bowel syndrome is a cause of both, and antispasmodics are available for treatment. Inflammatory bowel disease is commonly treated with anti-inflammatory drugs, either locally or systemically.

11.1 Gastric acid-related conditions

Learning objectives

You should:

- be able to explain the control of acid secretion in the stomach

- be able to explain how drugs can affect acid secretion and the types of drug used, giving examples

- know the role of *Helicobacter pylori* in acid-related diseases

- be able to describe the regimens used for *H. pylori* eradication.

Clinical sketch

A 28-year-old man goes to his GP complaining of pain in his epigastrium. The pain occurs whenever he eats spicy foods, but also at other times and, in particular, wakes him up at night.

Comment: As many as one in 10 of all GP consultations are for dyspepsia; this is an indication of epigastric pain for which it is often difficult to work out from the history what the exact cause is: Causes include peptic ulcer disease, reflux oesophagitis or more serious pathologies such as gastric cancer. In at least half of all cases of dyspepsia there is no clear pathological cause. Treatment policies include early endoscopy for all patients, Helicobacter pylori screening to identify patients for endoscopy or specific treatment, or simple empirical treatment. In a young man presenting for the first time like this, simple empirical treatment is probably the best option.

Control of gastric acid secretion

Gastric acid serves many purposes, including providing an optimal environment of proteolytic enzymes to work and enhancing the sterility of stomach contents. It is controlled by CNS and local endocrine effects.

Acid secretion is increased by:

- the vagus nerve secreting acetylcholine
- local nerve endings secreting histamine, which acts on histamine type II receptors
- Gastrin secreted by the antrum of the stomach.

Acid secretion is decreased by:

- prostaglandin receptors on the luminal surface of the cell.

All of these mechanisms act ultimately via the 'proton pump' (Fig. 40). Gastrin provides a negative feedback system: an acid environment in the stomach decreases gastrin output, shutting down acid secretion, while an alkaline environment (e.g. after eating) stimulates acid secretion.

Drugs and gastric acid
Drugs may:

- buffer acid secretion: antacids
- decrease acid secretion by

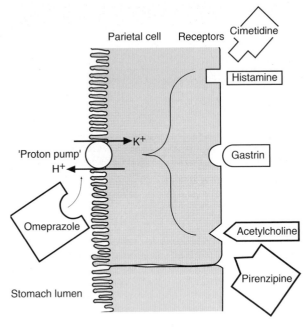

Fig. 40 The pharmacology of acid secretion.

—blocking acetylcholine receptors
—blocking histamine H_2 receptors
—stimulating prostaglandin receptors
—blocking the final common pathway of all of these mechanisms, i.e. the proton pump.

The principal pathological conditions in which it is useful to reduce acid secretion are:

- simple dyspepsia
- peptic ulcers
- gastro-oesophageal reflux
- Zollinger–Ellison syndrome.

Peptic ulcers

In peptic ulcers, the balance between protective elements (mucus secretion, gastric blood flow and harmful elements (acid, exotoxins, drugs) is deranged.

Duodenal ulcers

These have:

- high acid output
- usually (95%+) associated with *Helicobacter pylori* infection
- no risk of malignancy.

The Zollinger–Ellison syndrome is a rare gastrin-secreting tumour that causes very high acid output.

Duodenal ulcers can be cured by acid suppressant therapy but have a very high relapse rate (90% at 12 months); this can be reduced by eradication of *H. pylori* (see below).

Gastric ulcers

These:

- often have low–normal acid output
- are related to *H. pylori* infection in 70% of cases
- carry a risk of malignancy
- can be related in some cases to use of non-steroidal anti-inflammatory drugs (NSAIDs; see Ch. 9).

Complications of peptic ulcers

- Pain
- Anaemia
- Severe bleeding
- Perforation
- Pyloric stenosis.

Helicobacter pylori and peptic ulcer

H. pylori is spread by the faeco-oral route. It is highly prevalent and is associated with 95%+ of duodenal ulcers and 70% of gastric ulcers. It is not clearly associated with non-specific dyspepsia nor with gastro-oesophageal reflux disease.

H. pylori colonises the antrum of the stomach, where it protects itself by secreting urease. This breaks down urea to ammonia and creates an alkaline microenvironment. Because it interferes with the normal control of acid secretion, acid output increases (Fig. 41). H.pylori also secretes exotoxins, directly damaging the mucosa.

Successful eradication of *H. pylori* heals duodenal ulcers and is associated with a very low relapse rate.

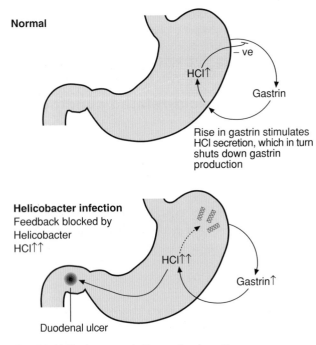

Fig. 41 *Helicobacter pylori* in peptic ulcer disease.

Regimens for *H. pylori* eradication

The usual treatment is with a proton pump inhibitor and two antibiotics. Bismuth-based regimens are possibly slightly superior in effectiveness but less convenient and less tolerated; consequently they form second-line use only.

Proton pump inhibitor regimen. This usually comprises high-dose omeprazole and two antibiotics (any two of clarithromycin, amoxicillin and metronidazole) for 1 week. Clarithromycin regimens are probably slightly more effective.

Bismuth-based regimen. This is usually *chelated bismuth* and two antibiotics (*metronidazole* or *tinidazole*, and either *amoxicillin* or *tetracycline*, all in high doses), usually for 2 weeks.

Clinical sketch

A 45-year-old woman had peptic ulcer disease diagnosed 2 years ago. She was treated with ranitidine for 12 months, which settled her symptoms, but now they have recurred.

Comment: Peptic ulcer disease is most commonly caused by Helicobacter pylori. *Simple acid suppression will allow the ulcer to heal but does not remove the underlying cause and relapse is likely, as in this patient.*

Clinical sketch

A 50-year-old man has peptic ulcer disease diagnosed as related to *Helicobacter pylori*. He is given an eradication course of treatment and his symptoms settle. However, a year later his symptoms recur and retesting shows the presence of *H. pylori*.

Comment: Reinfection with H. pylori *occurs at the rate of about 1% per year. The alternative explanation in this patient is that eradication therapy was unsuccessful, either because the patient had resistant* H. pylori *or (as is frequently the case) the patient was not compliant with the full course of therapy to eradicate the infection.*

NSAIDs and peptic ulcers

NSAIDs (see Ch. 9) may cause peptic ulcer (especially gastric) by decreasing local prostaglandin secretion in the gastric mucosa and hence reducing mucosal blood flow, mucus secretion and other protective factors. This may occur regardless of the route of administration of the NSAID. Many NSAIDs may also have a direct irritant effect on the gastric mucosa.

Appropriate treatment is withdrawal of the NSAID if possible; if necessary, antisecretory drugs (see below) or the prostaglandin analogue *misoprostol* may be used.

Clinical sketch

A 72-year-old woman taking diclofenac for her arthritis presents to hospital with haematemesis (vomiting blood).

Comment: Irritant drugs such as non-steroidal anti-inflammatory drugs (NSAIDs) can also cause peptic ulcer disease or can flare up existing peptic ulcer disease. These gastrointestinal complications are among the most serious for NSAIDs. It may occur without any prior warning of dyspepsia and present with a serious complication, as in this case. This patient needs to have her NSAID withdrawn and needs an urgent endoscopy. She may also require blood transfusion or even surgery if the bleeding fails to stop spontaneously. She should avoid NSAIDs in the future. Many patients receive acid-suppressant drugs such as proton pump inhibitors with their NSAIDs because they are considered to be at risk of such complications. A better approach, however, would be careful selection of those patients who receive NSAIDs, which are commonly overused.

Gastro-oesophageal reflux

Gastric contents regurgitate into the oesophagus in some patients with an incompetent gastro-oesophageal sphincter, causing heartburn or severe pain. In severe cases, complications such as erosions, bleeding and stricture may occur. Management involves general measures (weight loss if obese, avoiding tight clothes around the waist, avoiding stooping, elevating the head of the bed to reduce nocturnal reflux) and, often, drug therapy.

Therapy includes:

- Antacids: particularly antacids combined with alginate, which coats the oesophagus and reduces the contact with acid.
- Antisecretory drugs: proton pump inhibitors are usually highly effective in severe cases. Long-term use may be necessary in some patients. Histamine H_2 blockers are effective in less severe cases.
- Prokinetic drugs. *Metoclopramide* and *domperidone* are discussed under antiemetics (see below) but both increase lower oesophageal sphincter pressure and increase gastric clearance, in addition to their central effects. *Cisapride* stimulates releases of acetylcholine to encourage motility in the stomach and elsewhere in the gastrointestinal tract but its use is limited because of a potential for dangerous interactions with other drugs, leading to cardiac arrhythmias.

Acid-modifying drugs

Antacids

Antacids are weak alkali used for symptomatic relief. They:

- neutralise the acid secreted by the parietal cells
- are not absorbed and so cause no systemic effects
- may also reduce the absorption of other drugs, e.g. tetracyclines or digoxin.

Examples

Aluminium hydroxide (tends to cause constipation) *or magnesium trisilicate* (diarrhoea). *Sodium bicarbonate* is sometimes taken as a popular home remedy for dyspepsia. It is not recommended because it is absorbed and if used in large amounts can cause systemic alkalosis.

Histamine receptor antagonists

These drugs act by antagonising histamine at H_2 receptors. They:

- decrease acid secretion, especially at night and during fasting
- heal almost all duodenal ulcers after 4–8 weeks: gastric ulcers heal more slowly and may require higher doses for longer. There is a high relapse rate unless *H. pylori* is treated also
- are also effective in reflux oesophagitis, but here high-dose long-term therapy is often necessary
- relieve symptoms in many patients who have dyspepsia without any clear organic lesion.

Many patients take H_2 receptor antagonists indefinitely, or in repeated courses.

Clinical sketch

A 47-year-old woman has severe reflux oesophagitis confirmed on endoscopy. Initial treatment with ranitidine is partly successful, but she continues to have a lot of pain.

Comment: In severe cases of reflux oesophagitis, proton pump inhibitors are more effective. In general, proton pump inhibitors decrease acid secretion to a greater extent than histamine H_2 blockers, even in a high dose. Such intense acid suppression is not always necessary in acid-related conditions.

Examples

Cimetidine and *ranitidine* are both well absorbed after oral administration, but both can also be given i.v. They are excreted unchanged by the kidney.

Adverse effects

Cimetidine has weak antiandrogen effects and occasionally causes gynaecomastia in long-term use. This is less common with ranitidine. Either may cause confusion and drowsiness in the elderly.

Interactions

Cimetidine inhibits drug-metabolising enzymes in the liver and may increase the effects and toxicity of many drugs (see Ch. 21).

Proton pump inhibitors

The H^+/K^+-ATPase enzyme ('proton pump') is irreversibly inhibited by these drugs, and so acid production ceases. Acid secretion can only resume when new enzyme has been formed. They:

- are the most effective acid suppressants: heal acid-related diseases faster and to a greater extent than other drugs
- have a high relapse rate in peptic ulcers unless *H. pylori* is eradicated
- form long-term therapy in reflux oesophagitis commonly
- are used, in high doses, to treat Zollinger–Ellison syndrome.

Examples

Omeprazole is metabolised by the liver. Because of the irreversible inhibition of the proton pump, its duration of action is considerably longer than its half-life and omeprazole is usually administered once per day. *Lanzoprazole* is similar. *Esomaprazole* is an isomer of omeprazole and is used for intermittent treatment of gastro-oesophagal reflux disease.

Adverse effects

- Headache
- Nausea, vomiting and diarrhoea.

Interactions

Omeprazole can inhibit some hepatic drug-metabolising enzymes.

Prostaglandin E_1 analogues: misoprostol

Prostaglandin E_1 decreases acid secretion by an action on a receptor on the surface of the parietal cell. It may have an effect in protecting the mucosa of the stomach, perhaps by increasing mucosal blood flow and mucus and duodenal bicarbonate secretion.

Example

Misoprostol is an analogue of prostaglandin E_1 with a half-life of 2 hours. It is well absorbed and is metabolised to active metabolites.

While misoprostol can heal peptic ulcers, H_2 blockers or proton pump inhibitors are better and easier to take. Misoprostol may have a role in the treatment and prophylaxis of ulcers caused by NSAIDs, and this is its main use. Prophylactic therapy may be advisable in patients at high risk (e.g. those who require a NSAID despite a previous history of peptic ulcer disease); its routine use in all patients taking NSAIDs is not justified.

Contraindication

In pregnant women, it may cause uterine contractions and miscarriages.

Adverse effects

- Crampy abdominal pains
- Diarrhoea.

Drugs with no effect on acid secretion

These drugs are believed to enhance the protective elements by forming a protective coating over the ulcer crater and allowing healing to occur underneath. They may also have a separate action in stimulating local prostaglandin release. They are not used often today.

Chelated bismuth

This has some activity against *H. pylori* infection and also protects the ulcer crater and allows healing.

It is given orally and a small quantity is absorbed; this is later excreted through the kidney.

Adverse effects

- Metallic taste
- Blackening of faeces
- Encephalopathy, if used in high doses for prolonged periods; bismuth should not be used repeatedly or for more than 2 months at a time.

Sucralfate

Sucralfate is an aluminum salt of sucrose. It heals peptic ulcers as effectively as histamine H_2 blockers but is less convenient.

It causes constipation.

Carbenoxolone

Carbenoxolone is a derivative of licorice. It stimulates gastric mucus secretion as well as protecting the ulcer. It is also used in treatment for reflux oesophagitis.

Adverse effect

Carbenoxolone has mineralocorticoid effects and may cause sodium retention and hypokalaemia; this could be serious in patients with cardiac failure.

11.2 Nausea and vomiting

Learning objectives

You should:

- understand the mechanisms that may case nausea and vomiting
- be able to describe the drugs that can be used to prevent or treat nausea and vomiting.

Clinical sketch

A 22-month-old child develops profuse diarrhoea. The mother is told this is infective gastroenteritis and goes to see her GP to ask for an antidiarrhoeal agent and an antibiotic.

Comment: The priority in treating a child with diarrhoea is maintaining hydration of the child; oral rehydration therapy (dilute solutions of essential salts) is the correct therapy. Children die from dehydration in infective gastroenteritis. The use of antibiotics or antidiarrhoeal agents is entirely inappropriate in this setting.

Clinical sketch

A patient with migraine is unable to take simple analgesics because of the associated nausea and vomiting from the migraine.

Comment: Combined use of analgesic and a simple antinauseant such as metoclopramide is appropriate. This also has effects overcoming the gastric stasis common in migraine treated with an analgesic.

Nausea and vomiting are common non-specific features of disease or drug toxicity and the cause should be diagnosed and treated where possible. Drugs to treat nausea and vomiting may be given orally or parenterally (i.m. or i.v.).

Vomiting is caused by activation of the vomiting centre in the brainstem, mainly via the vagus nerve. The vomiting centre is also influenced by the vestibular apparatus, by the cerebral cortex, by afferents from the gastrointestinal tract and by the chemoreceptor trigger zone, through muscarinic and histamine (H_1) receptors. The chemoreceptor trigger zone is another region of the brainstem and is activated by afferents (often D_2 dopaminergic) similar to those of the vomiting centre. In addition it is activated by toxins, including drugs.

Antiemetics

Antiemetics may act in several different ways (Fig. 42).

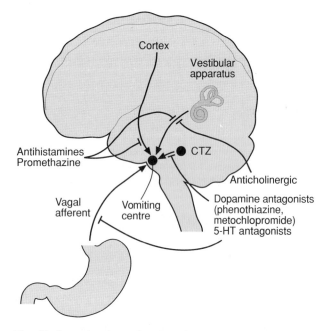

Fig. 42 Central actions of antiemetics.

Anticholinergic drugs. These act on the vomiting centre especially but also affect the gastrointestinal tract directly, for example *hyoscine*. Adverse effects include dry mouth, occasionally confusion and agitation.

Antihistamines. These act on H_1 receptors in the vomiting centre and also have weak anticholinergic and sedating effects. Newer non-sedating antihistamines are not effective. The antihistamines are frequently used to treat motion sickness or vestibular disease (often inappropriately in the elderly). Example: *promethazine*.

Phenothiazines. In addition to anticholinergic, sedative and H_1-blocking effects, the phenothiazines also block dopamine receptors in the chemoreceptor trigger zone. Example: *prochlorperazine*.

Adverse effects include parkinsonism (see Ch. 6 for fuller description).

Dopamine receptor antagonists. *Metoclopramide* acts in the chemoreceptor trigger zone and has direct effects on the gastrointestinal tract (see above). It is given orally or parenterally for most causes of vomiting, although it is not effective for motion sickness.

Adverse effects include acute extrapyramidal reactions, such as oculogyric crisis, especially in children (treat with parenteral anticholinergic such as benztropine). Increased prolactin concentrations and gynaecomastia can occur in prolonged use.

Domperidone is similar to metoclopramide but is less likely to cause extrapyramidal reactions; it can, however, cause cardiac arrhythmias when given parenterally in high dose.

5-Hydroxytryptamine (5-HT) antagonists. *Ondansetron* is one of several $5\text{-}HT_3$ antagonists, which are very effec-

tive in treating severe nausea and vomiting, particularly after anticancer chemotherapy but also postoperatively. It is reserved for cases where other drugs are ineffective.

Adverse effects include constipation and headache.

11.3 Disorders of the bowel

Learning objectives

You should:

● be aware that disorders of the bowel are common, often resolve without treatment and can be secondary to drug therapy, and inflammatory conditions as well as infections

● know the main treatment possibilities and when to use them.

Disturbances of bowel habit are common and often resolve spontaneously without treatment. The cause should be identified if possible and treated as necessary. Bowel disturbance may be an adverse effect of many drugs (e.g. opiates, tricyclics for constipation, antibiotics for diarrhoea).

Treatment of constipation

Constipation can often be treated effectively with dietary modification, with increased fibre and fluids; and with careful education of the patient. Only if this fails should laxatives be used, adjusting the dose to achieve the desired effect (Fig. 43). In order of preference:

1. the bulking agents
2. osmotic laxatives
3. stimulant drugs (reserved for intermittent use)
4. The faecal softeners (used less often).

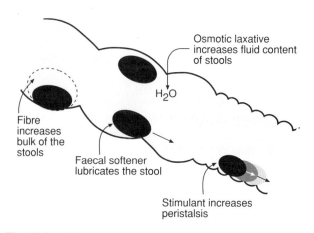

Fig. 43 Laxatives.

Bulking agents

Bulking agents absorb water, swell and increase the bulk of the stool. This increased bulk stimulates normal peristalsis and hence defaecation. They may take a few days to act fully and may cause flatulence and crampy abdominal pain at first. They are given orally.

Examples: *bran, ispaghula.*

Osmotic laxatives

The osmotic laxatives reduce absorption of water from the bowel. This softens the stool and increase its bulk, stimulating peristalsis.

Lactulose is a disaccharide that is broken down by colonic bacteria to acetic and lactic acid, which cause the osmotic effects. Polyethylene glycols are non-absorbed inert compounds. Both are taken orally. Adverse effects include abdominal pain and flatulence. *Phosphate* or *magnesium* salts are used as enemas.

Stimulants

Stimulants are drugs used to stimulate peristalsis and are indicated for severe chronic constipation or where a more rapid effect (within 6–8 hours) is required. They may cause atony of the bowel if used chronically, creating a vicious cycle of laxative use/constipation/laxative use for the patient. Stimulants are usually given orally.

Examples: *senna, bisacodyl, castor oil.*

Faecal softeners

The faecal softeners lubricate and soften the stool and are usually given orally.

Examples: *liquid paraffin.* (There is a risk of aspiration lipoid pneumonia with liquid paraffin.)

Treatment of diarrhoea

In treating diarrhoea, especially in children, it is vitally important to replace fluid and electrolyte losses. Since most cases of diarrhoea are self-limiting, this is often all that is necessary, and the use of specific antidiarrhoeal drugs is often inappropriate.

Antimotility drugs

Antimotility drugs reduce peristalsis by stimulating opioid receptors in the bowel. An adverse effect is constipation.

Examples: *loperamide, diphenoxylate* are pethidine derivatives that act only in the bowel. Diphenoxylate is often combined with atropine. *Codeine phosphate* and *morphine* (Ch. 7) are occasionally used also.

Adsorbents

Some drugs absorb water without increasing stool bulk, so making the stool firmer and smaller, for example *kaolin.*

Irritable bowel syndrome

Irritable bowel syndrome is common (30% of women, 15% of men) and is caused by dysmotility of the bowel. It overlaps in some cases with simple dyspepsia.

Symptoms include intermittent diarrhoea and constipation, and abdominal pain.

Treatment is symptomatic.

Antispasmodics

Anticholinergic drugs decrease bowel motility by reducing peristalsis and are used orally to treat painful spasm of the large bowel.

Examples: *mebeverine*, which has little systemic anticholinergic effect; *propantheline*, which has more systemic effects and which is also used parenterally to relieve severe pain associated with spasm, e.g. in biliary colic.

Inflammatory bowel diseases

The cause of the chronic inflammatory diseases is not known. Ulcerative colitis affects the large bowel; Crohn's disease affects mainly the small bowel but also the large bowel and other parts of the gastrointestinal tract. Both diseases typically undergo exacerbations and remissions.

The aim of treatment is to resolve the acute episodes and prolong remissions. In addition to drug therapy, treatment involves correction of any nutritional deficiencies (enteral feeding may be effective in Crohn's) and sometimes surgery for complications or severe uncontrolled disease.

Anti-inflammatory drugs

Drug treatment is with anti-inflammatory drugs, especially the corticosteroids, which are used systemically in severe acute attacks (e.g. *prednisolone* or *hydrocortisone*) (see Ch. 12). They may also be given locally by means of enemas for less severe acute attacks involving the large bowel, or as maintenance therapy. Other anti-inflammatories such as *azathioprine* or *cyclosporin* (see Ch. 9) are also occasionally used.

Infliximab is a monoclonal antibody which inhibits the actions of the inflammatory cytokine tumour necrosis factor α. It is used in refractory Crohn's disease (also in rheumatoid arthritis).

Aminosalicylates

5-Aminosalicylate (5-ASA) is the active drug, effective in treatment and maintenance of colonic disease in ulcerative colitis or Crohn's disease.

Sulfasalazine is a complex of a sulphonamide, *sulfapyridine* (*sulphapyridine*), and 5-ASA. The complex is taken orally or rectally and is broken down by bacteria in the large bowel to release the 5-ASA. It is also used as a disease-modifying drug in rheumatoid arthritis (see Ch. 9).

Mesalazine is another name for 5-ASA and can be given orally or rectally as an enema.

Olsalazine is two molecules of 5-ASA combined, given orally.

Adverse effects

Adverse effects are mainly because of the sulfapyridine (sulphapyridine) content: headache, nausea and vomiting, rashes and occasionally blood dyscrasias and renal dysfunction. Infertility in males can occur because of decreased sperm count.

Adverse effects of 5-ASA: diarrhoea, occasionally blood disorders (patients should be advised to report any purpura, unexplained bruising or sore throat or fever and a full blood count should then be done).

11.4 Gallstones

In the developed world, gallstones are usually made of cholesterol.

Bile acids

Bile acids may be used to gradually dissolve cholesterol gallstones. This is only suitable for small stones, as 3–6 months of treatment is required. Recurrence is common. Bile acid treatment for gallstones is generally reserved for patients who are unfit for surgery. Diarrhoea is an adverse effect.

Examples: *chenodeoxycholic acid, ursodeoxycholic acid*.

Self-assessment: questions

Multiple choice questions

1. In duodenal ulcers:
   a. *H. pylori* is present in almost all cases
   b. Relapse after treatment with cimetidine is rare
   c. *H. pylori* secretes a urease enzyme
   d. Basal acid secretion is increased
   e. Attempts to eradicate *H. pylori* are rarely successful

2. In conditions where gastric acid secretion causes symptoms:
   a. Antacids are mainly used for symptomatic relief
   b. H_2 receptor antagonists block all acid secretion
   c. Ranitidine may commonly cause drug interactions
   d. The final common pathway of all stimuli to acid secretion is the proton pump
   e. Omeprazole is very effective in reflux oesophagitis

3. In treating peptic ulcer disease:
   a. Misoprostol is used to treat the gastrointestinal adverse effect of NSAIDs
   b. All patients taking NSAIDs should also take misoprostol
   c. Chelated bismuth can be used to treat acute peptic ulcer
   d. Long-term bismuth is used to maintain remission in peptic ulcer disease
   e. Sucralfate may cause diarrhoea

4. In the treatment of gastro-oesophageal reflux:
   a. Metoclopramide may enhance drug absorption
   b. Metoclopramide may cause severe dystonic reactions
   c. Hyperprolactinaemia is a result of taking antidopaminergic drugs
   d. Domperidone increases large bowel motility
   e. Cisapride may cause anticholinergic adverse effects

5. Drugs used to treat nausea include:
   a. Ondansetron
   b. Prochlorperazine
   c. Bromocriptine
   d. Atropine
   e. Dexamethasone

6. Bowel disturbance may arise as a result of treatment with:
   a. Disopyramide
   b. Omeprazole
   c. Erythromycin
   d. Iron salts
   e. Morphine

7. In treating disturbances of bowel motility:
   a. Rehydration is more important than using antidiarrhoeal drugs
   b. Sulfasalazine is used to treat irritable bowel syndrome
   c. Corticosteroids are the main anti-inflammatories used to treat acute ulcerative colitis
   d. Steroids are always used topically in inflammatory bowel disease
   e. Overdose of diphenoxylate may be treated with naloxone

Case history questions

Case history 1

A patient complaining of upper abdominal pain is found by endoscopy to have a duodenal ulcer. Antral biopsies show *Helicobacter pylori*.

1. Should this patient receive treatment to eradicate *H. pylori* on first presentation?
2. If so, what treatment should be given to eradicate *H. pylori*?
3. What treatment might be given to heal the peptic ulcer?
4. If therapy to eradicate *H. pylori* is not given, what are the risks of recurrence?
5. The patient later develops osteoarthritis of the knee; should he be given a non-steroidal anti-inflammatory drug (NSAID)?

Case history 2

A patient has gastro-oesophageal reflux proven on endoscopy.

1. Apart from non-pharmacological treatments, what drugs might be considered?
2. How might metoclopramide be helpful?
3. What drugs might aggravate this condition?
4. How should severe cases be treated?
5. What are the adverse effects of omeprazole?

Case history 3

> An elderly patient resident in a nursing home is constipated, i.e. no bowel motion passed for 5 days.

1. What drugs might exacerbate constipation?
2. What other causative factors should be considered in this patient's constipation?
3. If dietary treatment is unsuccessful in this patient, what drug treatment should be considered?
4. What are the harmful effects of long-term use of senna or other stimulant laxatives?
5. What drug therapies might be useful in acute severe constipation?

Short note questions

Write short notes on:

1. Treatment of *Helicobacter pylori* infection.
2. Acid-suppressant drugs.
3. Drugs in the treatment of reflux oesophagitis.

Extended matching items question

Theme: gastrointestinal disorders
Options

A. Octreotide
B. Omeprazole
C. Cimetidine
D. Clarithromycin
E. Ranitidine
F. Metronidazole
G. Lactulose
H. Lansoprazole
I. Metoclopramide
J. Erythromycin
K. Barium preparations
L. Loratidine

Read 1–6 below and choose the most appropriate answer from options A–L. Each option may be used once, more than once or not at all.

1. Select three drugs that might be used together in the eradication of *Helicobacter pylori*.
2. Select a drug that might be used as an antiemetic.
3. Select a drug that binds to histamine H_2 receptors.
4. Select a drug that increases gastric motility.
5. Select a drug that might be used to treat constipation.
6. Select a drug that might be used to treat oesophageal varices.

Self-assessment: answers

Multiple choice answers

1. a. **True**. Its association with gastric ulcers is less certain.
   b. **False**. Relapse is frequent since the cause of the peptic ulcer, the *H. pylori* infection, persists.
   c. **True**. This is how it protects itself from stomach acid.
   d. **True**. As a result of blockage of negative feedback on gastrin.
   e. **False**. Triple therapy with bismuth and antibiotics is successful in about 90% of cases.

2. a. **True**. Very high but unpalatable doses can be used to heal ulcers also.
   b. **False**. Acid production is reduced by about 70–80%.
   c. **False**. Cimetidine, however, does, because of its effects on liver enzymes.
   d. **True**. Hence omeprazole is the most effective of all antisecretory drugs.
   e. **True**. Again, omeprazole is the most effective treatment.

3. a. **True**. By replacing the decreased mucosal prostaglandins.
   b. **False**. It is unnecessary in many patients, has adverse effects of its own and adds considerably to the costs.
   c. **True**. Less widely used today because it has to be taken four times per day compared to once per day for the H_2 receptor antagonists.
   d. **False**. There would be a serious risk of bismuth encephalopathy.
   e. **False**. Sucralfate tends to cause constipation.

4. a. **True**. For instance, used with paracetamol in patients with migraine.
   b. **True**. Especially in children or young women.
   c. **True**. Because dopamine inhibits prolactin release from the pituitary.
   d. **False**. Domperidone may stimulate upper gastrointestinal motility, but not lower.
   e. **False**. Cisapride is procholinergic, not anticholinergic.

5. a. **True**. A 5-HT_3 antagonist.
   b. **True**. Widely and perhaps excessively used.
   c. **False**. Bromocriptine is a dopamine agonist, and its adverse effects include nausea.
   d. **False**. Although the anticholinergic hyoscine is used.

e. **True**. Especially after anticancer chemotherapy.

6. a. **True**. Anticholinergic, so may cause constipation.
   b. **True**. Diarrhoea.
   c. **True**. Diarrhoea, and so may many other antibiotics.
   d. **True**. Constipation.
   e. **True**. Constipation.

7. a. **True**. Often forgotten.
   b. **False**. Sulfasalazine is used to treat inflammatory bowel disease of the colon.
   c. **True**. Topically or systemically.
   d. **False**. Systemic steroids are used in severe cases.
   e. **True**. Diphenoxylate is an opioid.

Case history answers

Case history 1

1. In general, current opinion is that he should not. The argument against treating all patients on first presentation is that the regimens used for eradicating *H. pylori* at present have a high incidence of adverse effects, and that eradication should be reserved for recurrent or complicated cases. The case for early treatment is becoming more widely accepted.
2. Triple therapy with bismuth, metronidazole, and amoxycillin or tetracycline is the standard therapy at present: many other, perhaps more acceptable, regimens are under study.
3. Eradicating the *H. pylori* is in addition to healing the ulcer, for which a wide range of drugs is available including H_2 receptor antagonists, chelated bismuth, omeprazole or sucralfate.
4. The recurrence rate at 1 year is 80–90%.
5. NSAIDs should be avoided wherever possible in patients with peptic ulcer disease. Patients with osteoarthritis often need only analgesia and not an anti-inflammatory, so paracetamol used regularly might be sufficent. If the patient had a true inflammatory arthropathy, a NSAID might be necessary and prophylactic therapy with misoprostol or ranitidine should be considered.

Case history 2

1. Drug treatment would normally be an antacid with alginate, drugs to suppress acid secretion, or prokinetic agents—or combinations of these.

2. Metoclopramide increases the tone of the lower oesophageal sphincter and increases gastric emptying.
3. Drugs with an anticholinergic adverse effect decrease lower oesophageal tone, as do smooth muscle relaxants (e.g. calcium-channel blockers).
4. The drug of choice in severe cases is omeprazole, which is exceedingly effective and may be needed for long-term maintenance in some patients.
5. Omeprazole may cause headache, diarrhoea and drug interactions. There are some theoretical concerns about the long-term safety of drugs that suppress acid secretion so profoundly, e.g. risk of gastric carcinoma because of failure to detoxify nitrosamines, but these remain unproved.

Case history 3

1. Drugs with anticholinergic adverse effects, such as tricyclic anticonvulsants or phenothiazines, also opiate analgesics.
2. Hypothyroidism and depression should be excluded. Other factors include poor diet (deficient in fibre), immobility and dehydration.
3. The first line of drug treatment is usually supplementation of fibre intake, either by diet or by use of a bulking agent, followed by an osmotic laxative and finally intermittent use of a stimulant laxative.
4. Atony of the bowel and laxative dependency.
5. Local treatment with suppositories (e.g. glycerin or bisacodyl) or by enema (e.g. phosphate enema) may be useful in acute severe cases: serious pathology, e.g. intestinal obstruction, should be excluded first.

Short note answers

1. This should mention regimens including 2 weeks with a proton pump inhibitor with two antibiotics. Reserve schemes should include mention of bismuth-based preparations in combination with antibiotics.
2. This should discuss histamine H_2 blockers, proton pump inhibitors and, for the very perceptive student, anticholinergics, although these are no longer used therapeutically.
3. This might describe antacids with alginates, histamine H_2 blockers and proton pump inhibitors. (PPIs). Description of the drugs alone would not suffice here; a student would also be expected to show an awareness of how the drugs are used, and which are the most effective approaches, etc. An alternative would be a step-up approach—using antacids, H_2 blockers if not resolved, and then PPIs if still not resolved—or a step-down approach—using high-dose PPIs to heal inflammation and then settling down to a maintenance dose, possibly given intermittently in mild cases. Both regimens have their advocates. In severely affected patients, PPIs are by far the most effective.

Extended matching items answer

1. D, B and F or H, D and F. These are standard regimens, a proton pump inhibitor with two antibiotics, for 2 weeks.
2. I Metoclopramide is a standard antiemetic.
3. C or E. (Loratidine binds to histamine H_1 receptors; see Ch. 10 on hypersensitivity.)
4. I or J (surprisingly). Metoclopramide increases gastric motility. So too does erythromycin, which seems to act at specific receptors. This is partly the basis of its common adverse effects. It is used as a gastric stimulant occasionally, for instance in patients with severe gastric stasis secondary to diabetic autonomic neuropathy.
5. G. Lactulose is the only one here used to treat constipation. It is better to treat constipation by dietary changes than by drugs, however.
6. A. Octreotide is used intravenously to stop bleeding from oesophageal varices.

12

Overview

Because hormones can have widespread and diverse effects, management of endocrine disorders is complex. Drugs can be used to replace deficiencies, to treat overactivity or to modulate secondary effects.

Diabetes mellitus is the most common endocrine disorder. Its complications are severe and can be reduced by good management. Insulin-dependent diabetics require insulin; non-insulin-dependent diabetics can be treated with oral hypoglycaemic drugs and also sometimes with insulin. Both groups are prone to complications that can be reduced by good diabetic control.

The thyroid gland can be over- or underactive. Treatment of overactivity depends largely on drugs, including radioiodine. Underactivity of the thyroid is generally easy to treat with thyroid replacement therapy.

Corticosteroids are widely used both as replacement therapy and especially as immunosuppressants. The major drugs and their uses are described. Their adverse effects are common and serious.

Sex hormone steroids are used for contraception and for hormone replacement therapy after the menopause, both to relieve symptoms and to prevent osteoporosis. Other drugs can also be used to prevent and treat osteoporosis, such as vitamin D, calcium salts and bisphosponates.

Lastly there are drugs to replace or modulate the range of peptide hormones from the pituitary gland.

12.1 Diabetes mellitus

Learning objectives

You should:

- be able to distinguish between the types of diabetes mellitus

- know the complications of diabetes mellitus

- understand the major elements of non-pharmacological treatment of diabetes mellitus

- be able to describe the drug regimens for insulin-dependent and non-insulin-dependent diabetes mellitus

- be able to describe the major drug classes used and give examples.

Diabetes mellitus (DM) is common, affecting about 1% of the population. In DM, the body becomes unable to regulate blood glucose, which rises, and the characteristic symptoms of polyuria, polydipsia and weight loss occur. DM is really two distinct disorders. DM of either type is associated with serious long-term complications, including neuropathy (damage to nerves), retinopathy (damage to the retina), nephropathy (DM is the commonest cause of chronic renal failure) and arterial disease (DM is a major risk factor for ischaemic heart disease). Treatment of DM aims to control the blood glucose, relieve symptoms, and reduce the severity and frequency of the complications. Good control reduces the risk of complications in both types of DM.

Non-insulin-dependent diabetes

Non-insulin-dependent DM (NIDDM):

- is more common (about 80% of all cases)
- occurs in middle-aged or elderly patients
- often has a family history
- is resistant at the cellular level to the effects of insulin.

A feature of the insulin resistance is the presence of high circulating concentrations of insulin. NIDDM is associated with obesity and hypertension.

Management

Treatment of NIDDM involves:

- patient education
- careful attention to diet
- weight loss if there is obesity
- in some patients, the use of oral hypoglycaemic drugs
  —*sulfonylureas* in non-obesity
  —*metformin* in obesity
  —combinations of drugs commonly required
- insulin if oral medication is unsuccessful; however, these patients are not 'insulin dependent' in that if they discontinue their insulin, they are not at risk of ketosis
- careful treatment of other cardiovascular risk factors
- NIDDM is a progressive disease: blood glucose control tends to deteriorate over time and requires increased therapy.

Insulin-dependent diabetes

Insulin-dependent diabetes tends to occur in younger patients. It:

- is caused by the autoimmune destruction of the beta cells in the islets of the pancreas, which produce insulin
- involves insulin deficiency, which prevents most cells from taking up glucose and forces them to metabolise lipids
- leads to ketosis and acidosis
- requires insulin therapy in addition to diet control
- without insulin, will result in the patient rapidly falling ill and possibly dying
- necessitates careful patient education
- requires careful treatment of complications/cardiovascular risk factors.

Insulin

Insulin is a peptide produced normally by the islet cells of the pancreas. It has a range of actions which depend on the type of cell (Fig. 44). It:

- allows the active uptake of glucose and its utilisation in muscle and fat cells
- stimulates synthesis of glycogen in the liver
- inhibits formation of glucose (gluconeogenesis) in the liver
- inhibits breakdown of lipids
- stimulates protein synthesis
- stimulates some cell ion transport mechanisms (e.g. Na^+/K^+-ATPase).

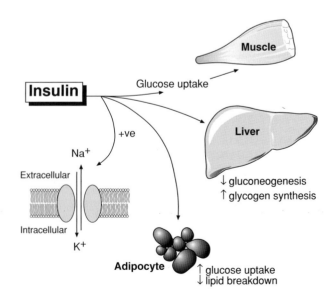

Fig. 44 Action of insulin.

Drugs used in the treatment of diabetes mellitas

Insulin

Insulin must be administered parenterally, usually by s.c. injection. It is metabolised by the liver and the kidney and has a half-life of 9–10 minutes. To extend its period of action, slow release preparations have been developed.

Formulations of insulin

Insulin preparations were originally derived from pigs (porcine insulin) or from cattle (beef insulin) and, as a result, antibodies sometimes developed. This was avoided by the development of highly purified porcine insulin. Now, however, most patients receive human insulin, produced either by biosynthesis (using genetic engineering to express the gene for human insulin in bacteria) or by chemical modification of the amino acid sequence of porcine insulin.

Human insulin is theoretically less immunogenic than porcine insulin but has no real advantage over the highly purified porcine insulins. Concerns that human insulin might cause hypoglycaemia more readily than earlier insulins seem unfounded now.

Insulins may be classified according to their duration of action as short, intermediate or long acting. Mixtures of these insulins are also available.

Short-acting preparations (e.g. soluble insulin) have a peak effect at about 1–2 hours when given s.c. and a duration of action of about 4–8 hours. They may also be given i.v.

Intermediate acting preparations (e.g., amorphous insulin zinc suspension) have insulin complexed with a zinc salt so that particles form. Insulin is then slowly released from these particles. The peak effect is at about 3–6 hours and the duration of action is about 12–24 hours.

Long acting preparations (e.g. crystalline insulin zinc suspension) have the insulin–zinc complex formed as crystals, which break down more slowly still. The peak action is at 5–12 hours and the duration of effect is 16–30 hours.

New very-short- and very-long-acting insulin analogues are becoming available. The former are used to avoid postprandial surge in blood sugar. The latter provide a more reliable and consistent 24 hour control of blood glucose than achieved with the existing long-acting formulations. *Insulin lispro* and *insulin aspart* are short-acting analogues; *insulin glargine* is a long-acting preparation.

Insulin regimens

Dose and choice of preparations must be determined for each patient individually. Patients may use a short-acting and an intermediate or long-acting preparation twice a day (before breakfast and the evening meal).

Clinical sketch

A 27-year-old man has been an insulin-dependent diabetic for the past 7 years. He is arrested by the police in the city centre one night, apparently confused and aggressive.

Comment: Hypoglycaemia is the most common adverse effect of insulin. The patient may be confused and aggressive or become rapidly unconscious. Failure to treat adequately can result in permanent brain damage or death. Knowledge of the previous history of diabetes mellitus in this patient gives the game away, but in any confused or unconscious patient, blood sugar should be checked as soon as possible.

Another popular regimen is a long-acting insulin once a day, supplemented around meal times with injections of soluble insulin, three times per day.

Many patients will monitor their blood glucose at home and make minor adjustments in dose accordingly.

Adverse effects

Hypoglycaemia is the most common and serious adverse effect; it is the result of an imbalance between glucose intake (e.g. missing a meal), glucose utilisation (e.g. unusual exercise) and insulin dose. The result is sympathetic activation (palpitations, anxiety and sweating) and neuroglycopenia (visual disturbance, drowsiness or aggression, coma). Treatment is by administration of carbohydrate orally to a conscious patient, or i.v. glucose or i.m. *glucagon* (a peptide hormone and physiological antagonist of insulin). Patients and their families should be trained to spot the warning signs and how to treat hypoglycaemia, including possibly administration of glucagon if the patient loses consciousness.

Lipodystrophy is the atrophy or hypertrophy of fat at the site of injection, less common with the newer insulin preparations.

Acute diabetic ketoacidosis may occur in newly diagnosed IDDM or may arise in IDDM if the insulin dose is inadequate for needs, e.g. during infection or other physiological stress. The patient will become seriously dehydrated, hyperglycaemic and acidotic. This is a serious condition and its treatment is described in Box 6.

Oral hypoglycaemic drugs

Sulfonylureas

The sulfonylureas stimulate release of endogenous insulin from the pancreas and so are only effective if the beta cells are functional. They may also have an extra-pancreatic effect in decreasing breakdown of insulin and increasing the density of insulin receptors on the cell, improving insulin sensitivity.

Glibenclamide is long acting (up to 24 hours) and is metabolised by the liver. *Gliclazide* (6–12 hours) and

It is important to carefully monitor the clinical state and serum biochemistry and to consider why the ketoacidosis might have occurred (e.g. infection, myocardial infarction, etc.). Treatment involves:

- rehydration: the fluid deficit may be as much as 5–12 litres
- insulin given as a slow i.v. infusion
- not usually necessary to treat the acidosis separately
- monitor serum K$^+$ level: may be high initially but supplementation needed as rehydration proceeds
- treat any underlying cause
- Beware of aspiration from gastric stasis.

tolbutamide (3–6 hours) are shorter acting and are more suitable for use in elderly patients for this reason. All are metabolised by the liver.

Repaglinide is not chemically a sulfonylurea but it acts in a similar way. Its action is very rapid but short lived. It is used to minimise the postprandial surge in blood glucose and is taken once or twice a day with main meals.

Adverse effects

- Hypoglycaemia
- Gastrointestinal upsets
- Hypersensitivity: rashes etc.
- Weight gain: stimulation of appetite can be a problem in obese patients.

Drug interactions. Sulfonylureas are heavily protein bound and their actions may be increased by other drugs (e.g. sulfonamides) that compete for the binding sites.

Biguanides

The biguanides are orally active agents that do not require functioning beta cells. They act by increasing peripheral utilisation of glucose and decreasing absorption of glucose from the gastrointestinal tract and gluconeogenesis. They do not cause hypoglycaemia and are excreted unchanged by the kidney. *Metformin* is the only drug of this class in use.

Adverse effects

- Gastrointestinal upsets are common; nausea, vomiting and anorexia
- Lactic acidosis can occur if metformin is used in patients with coexisting liver or renal disease or congestive cardiac failure.

Glitazones

The glitazones are a new class of oral hypoglycaemic drug. They act by increasing cell sensitivity to insulin. They are used in combination with either a sulfonylurea or metformin when either of these alone is insufficient to control blood glucose. The long-term effects of these drugs are not yet known. Examples of glitazones are pioglitazone and rosiglitazone.

Adverse effects

- Hepatitis
- Weight gain
- Fluid retention and heart failure.

12.2 Thyroid disease

Hyperthyroidism

Excessive activity of the thyroid gland most often results from an autoimmune condition, **Graves' disease**, in which autoantibodies stimulate the thyroid cells. Graves' disease tends to undergo spontaneous remission in time, and treatment does not cure the condition but rather suppresses the hyperthyroidism until a remission occurs. Some patients will experience only one episode: about half will experience repeated episodes and may need a more definitive procedure such as radioactive iodine or surgery (Fig. 45).

Hyperthyroidism can also result (in older patients) from autonomous overactivity of a single toxic adenoma, or from a toxic multinodular goitre. In these cases,

A 58-year-old woman presents with weight loss, tremor and palpitations. She is diagnosed as hyperthyroid based on raised plasma thyroxin concentrations and low thyroid-stimulating hormone (TSH). She is treated initially with carbimazole for 6 months. This initially achieves control, but when the drug is withdrawn she relapses.

Comment: Grave's disease is an autoimmune cause of hyperthyroidism. Long courses of carbimazole (12 to 18 months) are often adequate to treat this. However, in an older patient, the more likely cause is a toxic nodule and although carbimazole will control the thyroid while it is taken, remission of the underlying disease is unlikely. This patient is likely to need radioiodine, surgery or long-term carbimazole.

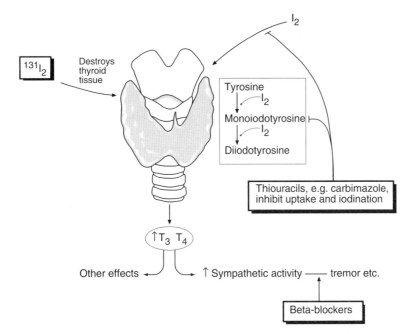

Fig. 45 Hyperthyroidism. T_4, thyroxine; T_3, triiodothyronine.

remission is less likely and long-term therapy or definitive procedure will probably be needed.

High circulating concentrations of thyroxine:

- suppress the release of thyroid-stimulating hormone (TSH) from the pituitary.
- increase metabolism: causing weight loss, anxiety, tremor, palpitations and diarrhoea.

In the elderly, these symptoms may be less clear and hyperthyroidism more difficult to diagnose.

Thyroid crisis

Thyroid crisis is severe sudden hyperthyroidism perhaps precipitated by physiological stress, surgery, etc. It comprises fever, tachycardia, dehydration and encephalopathy. Treatment is given in Box 7.

Box 7 Treatment of thyroid crisis

Symptoms:
- fever
- tachycardia
- dehydration
- encephalopathy.

Treatment:
- i.v. fluids
- beta-blockers
- iodine solution
- corticosteroids
- carbimazole or propylthiouracil.

Drugs used to treat hyperthyroidism

Thiouracils

The thiouracils inhibit the formation of thyroxine by inhibiting the uptake of iodine by the thyroid, the iodination of tyrosine and the coupling of iodinated tyrosine to form thyroxine (Fig. 45).

Carbimazole may have additional properties, influencing the immunological disorders in Graves' disease and increasing the likelihood of remission. Carbimazole is metabolised to methimazole (which is used widely to treat hyperthyroidism in the USA and Europe). If it is given to pregnant women, carbimazole can cross the placenta and can result in fetal hyperthyroidism or goitre.

Carbimazole is given in high doses initially until the patient becomes euthyroid (usually 4–8 weeks) then gradually reduced over 12 months, while monitoring symptoms and thyroid function tests. Repeated courses or continuous therapy will be necessary in some patients.

Some endocrinologists combine thyroxine with carbimazole once the patient is euthyroid (blocking-replacement regimen), which may achieve better results than with carbimazole alone.

Adverse effects

- **Neutropenia.** Carbimazole may cause neutropenia which, if treatment is not stopped, may develop into full agranulocytosis. This may arise suddenly, and patients must be carefully warned to report any evidence of infection, such as a sore throat, immediately. A full blood count should then be checked straightaway and if there is any evidence of neutropenia, the carbimazole should be withdrawn.

- Allergy with rash and fever can occur.
- Hepatitis and arthralgia may rarely occur.

Propylthiouracil is similar to carbimazole but is less likely to cause agranulocytosis.

Non-specific beta-blockers

Non-specific beta-blockers, such as *propranolol* (Ch. 3) are usually given (if there are no contraindications) to improve many of the sympathetically mediated symptoms at the start of treatment before the thiouracils have reached their full effect.

Potassium iodide or iodine solution

Paradoxically, iodide/iodine causes an immediate reduction in the plasma thyroid hormone concentrations, as well as inhibiting thyroxine formation. The vascularity of the gland is also decreased. The effect is transient, lasting only 3–4 weeks, but is valuable in managing patients awaiting thyroid surgery or in thyroid crisis (see below).

Radioactive iodine

Isotopic ^{131}I is well absorbed and concentrated in the thyroid where it causes permanent damage to the hormone-producing tissue. A single oral dose is usually effective. Standard antithyroid therapy is used before and after ^{131}I administration since ^{131}I takes 4–6 weeks to work. Radioactive iodine is used in patients who have failed to respond to medical therapy or who have relapsed, or increasingly as first-line therapy for hyperthyroidism, especially in the elderly.

There is a very high incidence of hypothyroidism subsequently, but treating hypothyroidism is easier than treating hyperthyroidism. There is no evidence of any risk of later malignancy or of genetic damage.

Hypothyroidism

Hypothyroidism may result from autoimmune thyroiditis (Hashimoto's), thyroidectomy, radioiodine treatment or, in some parts of the world, from iodine deficiency. Rarely, it may be part of hypopituitarism.

The patient is most often elderly and female and may have:

- tiredness and lethargy
- coarsening of the skin and hair
- bradycardia
- constipation
- menorrhagia
- slowing of the tendon reflexes.

The concentration of free thyroxine in the blood is reduced, while that of thyroid-stimulating hormone from the pituitary is usually greatly increased.

Drugs used to treat hypothyroidism

Treatment is by levothyroxine, given orally. The dose is adjusted according to patient symptoms and in response to the concentration of thyroid-stimulating hormone, which should be maintained within the low normal range.

Adverse effects

The adverse effects are those of overdose, mimicking hyperthyroidism.

In patients with ischaemic heart disease, levothyroxine should be started in a low dose and should be increased very slowly; otherwise, an attack of angina or a myocardial infarction may be precipitated.

12.3 Corticosteroids

Learning objectives

You should:

- be able to describe the uses of glucocorticoid and mineralocorticoid drugs as replacement and as therapy and know their adverse effects
- be able to name examples of the major glucocorticoids and mineralocorticoids used.

Corticosteroids are hormones produced in the cortex of the adrenal gland: they may be broadly defined as **glucocorticoids** (major effect on inflammation and glucose metabolism) or **mineralocorticoids** (major effect on Na^+/K^+).

Glucocorticoids. the natural glucocorticoid is hydrocortisone (cortisol), produced under the control of the hypothalamus, which secretes corticotrophin-releasing factor to stimulate the pituitary to secrete **adrenocorticotrophic hormone** (ACTH). This is termed the hypothalamic–pituitary–adrenal (HPA) axis (Fig. 46).

Mineralocorticoids. Although hydrocortisone has some mineralocorticoid effects, the major natural mineralocorticoid is **aldosterone**, produced in response to the renin–angiotensin–aldosterone (RAA) axis (see Ch. 3).

These hormones or synthetic derivatives can be given as drugs. These are powerful drugs with serious adverse effects and should be reserved for conditions where replacement is necessary, where other drugs have failed or where the illness is so severe that the benefits of treatment outweigh the risks. Corticosteroid drugs often show a mixture of both glucocotricoid and mineralocorticoid activity.

Glucocorticoids

Glucocorticoids bind to receptors in the cytoplasm. The complex is transported into the cell nucleus, where it

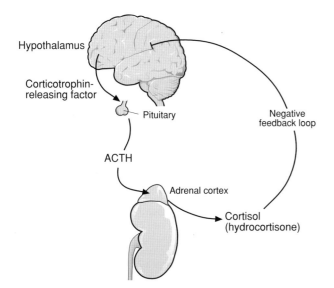

Fig. 46 The hypothalamic–pituitary–adrenal axis. ACTH, adrenocorticotrophic hormone.

binds to steroid-responsive elements on DNA to encourage new protein synthesis. The protein produced may have several effects; the best described is **lipocortin**, which in turn inhibits phospholipase A_2 and hence the release of **arachidonic acid**. This decreases activity in the cyclo-oxygenase and lipo-oxygenase pathways of production of inflammatory mediators. Corticosteroids do not appear to act for 12–18 hours and their action lasts for 24–48 hours after they are stopped.

Roles of glucocorticoids

1. Glucocorticoids are released in times of physiological stress. If absent, the patient may experience an Addisonian crisis, with hypotension, shock and death, when faced with physiological stress such as infection, etc.
2. Glucocorticoids are important in carbohydrate and protein metabolism; they promote gluconeogenesis, the formation of glycogen in the liver. Peripheral utilisation of glucose is decreased and the blood glucose may increase. Protein catabolism is increased, breaking down muscle and the matrix of bone.

Therapeutic uses

- Replacement therapy. In patients with adrenocortical insufficiency either caused by disease of the adrenal gland (autoimmune, Addison's disease), destruction or removal of the gland or pituitary failure.
- Anti-inflammatory effect. Glucocorticoids may be used (systemically or topically) to reduce inflammation in many conditions (e.g. asthma,

Clinical sketch

A 26-year-old woman presents with acute ulcerative colitis with rectal bleeding and extensive mucus production and diarrhoea.

Comment: Immediate treatment of such a patient includes supportive therapy (i.v. fluids, transfusion, etc. as required) and immunosuppression with corticosteroids. These will be administered systematically initially, but as the patient improves may change to topical application in the form of enemas. Topical application limits (but does not prevent) systematic exposure and reduces the risk of systemic side effects.

inflammatory bowel disease, eczema and other skin conditions, glomerulonephritis, treatment of hypersensitivity, arteritis). They are usually started at high doses and then reduced to the lowest level at which disease activity is suppressed, or withdrawn altogether if possible. Wherever possible, topical treatment is preferable to systemic so that adverse effects are minimised.

- Chemotherapy. Glucocorticoids are also used as part of chemotherapy for acute leukaemias and Hodgkin's lymphoma (see Ch. 15).

Glucocorticoid drugs

Glucocorticoids are well absorbed after oral administration and broken down by liver metabolism. Because of the time to achieve any clinical effect, the use of i.v. rather than oral glucocorticoids is often unnecessary.

Hydrocortisone is used orally in low doses (20–30 mg/day) for replacement therapy in adrenal insufficiency. It is used in high doses (400–1200 mg/day) parenterally to treat severe acute allergy or asthma or in inflammatory bowel disease. It is used topically as enemas in inflammatory bowel disease and as creams in skin conditions such as eczema.

Prednisolone is about five times more potent than hydrocortisone as a glucocorticoid but has less mineralocorticoid action. It is used orally for acute asthma, hypersensitivity or other serious systemic inflammatory conditions (40–60 mg/day initially, reducing to 5–10 mg/day for maintenance).

Methylprednisolone is a derivative of prednisolone that can also be given parenterally and is used especially in treating transplant rejection.

Dexamethasone is about 20 times more potent than hydrocortisone but with little mineralocorticoid effect. It is given orally or parenterally for its anti-inflammatory effects, particularly in the treatment of cerebral oedema.

Beclometasone and budesonide are very potent glucocorticoids used topically by inhalation to treat asthma (Ch. 10). Many other potent fluorinated glucocorticoids are used in skin conditions.

Tetracosactrin, a synthetic analogue of ACTH, was used by injection in the hope that the adrenals would not be suppressed: in practice, this advantage was slight and the clinical response to tetracosactrin was so variable that this has been largely abandoned. It is used in tests of pituitary–adrenal function.

Mineralocorticoids

Mineralocorticoids affect Na$^+$ balance and cause Na$^+$ and water retention and increase Na$^+$ reuptake in the distal tubule in exchange for K$^+$.

Aldosterone is not used therapeutically. An analogue, *fludrocortisone*, is used in replacement therapy for patients with adrenal insufficiency. It has effectively no glucocorticoid activity.

Adverse effects of corticosteroids

The adverse effects of corticosteroids (Fig. 47) are serious and common in clinical use. The frequency of adverse effects is related to the dosage, duration of use and relative glucocorticoid/mineralocorticoid effects, e.g. hydrocortisone will have few adverse effects when used in low doses for replacement therapy but will have both glucocorticoid and mineralocorticoid adverse effects when used in high doses. Dexamethasone, however, will have mostly glucocorticoid adverse effects. Topical therapy should be used wherever possible to minimise systemic adverse effects.

Clinical sketch

A 66-year-old man has chronic constructive pulmonary disease. He has been treated with a range of medication including oral corticosteroids for many years. He presents with sudden onset of severe back pain. On examination, he is centrally obese with high blood pressure and bruising of the skin.

Comment: This patient demonstrates many of the adverse effects of long-term corticosteroids. The immediate diagnosis is probably a crush vertebra owing to osteoporosis caused by the corticosteroids. The other manifestations are the hypertension, the truncal obesity and easy bruising. The risks and benefits of long-term corticosteroid therapy need to be weighed carefully. Any patient on more than 7.5 mg prednisolone or equivalent for 6 months should have their bone mineral density monitored and if appropriate should receive bisphosphonate therapy.

Glucocorticoid adverse effects

- Impaired glucose tolerance or sometimes diabetes mellitus
- Osteoporosis, especially of the vertebrae and in the elderly

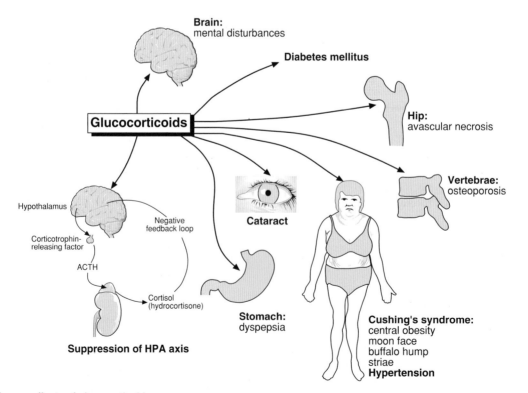

Fig. 47 Adverse effects of glucocorticoids.

- Cushing's syndrome, with characteristic appearance of moon face, buffalo hump, striae, as well as muscle wasting and thinning of the skin and poor healing
- Immune suppression: there may be reduced resistance to infections such as tuberculosis
- Growth suppression in children: the original disease state may be more relevant in causing growth suppression than the glucocorticoid
- Mental disturbances: euphoria, agitation or depression
- Cataract
- Striae and thinning of the skin: this may be a particular problem with topical use of potent glucocorticoids
- Dyspepsia: common; peptic ulceration may occur but whether this is caused by glucocorticoids is not certain
- Avascular necrosis of the hip
- Adrenal suppression: administering glucocorticoids suppresses the HPA axis; if used in high doses for prolonged periods, the adrenal glands may atrophy. This is also possible but less likely after topical use. To avoid this, it is important to use low doses for as short a time as possible.

Withdrawal of treatment after long-term glucocorticoid use. This must be gradual (perhaps over several months) to allow the HPA to recover. Otherwise the patient may experience an Addisonian crisis. Similarly, in patients who have received glucocorticoids for prolonged periods, adrenal insufficiency may occur during physiological stress, e.g. during surgery or after an accident. If such a reaction is suspected, an increased dose of hydrocortisone should be administered. All patients prescribed glucocorticoids should be warned of these dangers and should be issued with a 'steroid card', giving details of dosage and possible complications.

Mineralocorticoid adverse effects

- Sodium and water retention, leading to hypertension.
- Hypokalaemia.

12.4 The reproductive steroids

Learning objectives

You should:

- be able to describe the use of combined and progestogen only contraceptives
- know the adverse effects and contraindications of each type of drug used, and give examples
- be able to describe the problems that may occur as a result of the menopause
- be able to describe the use of hormone replacement therapy and the drugs used (including the selective oestrogen receptor modulators)

The steroid hormones of the reproductive system are of three broad types:

- oestrogens, produced by the ovary and also in adipose tissue
- progesterone, also produced by the ovary
- testosterone, produced by the testis.

Contraception and steroid hormones

The most common therapeutic use of the sex hormones is in oral contraceptives. These are of two types (Fig. 48):

- oestrogen–progestogen combinations (the combined pill)
- progestogen-only pill (minipill).

Oestrogen–progestogen combinations

These act by inhibiting ovulation. Oestrogen inhibits release of follicle-stimulating hormone (FSH) from the pituitary; progestogen blocks luteinising hormone (LH) release. Both are taken for 21 days and then stopped for 7 days before resuming the cycle. During the withdrawal period, there is uterine bleeding similar to menstruation. The tablet should be taken at the same time every day; if missed for more than 12 hours, the contraceptive effect may be lost. Therapy should be started on the first day of a cycle so as to provide contraceptive cover for that cycle; if started later, barrier contraceptives should also be used for that cycle. The failure rate is about 1 per 100 woman-years or less.

Examples

There are a wide variety of preparations available.

The oestrogen most commonly used is the synthetic *ethinylestradiol* in doses between 50 and 20 µg (the natural oestrogens undergo extensive first-pass metabolism and are unsuitable). Lower dose pills are now recognised as being as effective and have fewer adverse effects.

The progestogen is usually *norethisterone* or *levonorgestrel*. These are derivatives of nortestosterone and may have androgenic effects. Other progestogenes without androgenic effects are also used including gestodene and desogestril.

The synthetic steroids are all:

- absorbed well
- eliminated by conjugation with glucuronide
- excreted in bile.

There is enterohepatic circulation, i.e. the conjugated oestrogen is broken down in the gut by bacteria and the free oestrogen is reabsorbed.

Other uses

The combined pill is sometimes used for cycle regulation in women with dysmenorrhoea or dysfunctional uterine bleeding.

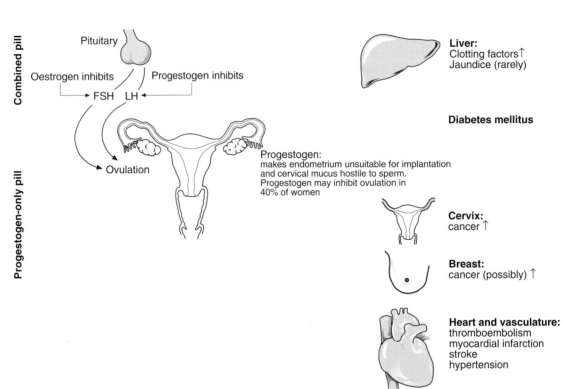

Action

Combined pill

Progestogen-only pill

Pituitary

Oestrogen inhibits   Progestogen inhibits

FSH   LH

Ovulation

Progestogen:
makes endometrium unsuitable for implantation
and cervical mucus hostile to sperm.
Progestogen may inhibit ovulation in
40% of women

Other effects

Liver:
Clotting factors↑
Jaundice (rarely)

Diabetes mellitus

Cervix:
cancer ↑

Breast:
cancer (possibly) ↑

Heart and vasculature:
thromboembolism
myocardial infarction
stroke
hypertension

Fig. 48 Action of the combined and progestogen-only oral contraceptives.

Clinical sketch

A 22-year-old woman wishes to go on the combined oral contraceptive. There is a family history of thromboembolic disorders in that her mother died from a pulmonary embolus postoperatively.

Comment: The risk of thromboembolic disorders is increased in women taking combined oral contraceptives by a factor of 3 or more. This is even higher in women who have a familial predisposition to thromboembolic disorders, possibly as a result of mutations in factor V or antithrombin III. It might be wise to screen this patient for such predispositions before initiating a combined oral contraceptive. There are alternatives available such as progestogen-based pills, implants or IUDs (intrauterine devices) which do not carry an increased risk of thromboembolic disorders.

Adverse effects

The most serious adverse effects involve the cardiovascular system.

- Venous thromboembolic disease, i.e. deep venous thrombosis or pulmonary embolism. The risk is approximately trebled by the combined pill to approximately 15/100 000 women-years

— more common with the higher oestrogen dose pills initially used and caused by a decrease in antithrombin III production and increase in fibrinogen production by the liver; this may be a particular risk around the time of surgery, and women having elective operations should discontinue the combined pill for 4 weeks before the operation and for 2 weeks after

— also more common with use of the newer progestogens, e.g. *gestodene* and *desogestrel*: about 25/100 000 women-years.

- Myocardial infarction and stroke: these are more common with higher oestrogen dose pills, in older women (>35 years), and smokers, probably because of the alteration of clotting factors and increased platelet aggregation.

- Hypertension: many women will experience a slight rise in blood pressure of little significance. In about 5–10%, the rise is greater and withdrawal of the combined pill may be necessary.

Other adverse effects are:

- malignant disease: the combined pill protects against endometrial and ovarian malignancy but is associated with an increased risk of cervical carcinoma and possibly breast carcinoma

- glucose intolerance and diabetes
- headache
- menstrual irregularity in the first months of treatment
- chloasma
- cholestatic jaundice, hepatic tumours: rarely.

Contraindications to the combined pill

- History of thromboembolic disease
- Liver disease
- Undiagnosed vaginal bleeding
- Hyperlipidaemia
- Breast, endometrial or hepatic carcinoma.

Use with caution

- Diabetes mellitus
- Smokers
- Older patients (aged over 35 years)
- Hypertensives
- Migraine sufferers.

The progestogen-only pill

The progestogen-only pill works by altering the cervical mucus and the endometrium so that fertilisation or subsequent implantation is unlikely. Ovulation is also inhibited in about 40% of women. The failure rate is higher than with the combined pill (about 2/100 woman-years) but it may be more suitable for patients with contraindications to estrogens.

The tablets are taken constantly with no breaks. They should be taken at the same time every day: if there is delay for more than 3 hours, the contraceptive effect may be lost.

Examples

The progestogens used are the same as in the combined pill, but in a lower dose, e.g. in the combined pill, *norethisterone* may be given in doses of 500–1000 µg/day while in progestogen-only pills, the dose is 350 µg/day.

Medroxyprogesterone is a depot progestogen given by injection: a single dose may provide contraception for 3 months. Levonorgestrel-releasing silastic rods are available, providing protection for up to 3 years. Levonorgestrel-releasing intrauterine devices provide very effective contraception for up to 5 years, reduce uterine bleeding and avoid systemic adverse effects.

Adverse effects of progestogens

- Menstrual irregularities
- Nausea and vomiting
- Breast discomfort.

Drug interactions

Drug interactions may be very important for both the combined and the progestogen-only pills as an unwanted pregnancy may occur. Enzyme inducers (see Ch. 1) decrease the action of the combined pill, as do some broad-spectrum antibiotics that interfere with enterohepatic circulation, e.g. amoxicillin.

Postcoital contraception

High doses of the combined pill can be given for two doses as a contraceptive for up to 72 hours after unprotected intercourse. Two doses of oral levonorgestrel are slightly more effective and cause fewer side effects. The earlier these are used, the more effective they are.

Dysfunctional uterine bleeding

The combined pill is sometimes used for cycle regulation in women with dysmenorrhoea or dysfunctional uterine bleeding.

Tranexamic acid reduces blood loss (see Ch. 5).

Danazol inhibits the release of pituitary gonadotrophins and is antiestrogen, antiandrogen and antiprogestogen. It is used to treat endometriosis and menorrhagia.

Adverse effects include gastrointestinal upsets and virilisation.

In severe cases of endometriosis, luteinising hormone-releasing hormone (LHRH) analogues may be used (see below).

Hormone replacement therapy

The menopause occurs at widely varying ages with a mean of 53 years. It is ovarian failure resulting in a fall in serum oestrogen levels and increased release of FSH/LH.

Clinical sketch

A 56-year-old woman presents to her GP complaining of hot flushes and vaginal dryness. It is 18 months since her last period. She is concerned about osteoporosis since she thinks she is menopausal.

Comment: The patient is probably menopausal, based on the symptoms and her age. It would be reasonable to prescribe hormone replacement therapy (HRT) for a period of 12 to 18 months to relieve her menopausal symptoms. However, if she is to be protected from osteoporosis she will need much longer therapy than this, at least 5 years. To achieve significant protection against hip fracture at its most common age in the early 80s, much longer than that is required. The patient should be given general lifestyle advice about what she can do to reduce her risk of osteoporosis, e.g. reducing smoking, increasing vitamin D and calcium intake and exercise in addition to considering long-term HRT. The benefits of long-term HRT need to be weighed against its possible disadvantages such as a possible increase in the risk of breast cancer.

The loss of sex hormone-dependent bone production hastens osteoporosis and there also is an increased risk of cardiovascular disease.

The main symptoms are vasomotor: not flushes, vaginal dryness. The use of hormone replacement therapy (HRT):

- treats symptoms (treatment needed for 6–12 months)
- avoids osteoporosis (treatment needed for 5–10 years or longer)
- May reduce cardiovascular disease (unproven as yet); overall, ischaemic heart disease is reduced compared with women not taking HRT but this may be a result of women with less risk of heart disease selectively receiving HRT.

Treatment

HRT is given as once daily oral doses, e.g. *conjugated equine oestrogens* or *oestradiol*.

Progestogens are unnecessary in women who have had a hysterectomy.

In women whose major problem is vaginal dryness, an estrogen cream applied to the affected area intermittently may be more appropriate than systemic therapy.

Adverse effects

- Increase in the risk of endometrial carcinoma: this can be avoided by giving progestogens in addition to the oestrogen for 10–12 days in every 28. This will cause a withdrawal bleed. Alternatively, continuous progestogen can be given — this usually results in amenorrhoea
- A probable increase in the risk of breast cancer in women who use long-term HRT (by 10–30%)
- Increased risk of thromboembolic disorders (despite the low dose of oestrogen used)
- Other oestrogen related effects as described above.

Contraindications

Contraindications to HRT are fewer than to the use of higher-dose oestrogens as contraceptives:

- thromboembolic disorders
- liver disease
- oestrogen-sensitive malignancy.

Hormone modulating therapy

Drugs that reduce the effects of oestrogens or progestogens in certain tissues are used in a number of indications: cancer, infertility, termination of pregnancy.

Selective oestrogen receptor modulators

The selective oe/estrogen receptor modulators (SERMs) have some oestrogen-like effects and some antioestrogen effects in different tissues. Examples are *tamoxifen*, *raloxifene*.

Tamoxifen

Breast cancer cells may have oestrogen receptors. Reducing oestrogen levels (by oophorectomy) is beneficial in about 60% of such cases, as well as in about 10% where oestrogen receptors are not identified.

Tamoxifen is an oestrogen receptor antagonist in breast tissue and is used to treat breast cancer. It may cause a response in about 30–40% of women. In other tissues, it has oestrogen-like activity: it can reduce osteoporosis, and stimulates the endometrium but is not used for these indications.

Adverse effects include hot flushes and gastrointestinal upsets. It may prevent development of breast cancer in high-risk patients

Raloxifene

Raloxifene has oestrogen-like activity in bones and is used to prevent osteoporosis but does not stimulate the endometrium. It may reduce the risk of breast cancer and possibly heart disease, though this is not yet proven. It does not treat menopausal symptoms. It may cause thromboembolic disease.

Other antioestrogens

Anastrozole prevents the formation of oestrogens from androgens in peripheral tissue by inhibiting aromatase enzymes. It is used in advanced breast cancer. *Aminoglutethimide* is a second-line therapy with similar effect. It also prevents the formation of hydrocortisone, which must be given with it to prevent an Addisonian crisis.

Luteinising hormone-releasing hormone and its analogues

LHRH is a peptide released in a pulsatile fashion by the hypothalamus. It stimulates LH release and hence oestrogen production in females or testosterone in males. LHRH analogues downregulate the LHRH receptors so that, after the initial surge of LH and oestrogen/testosterone, LH release falls off and oestrogen or testosterone fall to very low levels.

Long-acting analogues of LHRH (e.g. *goserelin*) can be given in slow-release depot injections to provide constant stimulation.

LHRH analogues are used to treat prostatic carcinoma and breast cancer. They are occasionally used for endometriosis.

Adverse effects include promotion of artificial menopause in male and female with secondary effects on bone etc. and tumour 'flush' on first administration in metastatic prostatic cancer.

Hormone modulation in infertility

Clomiphene

Clomiphene is an oestrogen antagonist at central receptors in the hypothalamus. By blocking these receptors, the normal negative feedback control on FSH and LH release is prevented. FSH/LH levels rise, stimulating ovulation and increasing the potential for fertilisation. The main adverse effect is the risk of overstimulation, and multiple pregnancy.

Gonadorelin

Gonadorelin is a synthetic LHRH given by intermittent injection to simulate pulsatile secretion to cause LH release in the treatment of infertility.

Hormone modulation in pregnancy or its termination

Oxytocin

Oxytocin is a peptide hormone from the posterior pituitary. It stimulates the uterus during labour. It is given i.v. to stimulate contractions during the active management of labour. It is given in combination with ergometrine i.m. during the third stage of labour to reduce the risk of postpartum haemorrhage.

Mifepristone

Mifepristone is a semisynthetic steroid used with prostaglandins to cause termination of pregnancy at up to 9 weeks. It acts as a progestogen antagonist, preventing endometrial maturation and increasing activity of the myometrium. The combination is effective in 95% of patients but may cause severe uterine pain and hypotension. The use of mifepristone is currently closely regulated and is confined to approved clinics.

Prostaglandins

Prostaglandins have significant effects on the uterus causing vasoconstriction and muscle contraction. *Dinoprostone* and *gemeprost* are used to cause abortion. *Carboprost* can be used to treat postpartum haemorrhage.

Androgens and antiandrogens

Testosterone is normally produced by the testis. Synthetic testosterone can be given in cases of deficiency: after orchidectomy or in primary deficiency states. In these patients, it will prevent osteoporosis and increase the libido. It is available as depot injections or as a patch, applied to skin.

Hormonal treatment of prostatic cancer

Prostatic cancer is treated using drugs or surgery to reduce the action of androgens:

- androgen production suppression
  - castration
  - Long-acting LHRH analogue (risk of tumour 'flare' when first used)
  - *flutamide*: blocks androgen formation probably by inhibiting androgen uptake or androgen binding to cytoplasmic/nuclear receptors; consequently it is a 'pure' antiandrogen with virtually no other hormonal effects

- testosterone receptor blocker: cyproterone
- combinations sometimes used
  - to prevent tumour flare
  - for long-term treatment in selected patients.

12.5 Other pituitary hormones

Learning objectives

You should:

- be able to list the major hormones produced by the pituitary gland
- be able to describe drugs used to replace or oppose them.

Antidiuretic hormone

Cranial diabetes insipidus (DI) is caused by a deficiency of antidiuretic hormone (ADH, also known as vasopressin). This is a peptide that is secreted from the posterior pituitary (cranial DI). It reduces the resorption of water in the renal collecting tubules and its absence leads to polyuria, polydipsia and dehydration with hypernatraemia.

Analogues of antidiuretic hormone

Treatment of deficiency of antidiuretic hormone is by synthetic analogues. *Desmopressin* is given as a nasal spray. The dose is adjusted according to effect. The major adverse effect is water intoxication if too much is used. *Arginine vasopressin* may be used parenterally. It may cause severe vasoconstriction and is used for this purpose in the treatment of bleeding from oesophageal varices.

Growth hormone disorders

Somatropin is a peptide analogue of human growth hormone. It is used parenterally in the treatment of short stature in growth hormone-deficient children and in growth hormone-deficient adults (e.g. after pituitary surgery).

Octreotide is a peptide analogue of somatostatin, a naturally occurring growth hormone antagonist. It is used to treat growth hormone excess in acromegaly and in gastrointestinal disease (Ch. 11).

Bromocriptine (dopamine agonist; see Ch. 6) can also be used to reduce secretion of growth hormone (and to reduce prolactin secretion in prolactinomas).

12.6 Calcium metabolism and osteoporosis

Learning objectives

You should:

- be able to describe the role of vitamin D in the metabolism of calcium in the body
- be able to describe the drugs used in the management of calcium and related bone disorders
- be able to describe the management of osteoporosis.

Vitamin D_2 (*ergocalciferol*, *calciferol*) is a fat-soluble vitamin that is formed in the skin on exposure to UV light. It may also be derived from the diet (dairy products). It is activated first in the liver and then in the kidney to 1,25-dihydroxycholecalciferol. It acts to:

- increase the serum Ca^{2+} by enhancing the absorption of Ca^{2+} from the gastrointestinal tract and the reabsorption of Ca^{2+} and phosphate from the renal tubule
- stimulate osteoclasts to increase bone turnover and release Ca^{2+}.

Deficiencies of vitamin D may be dietary (especially in vegetarians and the elderly) or be the result of malabsorption, liver disease or renal disease. The clinical result is **osteomalacia** (known in children as rickets).

Ergocalciferol

Ergocalciferol is used orally in vitamin D-deficiency states, malabsorption, liver and renal disease (in which very high doses may be required) and hypoparathyroidism. Its use in osteoporosis is controversial. 1α-*hydroxycholecalciferol* is a more potent analogue.

Adverse effects

Hypercalcaemia may occur; careful monitoring of serum Ca^{2+} is necessary.

Osteoporosis

Osteoporosis is the loss of trabecular bone, leading to weakening of bone and possible fractures. It can occur as an adverse effect of some drugs (e.g. corticosteroids, heparin) but more commonly is a result of age. Peak bone density occurs in the mid to late 20s; thereafter bone density declines. In women, sex hormone-dependent bone (approximately 15% of bone in vertebrae, hip, wrist) declines rapidly at the menopause. Women are, therefore, more vulnerable to osteoporosis than men. This may be avoided by oestrogen replacement. Other factors predisposing to osteoporosis are cigarette smoking, alcohol abuse and liver or renal disease. Weight-bearing exercise is protective.

Patients at high risk

- Elderly
- Women, especially if in early menopause
- Smokers
- Alcohol abusers
- Long-term steroid users (more than 7.5 mg prednisolone/day for 6 months).

Prevention

- Exercise, prevent any preventable risk factors
- Calcium intake and vitamin D: dietary intake often inadequate in the elderly; supplementation trials (approximately 1200 mg calcium in the form of calcium carbonate and 800 units ergocalciferol) show reduced risk of fracture
- HRT or raloxifene therapy in women.

Treatment of established osteoporosis

- Calcium/vitamin D
- HRT
- bisphosphonates.

Bisphosphonates

The bisphosphonates bind to hydroxyapatite crystals in bone and reduce the breakdown of bone. Some inhibit osteoclasts (break down bone) and osteoblasts (build up bone) (e.g. *etidronate*); others are just selective for osteoblasts (e.g. *alendronate*).

Bisphosphonates are used to treat:

- Paget's disease of the bones
- Hypercalcaemia of malignancy
- severe osteoporosis complicated by vertebral fractures
- Corticosteroid-induced osteoporosis (in combination with calcium salts).

Examples: *etidronate* (oral or i.v.), *pamidronate* (i.v. only), *clodronate* and *alendrate* (oral only).

Adverse effects

- Gastrointestinal upsets
- oesphageal ulceration (alendronate only)
- hypocalcaemia.

Some drugs also inhibit osteoblasts and fractures may occur. Etidronate is used intermittently in osteoporosis to avoid this.

Calcitonin

Calcitonin is a peptide secreted by the C cells of the thyroid that lowers serum Ca^{2+} by decreasing bone turnover and increasing excretion of Ca^{2+} through the kidneys. It is used to treat Paget's disease. Its adverse effects include flushing of the face and nausea.

Self-assessment: questions

Multiple choice questions

1. Drugs that may impair glucose tolerance include:
   a. Bendroflumethiazide
   b. Prednisolone
   c. Oral contraceptives
   d. Enalapril
   e. Benzylpenicillin

2. Carbimazole:
   a. Is a prodrug
   b. May cause hypothyroidism
   c. May cause thrombocytopenia
   d. Blocks iodine uptake in the gastrointestinal tract
   e. Treatment is rarely followed by relapse

3. In treating hyperthyroidism:
   a. High-dose potassium iodide is useful in the long-term treatment of hyperthyroidism
   b. Patients may be treated with ^{131}I while still taking carbimazole
   c. There is a high risk of hypothyroidism in patients treated with [131]I
   d. Hypothyroidism may be treated with dietary iodine supplements
   e. Treatment of hypothyroidism is best monitored by measuring serum thyroxine

4. Insulin:
   a. Is formed in the liver
   b. Insulin tends to increase body weight
   c. In patients treated with insulin, diet is unimportant
   d. Human insulin is more likely to cause hypoglycaemia than porcine insulin
   e. Good control of insulin-dependent diabetes mellitus (IDDM) results in a decreased risk of serious complications

5. The following statements are correct:
   a. IDDM is more common than non-insulin-dependent diabetes (NIDDM)
   b. Patients with IDDM should change their treatment only on the advice of their doctor
   c. Hypoglycaemia is the most common adverse effect of insulin
   d. Soluble insulin may be given i.v.
   e. In hypoglycaemia, high-dose, i.m. glucose should be given

6. The following statements are correct:
   a. In diabetic ketoacidosis, dehydration may be life theatening
   b. Acidosis always requires urgent treatment with i.v. sodium bicarbonate
   c. Crystalline insulin is used for its long duration of action
   d. Patients treated with insulin can monitor their own blood glucose
   e. Antibodies to insulin are more common with porcine than with human insulin

7. Concerning oral hypoglycaemics in NIDDM:
   a. Sulphonylureas can be used to treat a patient who has developed diabetes mellitus because of pancreatitis
   b. Chlorpropamide is appropriate for elderly patients
   c. Sulphonylureas are not the drug of choice in obese patients with NIDDM
   d. Metformin may cause lactic acidosis in some patients
   e. Hypoglycaemia is a common adverse effect of oral hypoglycaemic drugs

8. Concerning calcium metabolism:
   a. Vitamin D causes calcium resorption from the kidney
   b. Vitamin D can be manufactured in the body
   c. Vitamin D is found in fresh fruit and vegetables
   d. Vitamin D and Ca^{2+} are used to treat hypoparathyroidism
   e. Etidronate stabilises bone and reduces hypocalcaemia in malignant disease

9. Systemic glucocorticoids may cause:
   a. Psychosis
   b. Opportunistic infections
   c. Osteomalacia
   d. Suppression of the renin–angiotensin–aldosterone axis
   e. Skin changes

10. Corticosteroids:
    a. Hydrocortisone has no mineralocorticoid effects
    b. Glucocorticoids are potent anti-inflammatory drugs
    c. Hydrocortisone is a naturally occurring hormone
    d. Adrenocorticotrophic hormone (ACTH) is often used to treat inflammatory disease
    e. Aldosterone can be given to treat adrenal insufficiency

11. Diseases in which corticosteroids are used include:
    a. Addison's disease

b. Conn's syndrome
c. Asthma
d. Cellulitis
e. Lymphoma

12. In contraception:
    a. The combined oral contraceptive (COC) may cause ischaemic heart disease
    b. The failure rate for the progestogen-only pill is lower than for the COC
    c. The progestogens used in the COC may have androgenic effects
    d. Enterohepatic circulation of oestrogen occurs
    e. COC may be involved in a variety of drug interactions

13. In contraception:
    a. Low-dose oestrogen COCs are less likely to cause thromboembolic disease than older high-dose preparations
    b. COC should never be used in women over the age of 35
    c. COC decreases the risk of uterine carcinoma
    d. COC should not be used in women who smoke
    e. The progestogen-only pill is safe in women with a history of thromboembolic disease

14. Postmenopausal hormone replacement therapy:
    a. Is contraindicated in women with ischaemic heart disease
    b. If given to patients with a uterus, should include a progestogen as well as an oestrogen
    c. If given long term, may decrease the risks of osteoporosis
    d. Decreases the risks of breast cancer
    e. Should not be started for at least a year after the last period

Case history questions

Case history 1

A 28-year-old woman presents with hyperthyroidism caused by Graves' disease.

1. What treatment or treatments would be appropriate as first line?
2. What possible adverse effects of treatment must she be warned about?

While being treated for hyperthyroidism, she becomes pregnant.

3. What are the risks to the fetus?

She is treated for 12 months, but on stopping therapy, she quickly relapses.

4. What treatment options should be considered now?
5. What drugs may interfere with the interpretation of thyroid function tests?

Case history 2

An obese 68-year-old woman with hypertension complains of thirst and polyuria and is noted to have glycosuria. Blood sugar analysis confirms that she is diabetic.

1. What are the main lines of treatment to recommend to this woman?
2. What maintenance drug treatment should be considered first line?
3. If this fails, what should be second line?
4. What drugs may have precipitated her diabetes?
5. When might insulin therapy be considered in such a patient?

Case history 3

A 25-year-old man presents with a 3-day history of vomiting, polyuria and thirst. There is no previous history. Urinalysis shows glycosuria and ketonuria, and blood glucose is high.

1. What is the diagnosis?
2. What treatment should he be given?
3. How are insulins administered?

He is treated for diabetes mellitus over the next 3 years. However, one day he is found unconscious.

4. What diagnosis should be considered first?
5. How should he now be treated?

Case history 4

A 58-year-old woman is given high-dose prednisolone for several months because of giant cell arteritis, an inflammatory disease. Her condition responds well to this.

1. What problems may arise if her prednisolone is suddenly stopped?

2. She complains of swollen ankles: why might this be?
3. What musculoskeletal changes might she experience?
4. What other adverse effects might she experience?

> She fractures her hip in a fall and requires surgery.

5. What complications might she suffer because of her therapy around the time of operation?

Case history 5

> A 19-year-old woman wishes to go on an oral contraceptive.

1. She is worried because she has heard that the combined oral contraceptive (COC) pill can cause cancer: what can you tell her?
2. She smokes: is this a particular problem?

> She is started on a combined oestrogen-progestogen pill: she telephones you 6 months later to say that she forgot to take her pill yesterday and to ask what she should do.

3. What is your advice?

> She complains of pleuritic chest pain 6 months later again.

4. What drug-related diagnosis should be considered?

> She later develops epilepsy and is treated with carbamazepine; she wishes to continue using an oral contraceptive.

5. Are there any problems with this?

Case history 6

> A 50-year-old woman develops irregular periods. She complains of hot flushes, about 3 months after her last period, as well as feeling tired and irritable. She asks whether she should have hormone replacement therapy (HRT).

1. What are the likely benefits to this patient of short-term (6 months) treatment with HRT?

2. She asks about osteoporosis, since there is a family history of fractured hips; what should you tell her about this and HRT?
3. There is also a strong family history of ischaemic heart disease. Would you expect HRT to increase or decrease the risks of this?
4. Are doses of oestrogen in HRT higher than in combined oral contraceptives?
5. She is concerned particularly about vaginal dryness. Will HRT help this?

Short note questions

Write short notes on:

1. The adverse effects of corticosteroids
2. The management of hyperthyroidism
3. Insulin regimens in the treatment of insulin-dependent diabetes mellitus
4. The treatment of established osteoporosis

Extended matching items question

Theme: endocrinology
Options

A. Ethinylestradiol
B. Gestodene
C. Flutamide
D. Levonorgestrel
E. Hydrocortisone
F. Aldosterone
G. Testosterone
H. Tamoxifen
I. Estradiol
J. Clomiphene
K. Goserelin
L. Finasteride

For each of the requirements in 1–8, choose the most appropriate option from A–L. Each option may be used once, more than once or not at all.

1. An oestrogen used in postmenopausal hormone replacement therapy.
2. A drug to decrease oestrogen production.
3. A drug with mineralocorticoid effect.
4. A drug used in contraceptive implants and intrauterine devices.
5. A drug used as an oestrogen antagonist in the treatment of breast cancer.
6. A drug used as an oestrogen in combined oral contraceptives.
7. A drug used as a progestogen in combined oral contraceptives.
8. A drug used to treat benign prostatic hypertrophy.

Self-assessment: answers

Multiple choice answers

1. a. **True**. This is a thiazide diuretic.
   b. **True**. Glucocorticoids cause a rise in blood glucose by several mechanisms.
   c. **True**. But not usually clinically significant.
   d. **False**. ACE inhibitors may even increase insulin sensitivity.
   e. **False**. No effect on the pancreas or peripheral cells.

2. a. **True**. Converted to thiamazole.
   b. **True**. If used in high doses for prolonged periods.
   c. **False**. May cause agranulocytosis.
   d. **False**. Blocks iodine uptake by the thyroid gland.
   e. **False**. Carbimazole does not reverse the underlying cause and relapse is common.

3. a. **False**. Short-term use only.
   b. **False**. Carbimazole would impede uptake of ^{131}I into the thyroid. The patient should be off carbimazole for several days beforehand.
   c. **True**. Whether caused by the ^{131}I or the natural history of the condition.
   d. **False**. Thyroxine is needed.
   e. **False**. Thyroid-stimulating hormone is the best measure.

4. a. **False**. Insulin is formed in the pancreas.
   b. **True**. Insulin tends to stimulate appetite.
   c. **False**. Diet is exceedingly important in all diabetics.
   d. **False**. There is no evidence of this.
   e. **True**. Although many patients even with poor control do not develop complications: there is still much to be understood about the cause of diabetic complications.

5. a. **False**. NIDDM is far more common.
   b. **False**. Patients should be sufficiently knowledgeable about their condition to adjust their dose of insulin by themselves.
   c. **True**. This may be life threatening.
   d. **True**. This is the only insulin that may be given in any way other than subcutaneously.
   e. **False**. High concentrations of glucose are very hyperosmolar and severe tissue necrosis would be likely. Glucose should be given either orally or, if the patient is unconscious, i.v.

6. a. **True**. The extent of the dehydration is commonly underestimated.
   b. **False**. Acidosis usually corrects itself when dehydration and hyperglycaemia are treated.

   c. **True**. Often in combination with a short-acting insulin.
   d. **True**. And may adjust their dose of insulin accordingly.
   e. **True**. But with purified porcine insulins, this is of little clinical importance.

7. a. **False**. Because sulphonylureas depend mainly for their action on stimulating release of endogenous insulin.
   b. **False**. Its half-life is so long that it may accumulate and cause dangerous hypoglycaemia in the elderly.
   c. **True**. Because by stimulating insulin release they may increase the appetite. Metformin is the drug of choice.
   d. **True**. In patients with liver or renal disease.
   e. **True**. For the sulphonylureas.

8. a. **True**. One of its major actions.
   b. **True**. In the skin, vitamin D can be formed from cholesterol by the action of UV light.
   c. **False**. Milk and other dairy products are the best sources.
   d. **True**. Since the effect of hypoparathyroidism is hypocalcaemia.
   e. **True**. Its major use.

9. a. **True**. Usually depression, occasionally mania.
   b. **True**. Because of immune suppression.
   c. **False**. Osteoporosis, not osteomalacia.
   d. **False**. This axis is not dependent on corticotrophin-releasing factor or adrenocorticotrophic hormone.
   e. **True**. Striae and easy bruising.

10. a. **False**. Fluid retention is a common adverse effect of hydrocortisone.
    b. **True**. Their major use.
    c. **True**. Usually known as cortisol, for some reason.
    d. **False**. In the past, yes, but rarely used today.
    e. **False**. If mineralocorticoid replacement is needed, fludrocortisone is used.

11. a. **True**. This is adrenocortical insufficiency.
    b. **False**. This is primary hyperaldosteronism caused by tumour-secreting aldosterone.
    c. **True**. Usually by inhalation.
    d. **False**. Might even exacerbate this by causing immune suppression.
    e. **True**. For Hodgkin's and some other types.

12. a. **True**. But less likely with low-dose estrogen types used today.

b. **False**. About 2/100 as opposed to 1/100 for the COC.

c. **True**. Some are testosterone derivatives, such as norethisterone or levonorgestrel. This is less likely for desogestrel or gestodene.

d. **True**. Important for its action.

e. **True**. With enzyme inducers and broad-spectrum antibiotics for instance.

13. a. **True**. Hence their widespread use today, while the high-dose pills are reserved for special circumstances.

b. **False**. However, the risks are undoubtedly increased, and other risk factors should be considered before using them in older women.

c. **True**. But may increase the risk of cervical and possibly breast cancer.

d. **False**. Although again the risk is increased and women should be warned against smoking, particularly in combination with other risk factors.

e. **True**. Although this is still mentioned as a contraindication in the data sheets of most of these drugs.

14. a. **False**. Probably even decreases risk of progression of ischaemic heart disease.

b. **True**. Otherwise there is a risk of endometrial carcinoma.

c. **True**. But therapy for 5–10 years is needed.

d. **False**. May increase the risks of breast cancer (controversial).

e. **False**. Vasomotor symptoms may start even before the last period and may be treated.

Case history answers

Case history 1

1. Carbimazole (perhaps with thyroxine added at a later stage when euthyroid again) and a non-specific beta-blocker (if not contraindicated).

2. The risks of agranulocytosis on carbimazole: she must be warned to return immediately if she develops any signs of infection, such as a sore throat, so that her white cell count can be checked.

3. The antibodies that cause hyperthyroidism in Graves' disease can cross the placenta and cause neonatal hyperthyroidism: carbimazole may cause a goitre in a fetus and this may lead to complications in the delivery.

4. The options are long-term carbimazole, surgery or radioiodine (even in someone so young, this is a safe treatment).

5. Oral contraceptives increase production of thyroid-binding globulin, giving rise to increased serum total thyroxine concentrations (but not free thyroxine or thyroid-stimulating hormone, which remain normal). Some heavily protein-bound drugs (such as phenytoin) can cause displacement of thyroxine from protein-binding sites and lower total (but not free) thyroxine.

Case history 2

1. Weight loss, diet and perhaps oral hypoglycaemics. She should be educated about life-style, smoking, etc.

2. Metformin is most appropriate in an obese patient.

3. Sulphonylureas might be considered second line, in addition to metformin. They should probably not be used alone, if avoidable, in an obese patient since they tend to stimulate the appetite.

4. Since she is hypertensive, thiazide diuretics might have been a precipitant; many other drugs, e.g. corticosteroids, are also possible. However, hypertension and diabetes are associated even in the absence of drug therapy.

5. Insulin should be considered if oral drugs fail to control her blood sugar, or during periods of intercurrent illness (e.g. infections etc.) or surgery, when her diabetes is likely to go out of control.

Case history 3

1. Diabetic ketoacidosis.

2. Intravenous fluids to rehydrate, i.v. insulin to lower the blood sugar and K^+ supplements as appropriate, depending on the serum K^+. The precipitating cause should be identified and treated where possible.

3. Soluble insulin may be given i.v., i.m. or s.c.; all others are given s.c. only. In the future, insulin by inhaler may be available.

4. Hypoglycaemia.

5. He should be treated without delay, even if the diagnosis cannot be immediately confirmed: i.v. glucose can be given by trained staff, but in the absence of these, i.m. glucagon can be given by someone with very little training.

Case history 4

1. She might experience an Addisonian crisis with hypotension, collapse and death, since her hypothalamic–pituitary–adrenal axis is almost certainly suppressed and will need some time to recover. She might also experience a flare up of disease activity.

2. Prednisolone has some mineralocorticoid effects and will cause Na^+ and fluid retention.

3. She is at risk of osteoporosis and muscle wasting.

4. Impaired glucose tolerance, Cushingoid appearance, immune suppression are the most common.

5. Risk of an Addisonian crisis unless given additional parenteral steroids before operation; poor healing of wounds, which may delay recovery afterwards.

Case history 5

1. The COC protects against endometrial and ovarian carcinoma but is associated with an increased incidence of cervical carcinoma. This may be caused by life-style rather than a direct drug effect. There may also be an increase in the incidence of breast carcinoma, although this is controversial.
2. She is at higher risk of myocardial infarction or cerebrovascular accident while taking a COC and smoking: she should be advised to stop smoking. However, in a young woman this would not be a contraindication to the COC.
3. If she is less than 12 hours late, she should take the pill as soon as possible and the next pill at the usual time. If more than 12 hours late, the pill may be ineffective: she should continue taking the pill as usual, but use additional barrier contraceptive methods for the next 7 days. If there were less than seven tablets left in the pack, she should begin the next pack without the usual 7-day break.
4. Pulmonary embolism.
5. Carbamazepine may induce liver enzymes and reduce the efficacy of the COC. She may need a high-oestrogen dose pill.

Case history 6

1. Improvement in vasomotor and other symptoms of the menopause: no prophylactic effects can be anticipated in such short-term therapy.
2. Osteoporosis is common in women as there is increased bone loss after the menopause. HRT given for periods of 5–10 years reduces this—but there are concerns that there may be an increased bone loss when HRT is stopped.
3. HRT probably decreases the risks of ischaemic heart disease.
4. The doses of oestrogen used in HRT are lower than in COC and, therefore, fewer adverse effects are to be expected.
5. Systemic HRT will improve vaginal dryness, but if this is the predominant symptom, the patient may prefer to use just a local vaginal oestrogen ointment.

Short note answers

1. This should include hypertension, impaired glucose tolerance and possibly diabetes mellitus. Also cover skin changes, truncal obesity, immunosuppression, mental disturbances, cataract and suppression of the hypothalamic–pituitary–adrenal axis and the potential problems that may arise if the steroid is withdrawn suddenly.
2. This should include drugs such as carbimazole and propylthiouracil, including their possible adverse effects, and also discuss the role of surgery and radioiodine in long-term treatment of resistant disease.
3. This should consider the use of a long-acting insulin once or twice a day with short-acting insulin twice or more times a day, in particular to cover mealtimes (expand on this a little bit).
4. This should include consideration of:
a. vitamin D and calcium
b. bisphosphonates if the patient is high risk and has demonstrated this, for instance by having an osteoporotic-related fracture
c. hormone-replacement therapy in women or use of selective oestrogen receptor modulator. Calcium and vitamin D can be considered for all patients, bisphosphonates for the high-risk patients and HRT or SERM for female patients who have other indications for these therapies as well.

Extended matching items answer

1. I. Oestradiol, a naturally occurring oestrogen, is the most commonly used. Synthetic oestrogens such as ethinylestradiol are avoided as it is thought that they might cause excessive stimulation of breast tissue.
2. K. Goserelin is a longacting LHRH analogue which decreases oestrogen (and testosterone) production by causing down-regulation and loss of sensitivity of LHRH receptors.
3. E. Hydrocortisone (aldosterone is a hormone and not a drug).
4. D. Levonorgestrel.
5. H. Tamoxifen is an oestrogen antagonist in breast tissue but an oestrogen agonist in some other areas such as bone and endometrium.
6. A. Ethinylestradiol, a synthetic oestrogen.
7. B or D. Levonorgestrel or gestodene are both used. Gestodene-containing pills are associated with an increased risk of thromboembolic disorders compared with pills containing the older progestogens such as levonorgestrel.
8. L. Finasteride inhibits formation of the active dihydrotestosterone and has antiandrogenic effects in the prostate (and some other tissues such as the scalp). Some other drugs named here (goserelin, flutamide) have antiandrogenic effects and are used in prostatic cancer but not in benign prostatic hypertrophy.

Antibiotics (antimicrobials)

Overview

Antibiotics are substances that kill or inhibit the growth of microorganisms. The first antibiotics were produced by and isolated from microorganisms but subsequently knowledge of these agents has been used to synthesise chemotherapeutic agents. Biochemical differences between the host and the pathogen have also been exploited to produce drugs with selective toxicity.

In this chapter the major antibiotics are described in terms of their mode of action, their therapeutic use and their adverse effects. The effect of microbial resistance to drugs is also covered. The antibiotic regimens used for tuberculosis and leprosy are also discussed.

13.1 Action and use of antibiotics

Learning objectives

You should:

- understand the broad principles governing use of antibiotics
- be able to describe the common mechanisms by which antimicrobials work
- know examples of an antibiotic working by each mechanism
- be able to outline mechanisms of microbial resistance to antibiotics and the implications of this for prescribing.

Antimicrobials are drugs used to treat infection. They may be:

- antibacterial (often called antibiotics, since many are derivatives of naturally produced chemicals)
- antiviral (Ch. 14)
- antifungal (Ch. 14)
- antiprotozoal (Ch. 14)
- anthelmintic (Ch. 14).

Antibiotics may either kill the microorganism (bactericidal) or may retard their growth (bacteriostatic) so that the body's own immune system can overcome the infection. In clinical use, this distinction is usually not important, but bacteriostatic drugs should not be used in

Clinical sketch

A patient presents with weight loss and fever, present for about 3 weeks. Examination reveals no clear cause of this and initial investigations including a chest radiograph are normal. The full blood count shows a slightly raised white cell count at 13×10^9/litre and the erythrocyte sedimentation rate (ESR) is raised at 52 mm/h. It is not clear what is wrong but the doctor prescribes broad-spectrum antibiotics.

Comment: This is bad practice. Patients such as this require investigation to identify the cause of the fever. The ESR and full blood count are non-specific markers of inflammation, most often caused by infection but a range of other causes are possible, such as malignancy or autoimmune disease. The prescription of broad-spectrum antibiotics will muddy the water and will delay diagnosis of the true cause. It might also lead to disastrous partial treatment of a condition such as infective endocarditis. A patient with a fever for this long requires investigation and a definitive diagnosis.

Clinical sketch

A 30-year-old patient who previously had rheumatic fever presents with fever, clubbing and splinter haemorrhages. The patient has the murmur of aortic incompetence. Blood cultures grow *Streptococcus viridans*.

Comment: This patient has infective endocarditis and will require intensive antibiotic therapy, typically (given the organism); with benzylpenicillin i.v. for 2 weeks, followed by oral amoxicillin for a further 2 weeks. For the first week, the patient might also be prescribed gentamicin, with monitoring of plasma concentrations. Infectious endocarditis is a serious illness, which will be fatal if not adequately treated.

immunosuppressed patients, nor in life-threatening diseases like endocarditis or meningitis.

Principles for prescribing antibiotics

Antibiotics are often abused, i.e. used excessively or inappropriately, for example to treat minor viral infections (especially in childhood). Broad principles for the use of antibiotics, therefore include:

1. Make a diagnosis of bacterial infection (fever alone does not always imply bacterial infection) and its site and consider the likely organisms, e.g. in lobar pneumonia, the likely organism is *Streptococcus pneumoniae*.
2. Wherever possible, and particularly in all serious infections, take appropriate specimens (blood, sputum, pus, urine, swabs) for culture and antibiotic sensitivity testing, and perhaps for microscopy and Gram staining. It is not always practical to do this.
3. Consider the need for antibiotic therapy at all, e.g. antibiotics are usually inappropriate in gastroenteritis or many skin infections.
4. If cultures have been taken, is there a need for urgent therapy before results are available? Empirical antibiotic therapy may be necessary in seriously ill patients but may prevent the confirmation of the diagnosis of infection later or the identification of the infecting organism. This may be particularly important when there is a subsequent failure to respond or only partial response to the chosen antibiotic.
5. Select the most appropriate drug, its dose and route of administration. Consider the following factors.

    a. The organism: what antibiotics is it sensitive to? This would ideally be based on microbiological sensitivity testing but may have to be a 'best guess' if the organism or its sensitivities are not known.
    b. The patient: age, allergy, renal or hepatic function, diminished resistance to infection (malnutrition, malignant disease, immunosuppression, including by drugs such as corticosteroids), pregnancy or genetic factors (may all influence choice of or response to antibiotics).
    c. The severity of the infection: this will influence the choice of drug and route of administration. Some antibiotics are not absorbed when given orally (e.g. aminoglycosides). In seriously ill patients, parenteral administration is more reliable.
    d. The site of infection: antibiotics often do not penetrate abscess cavities well, and abscesses in general require drainage in addition. Some antibiotics may not penetrate to the site of infection (e.g. aminoglycosides are inappropriate for meningitis).

    e. The presence of foreign bodies: such as a prosthetic heart valve or a piece of glass in a skin wound, again likely to diminish or prevent response to antibiotics.

6. Monitor success of therapy clinically, or microbiologically by repeated cultures as appropriate. Some antibiotics with serious concentration-related toxicity also require monitoring of plasma concentrations (e.g. gentamicin).
7. Combinations of antibiotics are occasionally used:

    a. where there is a mixed infection, e.g. in peritonitis
    b. where the two antibiotics can produce a greater effect than one alone (synergism), e.g. penicillin and gentamicin in treating infective endocarditis
    c. where the infecting organism is not known and broad-spectrum cover is required urgently, e.g. septicaemia
    d. to prevent the development of resistance to one antibiotic, e.g. in tuberculosis.

8. Antibiotics may also be used occasionally for prophylaxis, i.e. to prevent the development of infection rather than to treat established infection. Examples are in some abdominal or orthopaedic surgery, in dental procedures for patients at risk of infective endocarditis, or in the close contacts of patients who have meningococcal meningitis. The duration of prophylactic use is brief (usually 24 hours or less), and the choice of drug is based on previous experience of what organisms are likely.

Reasons not to use antibiotics without consideration:

- risk of missing alternative diagnosis
- adverse reactions
- promotion of antibiotic resistance
- expense.

Sites of action

Antibiotics may act at different sites (Fig. 49):

- by inhibiting formation of the bacterial cell wall, e.g. penicillin and cephalosporins
- by inhibiting bacterial protein synthesis, e.g. tetracyclines, aminoglycosides, erythromycin, chloramphenicol
- by inhibiting nucleic acid synthesis, either at an early stage, e.g. sulphonamides, trimethoprim, or later, e.g. ciprofloxacin, rifampicin
- by altering the permeability of cytoplasmic membranes, e.g. amphotericin (an antifungal, see Ch. 14).

Antimicrobial resistance

The increased use of an antibiotic encourages the emergence of resistant strains of bacteria. There are geographic variations in antibiotic resistance depending on local prescribing trends. For safe empirical therapy, it is important to know the local patterns of resistance and help should be sought from a microbiologist. The reasons for resistance vary. Some antibiotics would never affect an organism because of its structure and their site of action. For example, Gram-negative bacilli are resistant to benzylpenicillin.

Mechanisms of resistance

Some bacteria acquire resistance. These traits may arise as new mutations or may be transferred from organism to organism by plasmids (DNA packages) either by conjugation or transduction, or by bacteriophage viruses.

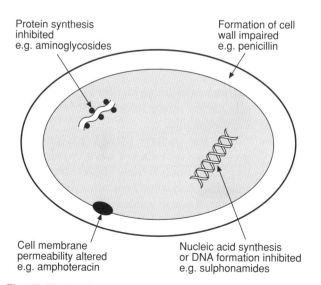

Protein synthesis inhibited e.g. aminoglycosides

Formation of cell wall impaired e.g. penicillin

Cell membrane permeability altered e.g. amphoteracin

Nucleic acid synthesis or DNA formation inhibited e.g. sulphonamides

Fig. 49 Modes of action of antibiotics.

Resistance can occur through a number of mechanisms:

- the production of an enzyme that breaks down the antibiotic, e.g. β-lactamase and many penicillins
- the cell membrane becomes impermeable to a drug, e.g. tetracyclines
- structural or biochemical alteration within the organism makes it less susceptible, e.g. alteration of ribosomal structure may lead to erythromycin resistance
- development of a pathway that bypasses the reaction inhibited by the antibiotic, e.g. a dihydrofolate reductase that is insensitive to trimethoprim inhibition.

13.2 Major antibiotics

Learning objectives

You should:

- be able to list the major classes of antibiotics, giving examples
- know their spectrum of activity
- know their adverse effects.

Antibacterial treatment

Choice of drug should be guided by a local formulary, as sensitivities and local policies may vary. Table 2 is a summary of typical first-line drugs that might be used to treat specific infections while awaiting culture and sensitivity results.

Table 2 Typical first-line drug therapy for infections while awaiting laboratory tests

Infection	First-line therapy
Respiratory tract	
Sore throat	Antibiotic not usually necessary
Tonsilitis	Phenoxymethylpenicillin or erythromycin
Sinusitis	Amoxicillin or erythromycin or doxycycline
Acute-on-chronic bronchitis	Amoxicillin or erythromycin
Pneumonia (healthy chest)	Amoxicillin and/or erythromycin
Pneumonia (COPD)	First-line amoxicillin and/or erythromycin; Second-line co-amoxiclav or oral cephalosporin or ciprofloxacin
Suspected 'atypical' pneumonia	Erythromycin
Tuberculosis	Rifampicin/isoniazid/pyrazinamide
Urinary tract	
Cystitis	Trimethoprim, nitrofurantoin
Pyelonephritis	Co-amoxiclav or ciprofloxacin
Pelvic inflammatory disease	Metronidazole and doxycycline, or co-amoxiclav
Skin	
Erysipelas	Amoxicillin
Cellulitis	Flucloxacillin (perhaps with amoxicillin)
CNS	
Meningitis	Initial blind therapy benzylpenicillin or cefotaxime
Abdominal sepsis	
Biliary tree	Injectable cephalosporin
Pseudomembranous colitis	Metronidazole or vancomycin orally
Peritonitis	Injectable cephalosporin and metronidazole
Endocarditis *Streptococcus viridans*	Benzylpenicillin with gentamicin
Streptococcus faecalis	Amoxicillin and gentamicin
Staphylococcus aureus or *S. epidermidis*	Flucloxacillin and gentamicin
Septicaemia	Injected cephalosporin or amoxicillin with gentamicin
Osteomyelitis	Flucloxacillin and fucidic acid

Penicillins

The penicillins contain a β-lactam ring and inhibit the formation of peptidoglycan cross-links in bacterial cell walls (especially in Gram-positive organisms). This weakens the cell wall and water enters the cell by osmosis, causing cells to burst. Penicillins are bactericidal but can act only on dividing cells and are not toxic to animal cells, which have no cell wall.

Pharmacokinetics
The penicillins are:

- poorly lipid soluble and do not cross the blood–brain barrier in appreciable concentrations unless it is inflamed (so they are effective in meningitis)
- actively excreted unchanged by tubular secretion in the kidney: this can be blocked by probenecid to potentiate penicillin's action and will require dose reduction in severe renal failure
- may be acid labile (i.e. broken down by the stomach acid and so inactive when given orally) or acid stable.

Resistance
Usually resistance is the result of production of β-lactamase in the bacteria, which destroys the β-lactam ring. It occurs in organisms such as *Staphylococcus aureus* (90% of strains), *Haemophilus influenzae* (15%), *S. pneumoniae* and *Neisseria gonorrhoea* (about 5–10%).

Examples
Benzylpenicillin (penicillin G) is acid labile and β-lactamase sensitive and is only given parenterally. It is the most potent penicillin but has a relatively narrow spectrum covering *Streptococcus pyogenes*, *S. pneumoniae*, *Neisseria meningitidis* or *N. gonorrhoea*, treponemes, *Listeria*, *Actinomyces* and many anaerobic organisms, e.g. *Clostridia* sp.

Phenoxymethylpenicillin (penicillin V) is acid stable and is given orally for minor infections; it is otherwise similar to benzylpenicillin.

Ampicillin is less active than benzylpenicillin against Gram-positive bacteria but has a broader spectrum including (in addition to those above) *Streptococcus faecalis*, *H. influenzae*, and some *Escherichia coli*, *Klebsiella* and *Proteus* strains. It is acid stable and is given orally or parenterally; it is β-lactamase sensitive.

Amoxicillin is similar but better absorbed orally. Amoxicillin is sometimes combined with *clavulanic acid*, which is a β-lactam with little antibacterial effect but which binds strongly to β-lactamase. It, therefore, blocks the action of β-lactamase and extends the spectrum of amoxicillin. The combination is called co-amoxiclav.

Flucloxacillin is acid stable and is given orally or parenterally. It is β-lactamase resistant and is used as a narrow spectrum drug for *S. aureus* infections.

Azlocillin is not acid stable and is only used parenterally. It is β-lactamase sensitive and has a broad spectrum, which includes *Pseudomonas aeruginosa* and *Proteus* species. It is used i.v. for life-threatening infections, especially in immunocompromised patients, in combination with an aminoglycoside.

Adverse effects

Adverse effects are relatively unusual.

- Allergy occurs in about 0.7% of patients, ranging from urticaria to potentially fatal anaphylaxis; patients should always be asked about a history of previous exposure and adverse effects.
  —rashes are common with ampicillin or amoxicillin (almost invariable if they are given in error to patients with infectious mononucleosis) and do not necessarily represent a true allergy.

  About 10% of patients have been told that they are allergic to penicillin. Allergy is generally overdiagnosed because of the potential serious effects of readministration and because usually there are alternative antibiotics—many patients with so called 'allergy' have had minor non-allergic adverse effects. However, it would be unwise to administer penicillin to any patient with a history of penicillin allergy, however uncertain.
- Superinfections (e.g. oral thrush caused by *Candida*).
- Diarrhoea: especially with ampicillin (20%), less common with amoxicillin, as it is better absorbed.
- Rare: blood dyscrasia or haemolysis; nephritis (ampicillin), hepatitis (co-amoxiclav, flucloxacillin).

Drug interactions

The use of ampicillin (or other broad-spectrum antibiotics) may decrease the effectiveness of oral contraceptives by diminishing enterohepatic circulation.

Cephalosporins

The cephalosporins also contain a β-lactam ring and are bactericidal. They are broad-spectrum antibiotics.

There are many different cephalosporins with varying side chains; these side chains alter the pharmacokinetics, spectrum of activity and β-lactamase resistance. Cephalosporins are relatively expensive and, although good alternatives to penicillins when a broad-spectrum drug is required, should not be used as first choice unless the organism is known to be sensitive. Some cephalosporins (e.g. cefotaxime) may be indicated for empirical use to treat life-threatening infections where the organism is probably sensitive.

Examples

Cefradine and cefalexin are well absorbed orally; cefradine can also be given parenterally. They are suitable for mostly Gram-positive organisms, such as *S. pyogenes*, *S. pneumoniae* and *S. aureus*, as well as some Gram-negative bacteria, although they are less effective in this than later cephalosporins. They are excreted by the kidney (reduce dose in renal failure).

Cefuroxime can be given parenterally or as an oral prodrug. It has a broader spectrum, including many Gram-negative bacilli.

Cefotaxime is given parenterally. It has an even broader spectrum, including many *Enterobacter*, *E. coli* and *Proteus* strains.

Adverse effects

- Allergy (10–20% of patients with penicillin allergy are also allergic to cephalosporins)
- Nephritis and acute renal failure
- Superinfections
- Gastrointestinal upsets when given orally.

Aminoglycosides

The aminoglycosides are bactericidal. They cause misreading of mRNA by the ribosome, leading to abnormal protein production. To enter the bacterium, aminoglycosides need to be actively transported across the cell membrane: this does not occur in anaerobic organisms, which are, therefore, resistant.

Clinical pharmacokinetics

The aminoglycosides are:

- poorly lipid soluble and, therefore, not absorbed orally: parenteral administration is required for systemic effect
- unable to enter the CNS even when the meninges are inflamed
- not metabolised
- excreted unchanged by the kidney (where very high concentrations may occur, perhaps causing toxic tubular damage) by glomerular filtration (no active secretion); their clearance is markedly reduced in renal impairment and toxic concentrations are more likely.

Resistance

Resistance can develop through acquisition of plasmid-determined inactivating enzymes and through changes resulting in decreased transport of aminoglycosides into the cells.

Examples

Gentamicin is the most commonly used, covering Gram-negative aerobes, e.g. enteric organisms (*E. coli*, *Klebsiella*, *S. faecalis*, *Pseudomonas* and *Proteus* spp.), and is also used in antibiotic combinations against *S. aureus*. It is not active against aerobic Streptococci. Gentamicin is often used blindly with other antibiotics in severe infections of unknown cause.

Streptomycin was formerly the mainstay of antituberculous therapy but is now rarely used in the developed world.

Tobramycin is used for pseudomonads and for some gentamicin-resistant organisms.

Topical use

Some aminoglycosides, e.g. gentamicin, may also be applied topically for local effect, for example in ear and eye ointments.

Adverse effects

The aminoglycosides have a narrow therapeutic window and toxicity is often related to plasma concentration. It is essential to *monitor plasma concentrations* (usually trough and peak, i.e. shortly before and after administration of a dose) to ensure adequate concentrations for bactericidal effect while minimising adverse effects, every 2–3 days during treatment.

- Nephrotoxicity: may cause renal failure
- Toxic to the 8th cranial nerve (ototoxic), especially the vestibular division
- Other adverse effects are not dose related and are relatively rare, e.g. allergies, eosinophilia.

Macrolides

The macrolides are broad-spectrum antibiotics to which resistance develops rapidly. They inhibit protein synthesis by binding to the ribosome and are bacteriostatic at usual doses but bactericidal in high doses.

Examples

Erythromycin is acid labile but is given as an enterically coated tablet; however, absorption is erratic and poor. It is given orally or parenterally. It is widely distributed in the body except to the brain and cerebrospinal fluid. Erythromycin is excreted unchanged in bile and is reabsorbed lower down the gastrointestinal tract (enterohepatic circulation). Its spectrum of activity includes *S. aureus*, *S. pyogenes* and *S. pneumoniae*. It is especially useful in these infections as an alternative to penicillins in allergic patients. In addition, it is specifically indicated in *Legionella pneumoniae*, *Mycoplasma pneumoniae* and *Chlamydia* infections.

Clarithromycin, and azithromycin are newer macrolides that may have fewer adverse effects. Their use is similar to that of erythromycin. In addition, clarithromycin is used to treat *Helicobacter pylori* (see Ch. 11).

Adverse effects

- Gastrointestinal upsets (common with erythromycin)
- Rarely hypersensitivity, or cholestatic jaundice.

Drug interactions

Erythromycin (and to a lesser extent clarithromycin) inhibits cytochrome P450 enzymes. This can increase the effect of a wide range of other drugs such as warfarin, cyclosporin, some antiepileptics, etc. (See Chapter 21.)

Clinical sketch

A patient with epilepsy takes carbamazepine. The patient is allegedly allergic to penicillin and when she develops her respiratory tract infection with fever and sputum she is prescribed erythromycin. Two days later the patient is drowsy and ataxic.

Comment: Erythromycin is a good choice for respiratory tract infections in patients who are allergic to amoiycillin or patients in whom atypical organisms such as Legionella or Mycoplasma are suspected. However, it does inhibit liver enzymes and they reduce metabolism of other drugs, such as carbamazepine, leading to toxic plasma concentrations of this drug.

Lincosamides; clindamycin

Clindamycin is chemically distinct to erythromycin but is similar in its mode of action and spectrum. It is rapidly absorbed and penetrates most tissues well, except the CNS. It is particularly useful systemically for *S. aureus* (especially osteomyelitis as it penetrates bone well) and anaerobic infections.

Adverse effects

Diarrhoea is common. *Pseudomembranous colitis* is a serious inflammation of the large bowel caused by a superinfection with a strain of *Clostridium difficile*, which secretes a toxin that damages the mucosal lining; this may occur after any antibiotic but is especially common after clindamycin, which severely limits its use.

Sulfonamides and trimethoprim

Sulfonamides are rarely used alone today. Trimethoprim is not chemically related but is considered here because their modes of action are complementary.

Sulfonamides

Sulfonamides are competitive antagonists of para-aminobenzoic acid (PABA), a precursor of folic acid that is essential for the synthesis of purine nucleotides for DNA and RNA. Animals do not manufacture folate, depending on absorbed folate and so are unaffected. The sulfonamides are bacteristatic and effective against Gram-positive and many Gram-negative organisms.

Trimethoprim

Folate is activated by the enzyme dihydrofolate reductase to tetrahydrofolic acid. Trimethoprim inhibits this enzyme in bacteria and to a lesser degree in animals. It is bacteristatic. Trimethoprim is well absorbed and excreted by the kidneys. It has a similar spectrum to the sulfonamides. It is widely used, especially for urinary tract infections and also for respiratory tract infections.

Co-trimoxazole

Co-trimoxazole is a combination of a sulfonamide (*sulfamethoxazole*) and trimethoprim. It blocks the same pathway at two different positions and is bactericidal. This combination is widely used in Europe and the USA, but in the UK is considered to have no advantage over trimethoprim alone while being more toxic.

Co-trimoxazole is the drug of choice for the treatment and prevention of pneumonia caused by *Pneumocystis carinii* in immunosuppressed patients.

Adverse effects

Gastrointestinal upsets can result from both components of co-trimoxazole.

Less common but more serious are effects of the components individually and as a combination:

- sulfonamides
  — allergy, rash, fever
  — agranulocytosis
  — Stevens–Johnson syndrome (a severe skin reaction)
  — haemolysis in patients with glucose 6-phosphatase deficiency
  — renal toxicity: sulfonamides may form crystals in an acid urine leading to tubular damage and severe renal impairment
  — inhibition of metabolism of other drugs
- trimethoprim
  — macrocytic anaemia
  — thrombocytopenia
- cotrimoxazole: aplastic anaemia (especially in the elderly).

Quinolones

The quinolones are effective but expensive antibiotics; and less expensive drugs are often equally effective, especially for minor infections. Resistance to quinolones is becoming more common and, in general, they are used as reserve drugs and not for first-line treatment.

Quinolones inhibit DNA gyrase and prevent recoiling of DNA after replication. This is bactericidal to dividing cells.

Examples

Nalidixic acid, the first quinolone identified, is used as a urinary antiseptic and for lower urinary tract infections as it has no systemic antibacterial effect.

Ciprofloxacin is a Fluoroquinolone with a broad spectrum against Gram-negative bacilli and *Pseudomonas* spp. It is given orally or i.v. to treat a wide range of infections, including urinary tract and respiratory infections (*Haemophilus, Branhamella*) as well as peritonitis (Gram-negative bacilli) and salmonellal infection. It is used as prophylaxis for the contacts of patients with meningococcal meningitis.

Adverse effects

- Gastrointestinal upsets
- Fluoroquinolones may block the inhibitory neurotransmitter GABA, and this may cause confusion in the elderly and lower the fitting threshold; they are also contraindicated in epileptics
- Allergy and anaphylaxis
- Tendonitis and possibly damage to growing cartilage: not recommended for pregnant women or children.

Drug interactions

Ciprofloxacin is a liver enzyme inhibitor and may cause life-threatening interactions with theophylline.

Tetracyclines

The tetracyclines are bacteriostatic and act by binding to the bacterial ribosome and interfering with protein synthesis.

Examples

Tetracycline, oxytetracycline have short half-lives, while *doxycycline* has a longer half-life and can be given once per day. These drugs:

- are not well absorbed
- bind avidly to heavy metal ions and so absorption is greatly reduced if taken with food, milk, antacids or iron tablets; they should be taken at least half an hour before food
- concentrate in bones and teeth
- are excreted mostly in urine, partly in bile
- are broad-spectrum, active against most bacteria except *Proteus* or *Pseudomonas*; resistance is frequent
- are specifically indicated for *Mycoplasma, Rickettsia, Chlamydia* and *Brucella* infections
- are widely used to treat acne, given either orally or topically.

Adverse effects

- Gastrointestinal upset
- Superinfection: candidiasis
- Discolouration and deformity in growing teeth and bones (contraindicated in pregnancy and in children under 12 years)
- Renal impairment (should also be avoided in renal disease).

Metronidazole

Metronidazole binds to DNA and blocks replication. It is well absorbed after oral or rectal administration and can also be given i.v. It is widely distributed in the body (including into abscess cavities) and is metabolised by the liver.

Use

Metronidazole is:

- active against anaerobic organisms (e.g. *Bacteroides*, *Clostridia*), which are encountered particularly in abdominal surgery
- used to treat psuedomembranous colitis (*Cl. difficile*)
- used against protozoa such as *Trichomonas*, *Giardia* and *Entamoeba* infections (Ch. 14)
- often part of the treatment of *Helicobacter pylori* (Ch. 11)
- used also to treat a variety of dental infections, particularly dental abscess.

Adverse effects

- Nausea, anorexia and a metallic taste
- Ataxia, caused by peripheral neuropathy
- Disulfiram-like reaction (Ch. 18): metronidazole inhibits alcohol dehydrogenase (an enzyme in the pathway metabolising alcohol) and patients receiving it who drink alcohol may experience unpleasant reactions (flushing, abdominal pain, hypotension) as acetaldehyde accumulates; patients taking metronidazole should be advised not to drink alcohol
- Possibly teratogenic if taken in the first trimester of pregnancy.

Drug interactions

Metronidazole may inhibit the metabolism of warfarin.

Nitrofurantoin

Nitrofurantoin is used as a urinary antiseptic and to treat Gram-negative infections in the lower urinary tract. It is taken orally and is well absorbed. It is excreted unchanged in the urine and is only antimicrobial when concentrated in the urine and so has no systemic antibacterial effect. It is ineffective in renal failure because of failure to concentrate. Resistance develops relatively quickly.

Adverse effects

- Gastrointestinal upsets
- Allergy (including pulmonary fibrosis)
- Polyneuritis.

Fucidic acid

Fucidic acid is active only against *S. aureus* (by inhibiting bacterial protein synthesis). It is not affected by β-lactamase. It is given orally or parenterally and can be used alone or with flucloxacillin to reduce the development of resistance. It is well absorbed and widely distributed, including to bone (useful in osteomyelitis). It is metabolised in the liver.

Adverse effects

- Gastrointestinal upsets
- Hepatitis and jaundice.

Vancomycin and teicoplanin

The glycopeptide antibiotics vancomycin and teicoplanin interfere with bacterial cell wall formation and are only effective against Gram-positive organisms. They are not absorbed after oral administration and must be given parenterally. Both are excreted by the kidney. Vancomycin and teicoplanin are used i.v. to treat serious or resistant *S. aureus* infections and for prophylaxis of endocarditis in penicillin-allergic patients.

Vancomycin is given orally to treat pseudomembranous colitis (see above).

Teicoplanin is similar.

Adverse effects

Although not an aminoglycoside, vancomycin has similar plasma concentration-dependent toxicity and monitoring of plasma concentrations is essential. This is not necessary for teicoplanin, which is much less toxic. Effects include:

- nephrotoxicity
- ototoxicity
- allergy
- histamine release (after rapid injection of vancomycin: 'red man syndrome').

Chloramphenicol

Chloramphenicol inhibits bacterial protein synthesis. It is well absorbed and widely distributed, including to the CNS. It is metabolised by glucuronidation in the liver.

Although chloramphenicol is an effective broad-spectrum antibiotic, its uses are limited by its serious toxicity. The major indication is to treat bacterial meningitis caused by *H. influenzae*, or *N. meningitidis* (initially in addition to benzylpenicillin or alone if the patient is penicillin allergic) or if the organism is unknown. It is also specifically used for *Rickettsia* (typhus).

Adverse effects

- A rare idiosyncratic aplastic anaemia (1/50 000), probably immunological in origin but often fatal
- Reversible bone marrow depression caused by its effect on protein synthesis in humans.

13.3 Antibiotics for mycobacterial infections

Learning objectives

You should:

- understand the significance of the increasing incidence of tuberculosis and the development of resistance
- be aware of the current drug regimens for tuberculosis and leprosy
- be aware of infections with atypical mycobacteria.

Mycobacteria spp. are intracellular pathogens that are resistant to host defences.

Tuberculosis

Tuberculosis (TB) is a major cause of death in many parts of the world (8 million new cases and 3 million deaths in 1996). In the developed world, TB is currently undergoing a resurgence, partly because of infection in immunosuppressed patients. *Mycobacterium tuberculosis* is an intracellular organism surviving inside phagocytes in a dormant form for many months. Consequently, therapy, needs to be prolonged.

Drug-resistant mutants are often present and will proliferate if only single drug therapy is used; hence several drugs are used simultaneously to avoid resistance.

Failure of therapy is most often the result of poor compliance with the drugs rather than drug resistance.

Regimens for treating pulmonary TB

Drug regimens will differ around the world, determined partly by bacterial resistance but mainly by economic factors. Currently recommended treatment in the UK is:

1. *Rifampicin* and *isoniazid* for 6 months
2. In addition, *pyrazinamide* and *ethambutol* for the first 2 months (quadruple therapy).

Some doubt the value of ethambutol and omit it.

Isoniazid

Isoniazid is bactericidal but its mode of action is unknown. It is the most active of the anti-TB drugs. It is well absorbed after oral administration and widely distributed, including into the CNS.

Isoniazid is acetylated by the liver prior to excretion; this shows **genetic polymorphism** (i.e. variation in metabolism owing to genetic differences producing enzymes of different activity) giving rise to fast and slow acetylators, which occur with different frequencies in different populations (see Ch. 1). Acetylation ability may affect efficiency and toxicity in an individual.

Adverse effects

- Peripheral neuropathy (occurs particularly in slow acetylators and is preventable by giving pyridoxine)
- Hepatitis
- Rashes
- Drug-induced lupus syndrome: a syndrome resembling systemic lupus erythematosus.

Drug interactions

Isoniazid is a liver enzyme inhibitor (caution with phenytoin and warfarin).

Rifampicin

Rifampicin inhibits RNA synthesis in bacteria but not in humans and is bactericidal. It is also a valuable broad-spectrum antibiotic but its use is restricted mainly to tuberculosis but also as prophylaxis for the contacts of patients with meningococcal meningitis, and the treatment of *Legionella pneumoniae* and resistant *S. aureus*.

Rifampicin is well absorbed after oral administration (best taken on an empty stomach) and is widely distributed. It is metabolised in the liver and excreted in bile.

Adverse effects

- Malaise, headache
- Fever, rashes
- Hepatitis
- Invariably, all body secretions (urine, tears, etc.) become an orange-red colour.

Drug interactions

Rifampicin is a potent liver enzyme inducer and may cause interactions with anticonvulsants, warfarin, oral contraceptives, etc.

Pyrazinamide

Pyrazinamide is bactericidal. It is well absorbed and widely distributed, in particular achieving good penetration of the CNS.

Adverse effects

- Hepatitis, especially if given at high doses; liver function tests should be monitored
- Hyperuricaemia.

Ethambutol

Ethambutol is bacteriostatic but its mode of action is unknown. It is excreted by the kidneys.

Adverse effects

Optic neuritis, which is dose related and rare.

Reserve drugs

Reserve drugs in TB include *Thiacetazone, ethionamide,* para-*aminosalicylate, capreomycin, streptomycin* which are also used in the treatment of atypical mycobacteria.

Leprosy

Leprosy is caused by infection with *Mycobacteria leprae.* A mixture of drugs are used to treat leprosy, depending on the type and severity of the infection and the local resistance patterns, e.g. *rifampicin* and *dapsone*. Dapsone is related to the sulfonamides and also inhibits folate metabolism (also used to treat dermatitis herpetiformis; see Ch. 16).

Adverse effects include haemolysis, gastrointestinal upsets and rashes.

Atypical mycobacteria

The atypical mycobacteria are environmental species that do not normally infect humans. They infect immunocompromised individuals causing pulmonary, skin, soft tissue infections and systemic infections. *M. avium intracellulare* (MAI) infection is a serious problem in HIV-positive patients. Treatment is difficult because they are often drug resistant but includes the reserve drugs listed for TB.

Self-assessment: questions

Multiple choice questions

1. The following antimicrobials should be avoided in pregnant women:
   a. Gentamicin
   b. Tetracycline
   c. Amoxicillin
   d. Nitrofurantoin
   e. Trimethoprim

2. In treating any infection:
   a. Cultures must always be taken first
   b. The clinical picture is of no help in deciding appropriate antibiotic therapy
   c. Superinfection implies infection with an organism resistant to antibiotics
   d. Antibiotic therapy may be standardised for all patients with each infection
   e. Combinations of antibiotics are sometimes useful

3. Failure to respond to an antibiotic may result from:
   a. Microbial resistance to the antibiotics used
   b. Inappropriate selection of antibiotics
   c. Immunosuppression of the patient
   d. Inappropriate route of administration
   e. Good blood supply to the area infected

4. Penicillins:
   a. Are highly lipid soluble
   b. Are excreted by glomerular filtration
   c. May all be destroyed by β-lactamase-producing bacteria
   d. Some may be given orally
   e. Are usually highly effective against streptococcal infection

5. Anaphylaxis:
   a. Should be treated with epinephrine (adrenaline)
   b. Is life threatening
   c. May occur within seconds or minutes of administration of a drug
   d. Usually occurs on first exposure to the drug
   e. Is caused by endotoxin release

6. Aminoglycosides:
   a. Cross the blood–brain barrier
   b. Are metabolised by the liver
   c. May cause ototoxicity
   d. Require plasma concentration measurement
   e. Are effective against anaerobic organisms like bacteroides

7. Erythromycin:
   a. May interact with phenytoin
   b. Is well absorbed after oral administration
   c. May cause nausea and vomiting
   d. May be used to treat *Legionella pneumoniae*
   e. Cross-allergy to penicillin may occur

8. Sulphonamides:
   a. May cause drug interactions by displacement from plasma proteins
   b. Inhibit nucleic acid formation in humans
   c. Co-trimoxazole may cause blood dyscrasias
   d. Co-trimoxazole may be used in the treatment of patients with AIDS
   e. Trimethoprim is more likely to cause adverse drug reactions than co-trimoxazole

9. Ciprofloxacin:
   a. Blocks protein synthesis
   b. Is the first choice drug for pneumonia
   c. May cause drug hypersensitivity
   d. Is effective against Gram-negative bacilli
   e. May cause interactions with theophylline

10. Tetracyclines:
    a. Are used to treat acne
    b. Should be taken with meals
    c. Should not be given to young children
    d. Bacterial resistance is rare
    e. Superinfection is common

11. Metronidazole:
    a. Is well absorbed
    b. Is effective in some protozoal infections
    c. Can be used to treat peptic ulcer disease
    d. May cause cerebellar damage
    e. May interact with ethanol

12. The antibiotic:
    a. Vancomycin is an aminoglycoside
    b. Vancomycin may be given orally to treat pseudomembranous colitis
    c. Fucidic acid and vancomycin are both effective against *Staphylococcus aureus*
    d. Chloramphenicol is widely used for respiratory tract infections
    e. Nitrofurantoin is used for Gram-negative septicaemia

13. In treating tuberculosis:
    a. Multiple drug therapy is usual
    b. Treatment for 1 month is considered adequate

   c. Isoniazid is metabolised at different rates in different races

   d. Isoniazid may cause hepatic failure

   e. Isoniazid may cause liver enzyme induction

14. In treating tuberculosis (TB):
   a. Rifampicin is only used against TB
   b. Rifampicin inhibits the metabolism of warfarin
   c. Rifampicin may cause the urine to change colour
   d. Pyrazinamide may cause hepatitis
   e. Patients about to start taking ethambutol should have their eyes checked first

Case history questions

Case history 1

> A 23-year-old woman presents with a urinary tract infection causing cystitis.

1. What general advice should be given to her?
2. What antibiotics should be considered?
3. If the woman was pregnant, how would this alter your choice of antibiotic?

Case history 2

> A 54-year-old alcoholic man with no fixed address is found to have tuberculosis with acid- and alcohol-fast bacilli seen in the sputum.

1. Is he infectious?
2. What drugs should be administered and in what regimen?
3. Do his social circumstances pose any problems?

Case history 3

> A 65-year-old man with a long history of chronic obstructive airway disease develops acute bronchitis: his doctor decides to prescribe an antibiotic.

1. What antibiotics would be appropriate first choices?

> A week later, the patient returns to the doctor complaining of severe diarrhoea.

2. What diagnosis should be considered?

3. If this diagnosis is confirmed, how should it be treated?

Short note questions

Write short notes on:

1. Drugs used in the treatment of tuberculosis.
2. Adverse effects of antibiotics.

Essay question

List some strategies that can be adopted to reduce the risks of bacterial resistance to antibiotics developing.

Extended matching items question

Theme: antibiotics
Options

A. Flucloxacillin
B. Ciprofloxacin
C. Cefotaxime
D. Nitrofurantoin
E. Trimethoprim
F. Aciclovir
G. Phenoxymethylpenicillin (Pen V)
H. Co-trimoxazole
I. Amoxicillin
J. Cefaclor
K. Erythromycin
L. Clindamycin
M. Oxytetracycline
N. Gentamicin

Which of these antibiotics would be the best choice in the following patients seen by their GP? There may be more than one reasonable option. Each option can be used once, more than once or not at all.

1. A 67-year-old man with an exacerbation of his chronic obstructive pulmonary disease who is coughing increased volumes of purulent sputum. He has just recovered from an exacerbation during which he was treated with amoxicillin without any adverse effects.
2. A 26-year-old pregnant woman with dysuria, frequency and a temperature of 38.5°C. The urine dipstick is positive for nitrites and leucocytes.
3. A 60-year-old man, previously well, with a lobar pneumonia. There is a history of allergy to penicillin.
4. A 65-year-old diabetic woman with redness, swelling and pain in her ankle. The clinical diagnosis is cellulitis.

Self-assessment: answers

Multiple choice answers

1. a. **True**. Aminoglycosides and vancomycin may cause 8th nerve damage in the fetus.
   b. **True**. Teeth and bone deformities may occur in the fetus.
   c. **False**. Widely used.
   d. **False**. May be used but should be avoided in late pregnancy or breast-feeding.
   e. **True**. Folate antagonist and possibly teratogenic.

2. a. **False**. This is an ideal but not always possible, e.g. in severely ill patients.
   b. **False**. The clinical picture often gives clues, e.g. a lobar pneumonia is most often caused by *Streptococcus pneumoniae* and benzylpenicillin is appropriate.
   c. **True**. At least to the antibiotic, which has led to the superinfection.
   d. **False**. Although broad guidelines may be given, each case must be judged on its own merits (as occurs elsewhere in medicine).
   e. **True**. For example in treating tuberculosis.

3. a. **True**. For example, penicillinase-producing *Staphylococcus aureus* will not respond to amoxicillin.
   b. **True**. For example, use of benzylpenicillin to treat a Gram-negative infection would be inappropriate.
   c. **True**. If the patient is known to be immunosuppressed, antibiotic regimens will need to be more sophisticated and aggressive to achieve cure.
   d. **True**. For example, oral antibiotics to treat a septicaemia.
   e. **False**. Poor blood supply to an infected area may prevent antibiotic transport to the site, and importantly will also lead to poor tissue inflammatory responses and healing.

4. a. **False**. They are preferentially water soluble.
   b. **False**. They are excreted actively in the renal tubule.
   c. **False**. For example, flucloxacillin.
   d. **True**. For example, amoxicillin, etc.
   e. **True**. Usually the drugs of first choice for this.

5. a. **True**. This is a physiological antagonist to histamine.
   b. **True**. If not treated promptly.

c. **True**. Particularly after parenteral administration.
   d. **False**. The patient must have been sensitised to the drug previously, but a history of exposure may be difficult to find; patients have unwittingly been sensitised to penicillin by penicillin in milk.
   e. **False**. Endotoxin release by bacteria is a factor in septicaemic shock. Anaphylaxis is caused by histamine and other inflammatory mediators.

6. a. **False**. Since they are poorly lipid soluble.
   b. **False**. They are excreted by the kidney: this is a general feature of drugs that are not lipid soluble.
   c. **True**. A major adverse effect.
   d. **True**. To avoid some of the dose-related adverse effects.
   e. **False**. Only effective against aerobic organisms.

7. a. **True**. Erythromycin is a liver enzyme inhibitor.
   b. **False**. Absorption is erratic.
   c. **True**. The most common adverse effect.
   d. **True**.
   e. **False**. Widely used to treat patients thought to be allergic to penicillin.

8. a. **True**. Although enzyme inhibition may also occur.
   b. **False**. Humans cannot manufacture folate and so are not affected.
   c. **True**. Especially in the elderly.
   d. **True**. To treat *Pneumocystis pneumoniae* infection.
   e. **False**. Trimethoprim is part of co-trimoxazole and is far less likely to cause adverse effects than the sulphonamide component.

9. a. **False**. Interferes with nucleic acid coiling.
   b. **False**. Not very effective against *Streptococcus pneumoniae*.
   c. **True**. Anaphylaxis and other reactions are recorded.
   d. **True**. This is its main use.
   e. **True**. By liver enzyme inhibition.

10. a. **True**. And probably its most common use.
    b. **False**. It will bind to heavy metal ions in the food and not be absorbed.
    c. **True**. Damage to teeth.
    d. **False**. Increasingly common.
    e. **True**.

11. a. **True**. And penetrates most tissues well.
    b. **True**. For example, amoebiasis.
    c. **True**. When peptic ulcer disease is associated with *Helicobacter* infection.
    d. **False**. May cause ataxia, but this is caused by peripheral neuropathy.
    e. **True**. The disulfiram reaction.

12. a. **False**. Although similar in its toxicity.
    b. **True**. Metronidazole is usually first choice on grounds of cost.
    c. **True**. Also flucloxacillin (the most widely used) and rifampicin.
    d. **False**. Considered too toxic for anything other than life-threatening indications.
    e. **False**. Nitrofurantoin is only effective after concentration in the urine.

13. a. **True**. To reduce resistance.
    b. **False**. Treatment for 6 months is usually the minimum for pulmonary tuberculosis.
    c. **True**. Genetic polymorphism.
    d. **True**. Especially in patients who are fast acetylators or who have their enzymes induced.
    e. **False**. Liver enzyme inhibitor.

14. a. **False**. Also used for *Staphylococcus aureus* and *Legionella pneumoniae*.
    b. **False**. Rifampicin is a liver enzyme inducer.
    c. **True**. Orange.
    d. **True**. This is rare at currently used doses.
    e. **True**. Since optic neuritis is a major adverse effect.

Case history answers

Case history 1

1. Copious fluid intake, rest and antipyretics as necessary.
2. Antibiotic choice will ideally be based on urine culture. Amoxicillin, trimethoprim or nitrofurantoin would all be reasonable choices. Ciprofloxacin should be a reserve drug.
3. Treating minor urinary tract infections is more important in pregnant women because of the increased risk of progression to pyelonephritis. Neither trimethoprim nor ciprofloxacin would be appropriate.

Case history 2

1. Yes: he should be isolated if possible for the first 2 weeks of treatment.
2. Rifampicin and isoniazid for 6 months: pyrazinamide and possibly ethambutol for the first 2 months also.

3. This patient's compliance with long-term medication might be poor. It might be appropriate to admit him to hospital for the duration of his treatment or to ensure in some other way that he takes his medication under observation.

Case history 3

1. Trimethoprim or amoxicillin or erythromycin would be appropriate.
2. The patient may have pseudomembranous colitis as a result of the use of broad-spectrum antibiotic. A stool sample should be sent for detection of the toxin, and a sigmoidoscopy performed.
3. Metronidazole is first choice, with vancomycin for resistant cases.

Short note answers

1. When asked to write a short note on any drug consider:
   a. its indications
   b. its mechanism of action
   c. its therapeutic use
   d. its adverse effects.

In this case, therefore, one would start by naming the major drugs (rifampicin, isoniazid, ethambutol and pyrazinamide) and for each include a mechanism of action where it is known. Discuss (in combination in this case) how all of the drugs are used together (rifampicin and isoniazid for 6 months, ethambutol and pyrazinamide for the first 2 months) and why. And finally consider the drugs' adverse effects, listing the major adverse reactions for each and their possible interactions. Here one would spend most time talking about rifampicin and isoniazid since they are the drugs used for the longest period and, therefore, the ones most likely to cause adverse reactions and interactions.

2. This is a very general question, but one should consider the patterns of adverse reactions to antibiotics which should include:

   a. hypersensitivity reactions, e.g. anaphylaxis to penicillin, drug fevers, fixed drug skin reactions, etc. These constitute the type B or bizarre adverse drug reactions (see Ch. 10). They are rare but potentially serious.
   b. reactions which might arise as a result of the augmented effect of antibiotics, i.e. antimicrobial killing leading to superinfection with *Candida* or *Clostridium difficile*; drug-induced diarrhoea, etc.
   c. The long-term environmental hazards of these drugs, for instance in promoting antibiotic resistance.

Essay answer

Make the following points:

1. Restricting drug use to confirmed indications and sensitive bacteria
2. Using drug combinations if treatment is to be prolonged
3. Avoiding unnecessarily prolonged treatment
4. Establishing a hierarchy of drug usage, with more potent drugs reserved for resistant cases.

Extended matching items answer

1. J best but B or E also reasonable. The likely organisms are *Streptococcus pneumoniae*, *Haemophilus influenzae* or *Branhamella* sp., or even all three. The last two in particular are showing increasing rates of resistance to amoxicillin. Amoxicillin is a reasonable first-line choice but this infection has occurred immediately after such treatment and is likely to be with a resistant organism, The options then are to use a cephalosporin with increased activity against Gram-negative organisms such as *Haemophilus* (e.g. cefaclor) or a fluoroquinolone such as ciprofloxacin or trimethoprim. The last two would not be good first-line choices since they do not have reliable effectiveness against *Streptococcus* spp. Since amoxicillin with its greater effectiveness against *Streptococcus* spp. has been used already in this case, we can assume that it is the *Haemophilus* or *Branhamella* spp. which is the culprit. Another alternative, not given here, is the combination of amoxicillin and clavulinic acid, co-amoxiclav.
2. J is the best choice. The concern in a pregnant woman is always about teratogenesis, i.e. causing fetal defects as a result of medication. Trimethoprim, ciprofloxacin and nitrofurantoin are, therefore, generally avoided. The safest option would be cefaclor. Co-amoxiclav would be a reasonable alternative; the resistance of the commonest organism causing urinary tract infection (*Escherichia coli*) to amoxicillin is too great to allow this to be used alone.
3. K is best; M would be a reasonable choice also. The organism in lobar pneumonia is usually *Streptococcus pneumoniae*. This is usually very sensitive to penicillin and, therefore, one might think that either phenoxymethylpenicillin or amoxicillin (because of its better absorption) would be favoured drugs. However, as this patient has a history of allergy to penicillin, it is safest to avoid these. About 10% of the population has some vague history of allergy to penicillin, although true incidence is much lower. Often this history of 'allergy' arises from non-allergic adverse effects, such as stomach upsets. However, it is safer to avoid these drugs completely. As there is a 10% cross-reactivity between penicillins and cephalosporins, it is probably better to avoid cefaclor also. This would normally have very good activity against *S. pneumoniae*. Some authorities would argue that in a life-threatening situation and where there is anything less than a clear history of full-blown anaphylaxis, it is reasonable to use a cephalosporin. However, this does not apply in this case when there are reasonable alternatives available.
4. Best answer is A. The likely organisms in cellulitis are *Staphylococcus aureus* and/or *Streptococcus pyogenes*. Treatment for these should be with flucloxacillin, possibly with amoxicillin in addition. Depending on the severity of the infection, it may be reasonable to treat these at home or it may be advisable to refer the patient to hospital for i.v. treatment.

Chemotherapy for fungi, viruses and protozoa

Overview

This chapter deals with drugs used in infections by fungi, viruses and protozoa. The fungi and protozoa are more similar to mammalian cells in structure and so can be harder to kill by pathogen-specific methods.

Fungal infections are usually confined to the skin, mucous membranes and nails but, in immunocompromised patients, can give rise to systemic disease. Topical antifungal agents are largely without toxicity but systemic agents can also damage the host.

Viruses cannot grow or propagate outside living cells and use host cell mechanisms to reproduce. Although they are most vulnerable at this stage, the antiviral drugs are often toxic to the host.

The protozoa have life cycles outside the human and most protozoan pathogens multiply in the human having been acquired by ingestion, inhalation or an insect bite. Protozoan infections are unusual in general medical practice.

14.1 Antifungal drugs

Learning objectives

You should:

- be able to describe the main 'syndromes' caused by fungal skin infections
- know the appropriate treatment for common fungal skin infections
- be aware that systemic fungal infections are mainly a problem in immunosuppressed patients
- know the main adverse effects of amphotericin, systemic imidazoles and flucytosine.

Fungal infections are usually confined to the skin, mucous membranes and nails: these conditions are frequent and the general physician should have a working knowledge of the drugs used. Most of these drugs are used topically and are largely without major toxicity. In contrast, systemic fungal disease is unusual in the immunocompetent patient. Systemic antifungal drugs is a specialist area: these drugs are toxic and difficult to use.

Superficial cutaneous and mucous membrane infections

Superficial fungal infections can be classified as **dermatomycoses** and **candidiasis**.

Ringworm (tinea). There are various types of dermatomycosis; the commonest are caused by tinea; tinea corporalis affects the body, tinea pedis ('athlete's foot') the feet and tinea cruris the groin. *All are equally common and easily treated. Identification of the fungus and drug sensitivity testing are neither practical nor necessary in the majority of cases.*

Clinical sketch

A woman brings her little boy to surgery because he has developed several raised, itchy, red lesions on his arms. They have a red raised edge. The doctor diagnoses **tinea corporis** and prescribes clotrimazole cream.

Comment: these infections are common and usually respond to topical treatment.

Clinical sketch

A woman brings her 6-month-old baby to surgery with 'nappy rash'. The red area is mainly in the skin folds and is probably caused by wet nappies left on too long, but there are 'satellite' lesions over convex surfaces. The GP feels that there is an element of candidal infection; she advises more frequent changes of nappy, and gives clotrimazole cream.

Comment: nappy rash may be caused entirely by infrequent nappy changes, leading to wet, ammonia-exposed skin. However Candida albicans *frequently superinfects such areas.*

Candidiasis. *Candida albicans* causes opportunist infections when the skin is damaged, when antibiotic treatment alters normal flora or when the immune system is compromised.

Onychia. Infections of the nails can be hard to treat with topical agents and a long course of oral griseofulvin may be required.

Drugs for fungal skin infections

Topical nystatin

Nystatin is too toxic for systemic use and is not absorbed from the gut. Nystatin is used topically for cutaneous, oral, oesophageal and vaginal infections with *C. albicans* and various dermatophytes. Nystatin is not beneficial against fungal nail infections. Because it is mainly used topically, adverse effects are unusual: very high oral doses can cause gastrointestinal upset.

Topical imidazoles

Miconazole and *clotrimazole* are relatively toxic compounds. However they are used topically for infections such as tinea and vaginal candidiasis. Under these circumstances, little drug is absorbed, and such topical use is usually safe. Allergic reactions are occasionally seen.

Systemic griseofulvin

Systemic griseofulvin is used for fungal nail infections, which respond poorly to topical applications; treatment must last for several months. Absorption of griseofulvin is very variable and is increased by fatty foods. Griseofulvin is relatively non-toxic but can occasionally produce **adverse reactions** including rashes, agranulocytosis, systemic lupus erythematosus-like syndromes and peripheral neuropathy. Griseofulvin induces hepatic drug-metabolising enzymes and can affect warfarin therapy. A course of griseofulvin may last for several months to achieve cure.

Terbinafine

Like griseofulvin, terbinafine is used systemically, mainly for onychia. Severe rashes have been reported and patients should be advised to stop the drug if they notice a rash. It can also cause hepatitis. It is more convenient than griseofulvin and a course lasts 2–6 months.

Systemic infections

The use of broad-spectrum antibiotics, which decrease the normal non-pathogenic bacterial flora on the body, and the increase in the population with reduced immune responses (from AIDS, immunosuppressant drugs, cancer chemotherapy) has led to an increase in systemic fungal disease. In the UK, the most common is systemic candidiasis, followed by cryptococciasis (meningitis or endocarditis), and aspergillosis (pulmonary).

Drugs for systemic infections

Imidazoles

Ketoconazole and *fluconazole*, though structurally similar to clotrimazole and miconazole, are less toxic. They may be given orally or parenterally for systemic infection. Both are well absorbed, but ketoconazole does not readily cross the blood–brain barrier, and fluconazole is preferred for fungal CNS infection. All are hepatotoxic and are hepatic enzyme inhibitors (and, therefore, prone to drug interactions).

Amphotericin

Amphotericin is not absorbed from the gut; its oral formulations are, therefore, for topical use only and are relatively free from adverse effects. It is given i.v. for life-threatening systemic fungal infections and then has frequent and severe toxicity. Rigors, fever and malaise are usual; renal failure, hepatic dysfunction and anaemia are common.

Flucytosine

Flucytosine is another toxic drug used for life-threatening systemic fungal infections. Bone marrow toxicity can be a major problem.

14.2 Antiviral drugs

Learning objectives

You should:

- know the main ways in which antiviral drugs work

- be able to describe some common syndromes caused by herpes simplex, herpes zoster, influenza and hepatitis viruses

- understand the concept of risk versus benefit in relation to the use of antivirus drugs

- know the principles of highly active antiretroviral therapy (HAART) for patients with HIV

Few of the vast number of viral infections are susceptible to drugs, and many of the available compounds suffer from variable efficacy, unacceptable toxicity or both. Viruses are more difficult 'targets' than bacteria: they are most vulnerable during reproduction, but all use host cell organelles and enzymes to do this; consequently, antiviral compounds are often as toxic to host cells as to the virus. Viruses have assumed increasing importance in the setting of immunosuppression—both drug induced and AIDS. For the most part, the use of antiviral drugs, particularly in patients with AIDS, is a specialist area, but the general physician needs a basic grounding.

Modes of action of antiviral drugs

Antiviral drugs act in a number of ways:

- inhibition of viral 'uncoating' shortly after penetration into the cell; such drugs are best used prophylactically, or very early in the disease course (e.g. amantadine)

- interference with viral RNA synthesis and function (e.g. ribavirin)

- interference with DNA synthesis by acting as analogues of pyrimidine or purine bases (e.g. idoxuridine, cytarabine and vidarabine)

- inhibition of viral DNA polymerase (e.g. aciclovir and gancyclovir)

- inhibition of reverse transcriptase (relevant only to retroviruses such as HIV, e.g. zidovudine)

- use of complex 'natural' antiviral defences (e.g. the interferons).

Influenza virus. Although influenza is often acute and self-limiting, it can give rise to high mortality rates. Antigenic shift allows the virus to 'escape' previous immunity or vaccine cover.

The hepatitis viruses. Viruses of different groups can cause hepatocellular damage. Hepatitis A is spread by the faecal-oral route and is common where sewage disposal is inadequate. Hepatitis B and C are spread in blood and body secretions (e.g. during sexual intercourse). Hepatitis B and C can lead to chronic liver disease and hepatocarcinoma.

Human immunodeficiency virus (HIV). Infection with HIV leads eventually to a depletion of CD4+ T cells and impaired immune responses. HIV-positive individuals are then at risk for a number of secondary infections; these form the acquired immunodeficiency syndrome (AIDS).

Clinical sketch

A man is troubled with frequent and debilitating cold sores: they make his lips split and are embarrassing. The GP gives him aciclovir cream.

Comment: Herpes simplex (cold sores) is a frequent indication for aciclovir. The drug should be applied as early after the onset of local discomfort as possible. Once ulceration has occurred its benefits are minimal.

Clinical sketch

A 30-year-old man is admitted with confusion and fever. The computed tomographic (CT) scan is suggestive of Herpes simplex encephalitis, and the cerebrospinal fluid shows a pleocytosis. Intravenous aciclovir is started and the patient gradually recovers. Polymerase chain reaction analysis confirms the organism later.

Comment: aciclovir may be life saving in herpes simplex encephalitis. It is important to maintain hydration since deterioration in renal function may occur in dehydrated patients.

A 50-year-old woman develops painful ulceration on the left side of her face. It involves her forehead, and her left eye is red and painful. She is admitted as an emergency where the ophthalmologist advises parenteral and topical aciclovir.

Comment: shingles (caused by Herpes zoster) involving the ophthalmic division of the Vth cranial nerve can involve the cornea, in which case sight may be threatened: specialist management is required.

Drugs used in viral infections

Herpes simplex and Herpes zoster infections

Aciclovir

Aciclovir is active against herpes simplex; it also has activity against herpes zoster, but less so. Aciclovir is metabolised to its active form by a viral enzyme and, therefore, targets virus-infected cells quite specifically. The drug may be used topically, orally and i.v. Little drug is absorbed from topical formulations, and the bioavailability of the oral drug is low (about 20%). Once in the body, aciclovir crosses the blood–brain barrier. It is mainly excreted in the urine as the unchanged drug; this renal excretion is impaired by probenecid (see Ch. 8). Adverse effects include:

- renal impairment: mainly with high i.v. doses in dehydrated patients
- local inflammation following extravascular administration
- encephalopathy: mainly at high i.v. doses.

Other drugs

Famciclovir is mainly used for Herpes zoster.

Influenza

Amantadine

Amantadine is taken orally and mainly eliminated by the kidney as the unchanged drug. Influenza A is a serious viral illness with a significant mortality rate, and amanta-

dine may be used in the prevention of influenza A (it has little activity against influenza B), postexposure, in defined individuals at high risk: with pre-existing cardiac or pulmonary disease or immunocompromised patients. It might also be given to 'key' health care workers in the setting of an epidemic.

Additionally, if it is started within 48 hours of symptoms, amantadine can reduce the duration and severity of influenza A. Adverse effects include acute CNS reactions. Relative contraindications include:

- epilepsy
- renal failure
- pregnancy: the drug is teratogenic.

Zanamivir

Zanamivir can be used within 48 hours of the onset of symptoms from either influenza A or B. Although patients with chronic lung disease are at grave risk from influenza (and would be among the patients who need protection), zanamivir can worsen bronchospasm and should be used with caution. Zanamivir is taken by inhalation of powder, using an 'inhaler device'.

HIV infection

There is no cure for HIV at present. Antiretroviral drugs are toxic but increase life expectancy. They should be used by experienced specialists.

- Treatment aims to reduce viral load and maintain this for as long as possible.
- Anti-HIV drugs should be started before the immune system is irreversibly damaged.
- Drug resistance is a major problem with monotherapy: standard treatment is now with drug combinations, so-called highly active antiretroviral therapy (HAART).
- HAART typically comprises two nucleoside reverse transcriptase inhibitors (NRTIs) with either a non-nucleoside reverse transcriptase inhibitor (NNRTI) or a protease inhibitor.

A 65-year-old cigarette smoker with chronic obstructive pulmonary disease was vaccinated against influenza by his GP but develops a febrile illness with severe rigors and myalgia. His chest is no worse than usual and there are no signs of pneumonia. The doctor diagnoses influenza and starts zanamivir as an 'inhaler'.

Comment: this drug may limit the effects of influenza and is indicated in high-risk patients. It may cause bronchospasm, so caution should be employed.

A 30-year-old homosexual man is diagnosed HIV positive after presenting with *Pneumocystis carinii* pneumonia (PCP). The PCP is treated with high-dose co-trimoxazole and he makes a slow recovery. His CD4$^+$ cell count is about 100×10^6 cells/l and his viral load is high. His physician starts highly active antiretroviral therapy (HAART) once he is better from the PCP.

Comment: HAART comprises a combination of antiretroviral drugs that work by different mechanisms: it is designed to avoid drug resistance (cf. tuberculosis). HAART has greatly increased life expectancy in AIDS but the drugs cause adverse effects.

- HAART is usually started when the patient is clinically well (i.e. after they have recovered from the presenting infection).
- HAART may be limited by toxicity, treatment failure or both.
- In addition to efforts to reduce HIV loads, management relies on the prevention and prompt treatment of superimposed infections such as tuberculosis and infections with *Streptococcus pneumoniae* and cytomegalovirus.
- The management of HIV is expensive: most HIV sufferers worldwide do not have access to such treatment.

Nucleoside reverse transcriptase inhibitors

HIV is an RNA virus capable of inducing the synthesis of a DNA transcript of its genome, which can then become integrated into the host cell's DNA, thereby allowing viral replication. Synthesis of the initial DNA transcript involves the enzyme reverse transcriptase. NRTIs resemble natural nucleoside substrates for the enzyme. These drugs are given by mouth. They are rapidly eliminated and must be taken more than once daily. Examples of these drugs, and their main adverse effects are:

Zidovudine (AZT): adverse effects include:

- bone marrow toxicity: about one third of patients develop severe anaemia or neutropenia
- polymyositis: muscle pain and tenderness
- headache and insomnia.

Didanosine (ddI): adverse effects include:

- pancreatitis
- peripheral neuropathy.

Zalcitabine (ddC): adverse effects include:

- peripheral neuropathy
- myalgia
- bone marrow toxicity.

Non-nucleoside reverse transcriptase inhibitors

Drugs such as *nevirapine* also inhibit reverse transcriptase but by a different mechanism to that of the NRTIs. This difference in mechanism of action is crucial in the avoidance of drug resistance. Adverse effects of nevirapine include:

- severe rashes
- hepatitis.

Protease inhibitors

Virus replication relies on the manufacture of new viral proteins, which are assembled into virus particles. The protease inhibitors interfere with this process. Again, this difference in mechanism of action is critical: HAART relies on the combination of differing drugs, and this reduces the risk of drug resistance. *Indinavir* and *ritonavir* are examples of this drug class. The main adverse effects are metabolic and include:

- hyperlipidaemia
- insulin resistance and hyperglycaemia
- lipodystrophy.

Cytomegalovirus (CMV) infection

CMV mainly causes disease in immunosuppressed patients. CMV retinitis is a common problem in people with AIDS.

Ganciclovir. This drug inhibits the DNA polymerase of CMV. Ganciclovir is used i.v. It causes severe adverse effects including neutropenia, thrombocytopenia and renal impairment.

Foscarnet. This drug has a wide spectrum of antiviral activity, working by inhibition of DNA polymerase. The drug is poorly absorbed from the gut and is usually given i.v. Elimination is mainly as unchanged drug in the urine. Foscarnet is indicated for life-threatening CMV infection. Adverse effects include renal impairment.

Viral hepatitis

Acute uncomplicated viral hepatitis is usually managed with supportive care. However both hepatitis B and C can cause chronic hepatitis. Chronic hepatitis B may be treated with *interferon-alfa* or *lamivudine*. Chronic hepatitis C may be treated with ribavirin, in combination with interferon-alfa-2b.

Interferons

Interferons are a natural part of the body's defence system. They have protective effects against human viral infections and have been studied in hepatitis B and C infections. Interferon is not indicated for patients with acute hepatitis B but has proven beneficial in chronic hepatitis B, where around 40% of patients show benefit. Only a few studies have evaluated the use of interferon in acute hepatitis C infection but treatment may decrease the likelihood of chronicity and should be considered. In chronic hepatitis C infection, treatment has been effective in achieving sustained viral eradication in up to 20% of patients. Adverse effects include fever, alopecia, anaemia and gastrointestinal upset.

Lamivudine

Lamivudine is an NRTI used in HIV disease. It can also be used for chronic hepatitis B infection. Its use tends to be limited by adverse effects such as:

- gastrointestinal upsets
- alopecia
- peripheral neuropathy.

Ribavirin

Ribavirin is effective against a wide range of DNA and RNA viruses. It probably works by interference with the 'capping' of viral mRNA. Ribavirin may be given by inhalation, orally or i.v. It is eliminated by both metabolism and renal excretion, with a terminal half-life of about 2 weeks. Other than hepatitis C, ribavirin may be used for severe respiratory syncytial virus (RSV) infections in young children (usually employed as an aerosol). Adverse effects include:

- dose-dependent bone marrow suppression
- gastrointestinal adverse effects.

14.3 Antiprotozoal drugs

Learning objectives

You should:

- Be aware of the protozoal infections likely to be seen in clinical practice
- Be able to list the drugs used to prevent and treat malaria.

Clinical sketch

A woman comes to the surgery asking for malaria prophylaxis for her 2 week visit to Kenya. The GP consults current guidelines on malaria prevention and stresses that (i) these drugs do not provide 100% protection, (ii) the patient needs to protect herself against mosquito bites (ideally by sleeping under an insecticide-dipped bednet), and (iii) she should seek medical advice for any influenza-like symptoms upon her return to Britain.

Comment: falciparum malaria is common in subSaharan Africa and can kill a non-immune patient within 24 hours of the onset of symptoms. Personal protection against bites and the use of chemoprophylaxis reduce risk.

The same woman develops fever, rigors and myalgia 2 weeks after her return from holiday. She is slightly confused. A blood film confirms *Plasmodium falciparum* infection. She is admitted to the local infectious diseases hospital and treated with i.v. quinine.

Comment: this is a medical emergency. Intravenous quinine is the drug of choice: resistance to quinine is unusual in Africa.

Clinical Sketch

A homosexual man presents with severe breathlessness. His chest radiograph shows midzone shadowing and *Pneumocystis carinii* pneumonia (PCP)

is suspected; he is found to be HIV positive with a low CD4 cell count. He is treated with high-dose co-trimoxazole.

Comment: PCP is a common AIDS-defining illness. If this man survives, he will need lifelong secondary prophylaxis with either co-trimoxazole or pentamidine.

Common protozoal infections include:

- malaria: a major cause of death in developing countries
- amoebiasis: causes dysentery and hepatic abscesses
- *Giardia lamblia*: causes diarrhoea and malabsorption
- *Pneumocystis carinii*: causes pneumonia mainly in immunosuppressed individuals
- toxoplasmosis: affects brain and eyes particularly; most common in immunosuppressed subjects.

There is a wide range of antiprotozoal drugs, the most important of which are summarised below. Some antibacterial drugs such as metronidazole are also used against some protozoa (e.g. in amoebiasis).

Atovaquone. This is a well-tolerated drug that can be used for *Toxoplasma gondii* infections (seen in AIDS) and for the treatment and prevention of malaria.

Quinine. Quinine is mostly used parenterally for severe malaria. At high dose, adverse effects are common but rarely serious if standard regimens are used: deafness, vertigo and nausea are common, and ECG abnormalities may occur. In overdose quinine is very dangerous.

Mefloquine. This is used for the treatment and prevention of malaria. Psychosis and seizures are well-reported adverse effects.

Chloroquine. Malaria parasites resistant to chloroquine are now widespread. It may be given for the prevention and treatment of malaria. Severe adverse effects are unusual with standard doses, but high doses given for many years can cause retinopathy. In overdose, chloroquine causes severe shock and arrhythmias.

Pyrimethamine. This is usually combined with a sulphonamide for the treatment of uncomplicated malaria or for toxoplasmic encephalitis in AIDS patients. The doses used for malaria are usually without severe toxicity but the high doses used for toxoplasmosis cause bone marrow suppression. This can be reversed using folinic acid.

Co-trimoxazole. This combination of trimethoprim and sulfamethoxazole is used at high dose for the treatment of PCP. Toxicity is quite common at such high doses.

Pentamidine. This drug has many effects on *P. carinii* and is mainly used as an aerosol in the treatment and prevention of PCP. The main adverse effect is hypoglycaemia, which is common at high dose.

Self-assessment: questions

Multiple choice questions

1. The following drugs reach high CNS concentrations when they are given by mouth:
   a. Nystatin
   b. Amphoteracin
   c. Ketoconazole
   d. Aciclovir
   e. Fluconazole

2. Aciclovir:
   a. Is as effective for herpes zoster as it is for herpes simplex infections
   b. Is effective for all herpes virus infections
   c. Must be metabolised before it becomes active
   d. Interacts with allopurinol
   e. Interacts with probenecid

3. In the management of an influenza A outbreak:
   a. Amantidine should be given prophylactically to whomever requests it
   b. Amantidine and zanamivir have clinical benefit, even if started late in the illness
   c. The available influenza vaccines are of little use
   d. Zanamivir is safe in patients with chronic obstructive pulmonary disease
   e. Amantidine is contraindicated in pregnancy

Case history questions

Case history 1

A 40-year-old man with a renal transplant takes ciclosporin as an immunosuppressant. He develops a painful rash on his trunk and thinks it might be shingles (herpes zoster). His doctor agrees and starts oral aciclovir. A week later the patient is very unwell with fever and breathlessness: he is admitted to hospital as an emergency.

1. What may have happened?
2. Were the doctor's actions appropriate and adequate?

Case history 2

A 30-year-old man presents with life-threatening pneumococcal pneumonia. He has oral candidiasis, retinal features of cytomegalovirus infection and a low CD4$^+$ cell count. After counselling, an HIV test is done: tragically this is positive.

1. How would you manage this man?

Case history 3

An 18-year-old has been back-packing in Kenya for 2 months. He took mefloquine every week while he was away but stopped it when he got back home. Two weeks after his return he presents with headache, fever, myalgia and sweats.

1. What should be done?

Self-assessment: answers

Multiple choice answers

1. a. **False**. Nystatin is not absorbed from the gut.
   b. **False**. Amphoteracin is not absorbed from the gut.
   c. **False**. Ketoconazole undergoes extensive first-pass metabolism and does not readily cross the blood–brain barrier.
   d. **False**. Aciclovir is poorly absorbed.
   e. **True**.

2. a. **False**.
   b. **False**. Aciclovir is very effective against herpes simplex, less so against herpes zoster and ineffective against Epstein–Barr virus and cytomegalovirus.
   c. **True**. Must be metabolised by thymidine kinase.
   d. **False**. Allopurinol (Ch. 9) inhibits xanthine oxidase and potentiates 6-mercaptopurine, an anticancer drug.
   e. **True**. Probenecid inhibits the renal tubular transport of some drugs including penicillin and aciclovir.

3. a. **False**. There are clear guidelines on the patient categories to whom amantadine may be offered (see the BNF).
   b. **False**. Both drugs have demonstrable effects if started within 48 hours of the onset of symptoms. Beyond then they are not of proven use.
   c. **False**. At risk patients should be offered vaccination annually.
   d. **False**. Zanamivir may worsen bronchospasm. However, patients with chronic airways disease are at particular risk from influenza and zanamivir has proven benefit against influenza.
   e. **True**. Amantadine is teratogenic.

Case history answers

Case history 1

1. Immunosuppressed patients are at risk of disseminated herpes, which can cause pneumonia and other systemic illnesses. Aciclovir is the drug of first choice, but its bioavailability is very low. The drug may be given i.v. (which would require hospital admission) to particularly high-risk patients.
2. The doctor should have known all of this, and he has failed to act vigorously enough in the circumstances.

Case history 2

The life-threatening pneumococcal pneumonia is the first and most pressing problem. It will require the full range of supportive care as well as appropriate antibiotics (guided by assessment of drug sensitivity) and oxygen therapy. The oral candidiasis will often not respond to topical drugs, like nystatin, in AIDS patients: fluconazole is probably the first-choice drug. CMV retinitis is very serious and threatens sight: ophthalmological advice is mandatory. Gancyclovir is the drug of first choice, but it must be given into a central vein as it causes phlebitis when given peripherally. HAART will be needed but should be postponed until the patient has recovered from his acute presentation.

Case history 3

Weekly chloroquine plus daily proguanil is a common regimen for antimalarial prophylaxis in east Africa: it probably gives no better than 55% 'protective efficacy'. This patient took weekly mefloquine, which probably has a protective efficacy of greater than 75%. Even so, there remains a risk of malaria transmission, and this diagnosis needs to be excluded *as an emergency*: non-immune patients may die within 24 hours of the onset of symptoms from falciparum malaria. If he does have parasites in his blood then he needs:

- emergency admission
- close monitoring of parasitaemia, blood sugar (hypoglycaemia is a complication), level of consciousness and haemoglobin
- oral treatment with quinine, three times daily for 7 days; there are concerns of additive cardiac toxicity when quinine is given to people with therapeutic mefloquine levels, and so daily ECGs would be wise.

15 Anticancer chemotherapy

Overview

Malignant disease accounts for a high proportion of deaths in industrialised countries. Chemotherapy is one of several treatment options. Treatment aims to give palliation, induce remission and, if possible, cure. Because chemotherapeutic drugs will also affect normal healthy cells, drug regimens form an important part of prescription, using courses of drugs with gaps to allow normal cells to recover and drug combinations. The latter approach also contributes to avoidance of drug resistance.

15.1 Principles of cancer treatment

Learning objectives

You should:

- understand the guiding principles underlying the use of anticancer drugs
- appreciate the benefit versus risk relationship with these drugs.

Prevention of malignant neoplasms continues to elude us because, despite strong epidemiological data linking certain high-risk activities (such as smoking) to cancer, changing the habits of a population is extremely difficult. Treatment options comprise **surgery**, **radiotherapy** and **chemotherapy**; the first two are outside the scope of this book.

Cancers may kill through the local effects of the primary lesion, such as compression of vital structures or invasion of major blood vessels, but more usually do so through organ 'failure' (e.g. liver, marrow, lung and brain) caused by metastases. The treatment of a patient with cancer may aim to:

- give palliation, for example prompt relief of unpleasant symptoms such as superior vena cava obstruction from a mediastinal tumour
- induce 'remission' so that all macroscopic and microscopic features of the cancer disappear, though disease is known to persist
- cure, for which all the cells of the clone must be destroyed.

The above options are ranked in increasing order of difficulty, and cure is often impossible with current drugs.

Unfortunately healthy cells, particularly those undergoing replication (e.g. those in the marrow, mucosa, skin and gonads), are also very susceptible to chemotherapeutic drugs, but *less* so than the malignant clone. A basic principle of anticancer therapy is that chemotherapy is given in *courses*, interspersed with 'gaps' of varying duration to allow recovery of normal cells (Fig. 50). Another principle of chemotherapy is the use of *drug combinations*: though different drugs have additive (sometimes synergistic) therapeutic effects, aspects of their toxicity need not be additive. This approach has the further benefit of reducing the risk of tumour cell resistance to a particular drug. Rather like tuberculosis (Ch. 13), malignant clones contain cells with inherent drug resistance, and use of one drug may allow this population to flourish.

The drug treatment of malignancy is a specialist area. Solid tumours are usually managed by multidisciplinary teams of surgeons and oncologists. Haematological

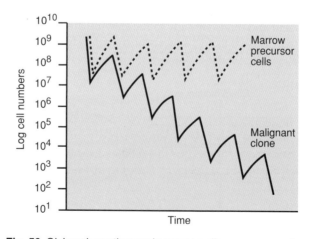

Fig. 50 Giving chemotherapy in courses allows recovery of normal cells.

malignancies are the province of haematologists. The general physician consequently needs no more than a grounding in the use of cancer chemotherapy.

15.2 Anticancer drugs

Learning objectives

You should:

- appreciate the importance of and be able to describe supportive care
- be able to list the main mechanisms of action of drugs used for malignancy
- be able to describe the therapeutic use of these drugs for a few common malignancies
- know the main adverse effects of the main drug groups

The clinical sketches in this chapter illustrate a few common malignancies—acute leukaemia, Hodgkin's disease, breast, prostate and lung cancer—and their chemotherapy.

Mechanisms of action of anticancer drugs

Alkylating agents

- These drugs 'transfer' their alkyl groups to cell components, thereby denaturing proteins.
- Examples include *cyclophosphamide* and *chlorambucil*.
- Toxicity is mainly dose related and affects rapidly growing cell types such as bone marrow, skin and mucous membranes and the gastrointestinal tract.

Antimetabolites

- These drugs 'mimic' a natural metabolite, thus impairing the efficiency of an essential biochemical path. For example *methotrexate* mimics dihydrofolic acid and binds strongly to the enzyme dihydrofolate reductase (Fig. 51), a mechanism that it shares with

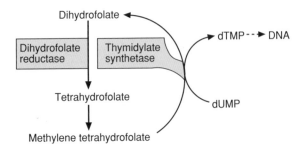

Fig. 51 The folate pathway. dUMP, uridylate; dTMP, thymidylate.

Clinical sketch: acute leukaemia

A 6-year-old girl presents with a short history of malaise, fever, bleeding gums and anaemia. She looks pale and has a temperature of 40°C but is otherwise normal: there is no organomegaly and no lymphadenopathy. Her haemoglobin is 9.0 g% (90 g/l), and she is both leukopenic and thrombocytopenic. Large numbers of primitive blasts are seen in the blood film; special staining reveals these to be lymphoblasts. She is given a blood transfusion and platelets, started on antibiotics and nursed in 'reversed barrier conditions'. Her haematologist starts cycles of combination chemotherapy including *vincristine*. After a stormy course, marked by many infections, she recovers. Five years later she is still in remission.

Comment: acute lymphoblastic leukaemia is the commonest childhood malignancy and responds well to chemotherapy. The prognosis is relatively good. Chemotherapy 'cocktails' vary, and their use is based on clinical trial data.

Clinical sketch: Hodgkin's disease

A 30-year-old man presents with fever and weight loss. Examination reveals cervical and axillary lymphadenopathy, and there is hilar adenopathy on his chest radiograph. Lymph node biopsy confirms Hodgkin's lymphoma. 'Staging computed tomographic (CT) scans' fail to show evidence of the disease below the diaphragm. After semen has been obtained and stored, his oncologist treats him with combination chemotherapy (including both *methotrexate* and *vincristine*) and radiotherapy. Five years later he is still disease free.

Comment: this young man did quite well considering that there were bad prognostic features including fever and weight loss. The prognosis of Hodgkin's disease very much depends on the stage at which it is caught. This man will probably want a family in due course, and the treatment has left him infertile: the stored semen samples are important.

---

the antimicrobial drug trimethoprim. However, whereas trimethoprim does not bind strongly to the human enzyme, methotrexate does. It thereby interferes with DNA synthesis.

- Examples include *methotrexate* and *6-mercaptoprine*.
- Toxicity is mainly dose related and affects rapidly proliferating tissues.

Plant alkaloids

- These are naturally occurring plant molecules. Mechanisms of action are variable but include effects on the cytoskeleton and on topoisomerase.
- Examples include *vincristine* and *vinblastine*.
- Adverse effects include bone marrow depression and neurotoxicity.

A 55-year-old, postmenopausal woman notices a breast lump and self-refers to the emergency breast assessment clinic. A fine needle aspiration is done the same day and breast cancer is confirmed. She is managed by a multidisciplinary surgical and oncological team. A segmental mastectomy is done and her axillary nodes are biopsied. Unfortunately, a metastasis is found in one of these local nodes. Postoperatively she is treated with cycles of chemotherapy (including *cyclophosphamide*, *methotrexate* and *doxorubicin*); she loses her hair and needs a wig. Thereafter, when she has recovered from initial treatment, she is started on *tamoxifen*. Unfortunately, 12 months later she presents with a pathological fracture and hypercalcaemia.

Comment: breast cancer affects around 10% of British women. It is treated with a combination of surgery and chemotherapy. The prognosis is relatively poor if there is lymph node disease, since distant metastases are common.

Clinical sketch: prostate cancer

A 70-year-old man presents with acute retention of urine: his prostate is large and hard, and biopsy confirms prostate cancer. The urologists do a subcapsular orchidectomy and he does well. Twelve months later he re-presents acutely with confusion and dehydration. He is markedly hypercalcaemic and his chest radiograph shows secondary deposits in his humeral head and several ribs. He is started on *goserelin* and *flutamide*.

Comment: goserelin is an expensive gonadorelin analogue that is beneficial in advanced prostate cancer. It can cause a 'tumour flare' soon after starting, and so an anti-androgen such as flutamide is usually given to prevent this.

Clinical sketch: Lung cancer

A 40-year-old smoker presents with cough and haemoptysis, and chest radiograph shows right upper lobe collapse and consolidation. Bronchoscopy reveals tumour in the right upper lobe bronchus and biopsies confirm this to be small cell carcinoma. The lesion is technically resectable and the patient's lung function is adequate: an upper lobectomy is done. Thereafter he is given combination chemotherapy (including *cyclophosphamide* and *doxorubicin*).

Comment: small cell tumours account for around 30% of lung cancer. They respond to chemotherapy but surgery is done where possible to 'debulk' the tumour. The prognosis is guarded.

Antibiotics

- These are products of microorganisms, just like the drugs used to combat infection. Their mechanisms of

action are variable but generally involve binding to host DNA.
- Examples include *daunorubicin*, *doxorubicin* and *bleomycin*.
- Adverse effects vary between drugs.

Hormonal agents

- Many common malignancies are hormone responsive (for example breast and prostate). These agents exploit this hormone-dependency.
- Examples include *tamoxifen*.
- Adverse effects vary between drugs.

An example of the alkylating agents: cyclophosphamide

Cyclophosphamide is well absorbed from the gut and widely distributed. It is metabolised in the liver to its active forms, which include a metabolite responsible for bladder toxicity. Most of a dose of cyclophosphamide is excreted as metabolites in the urine. Adverse effects include:

- marrow suppression: severe, dose related and often of long duration
- gonadal failure
- pulmonary fibrosis
- cystitis is a common problem caused by drug metabolites; this is usually avoided by co-administration of *mesna*, which protects the bladder epithelium
- carcinogenesis
- gastrointestinal upset is common and nausea may be severe
- cardiac toxicity, manifesting as arrhythmias and/or heart failure, may be seen at high doses.

An example of the antimetabolites: methotrexate

Methotrexate is also used in low dose as an immuno-suppressive in rheumatoid arthritis (Ch. 9).

Methotrexate may be given orally (it is well absorbed by an active uptake mechanism), i.v. or intrathecally. The drug is cleared unchanged, by renal excretion. Caution is needed in patients with renal impairment. Adverse effects include:

- marrow suppression, which manifests as agranulocytosis, thrombocytopenia and (to a lesser extent) anaemia; folinic acid has a useful therapeutic role
- mucositis, comprising ulceration and impaired function of the oral and intestinal mucosa; symptoms include stomatitis, nausea, diarrhoea and weight loss
- hepatitis, which varies between mild and life threatening

- neurotoxicity, particularly with the high local concentrations achieved with repeated intrathecal administration.

Drug interactions

Methotrexate increases the toxicity of fluorouracil, cytarabine, 6-mercaptopurine and 6-thioguanine.

Example of the plant alkaloids: vincristine

Vincristine must be given i.v. and causes necrosis if it extravasates. Vincristine readily crosses the blood–brain barrier, whereas vinblastine does not. It is cleared by hepatic metabolism. Adverse effects include:

- neurotoxicity: this is more severe and frequent with vincristine than vinblastine; the effects may comprise peripheral neuropathy, cranial nerve lesions, autonomic dysfunction and seizures
- gastrointestinal problems are common but usually mild; however, paralytic ileus may occur
- marrow suppression is not usually marked.

Examples of the antibiotics: doxorubicin and bleomycin

Doxorubicin is not absorbed from the gut and must be given i.v. It is extensively metabolised (some metabolites retain activity) and mainly excreted in the bile. Enterohepatic circulation occurs (see Ch. 1). It should be used with caution in patients with liver function impairment.

Bleomycin may be given i.v., i.m. or may be instilled into cavities (such as pleura or peritoneum). Bleomycin does not cross the blood–brain barrier but is otherwise widely distributed. It is mainly excreted unchanged, and renal impairment prolongs the half-life.

Adverse effects of doxorubicin include:

- marrow suppression, usually of short duration
- severe or total hair loss
- cumulative cardiac toxicity; this manifests as congestive cardiac failure and is usually avoided by careful recording of the cumulative dose given.

Adverse effects of bleomycin include:

- pulmonary fibrosis, which may affect 10% of patients; this is dose related and is more common in older patients
- anaphylactoid reactions
- mucositis, which may be severe
- marrow suppression: unlike most other anticancer drugs, bleomycin causes little myelosuppression, though it may be seen in patients with renal failure and drug accumulation.

Example of hormone therapy: tamoxifen

Tamoxifen is an oestrogen receptor modulator used for breast cancer. It is an oestrogen antagonist in breast tissue (see Ch. 12). It is taken orally in divided daily doses. Unlike the drugs described above, tamoxifen is well tolerated. Adverse effects include:

- hot flushes
- nausea
- fluid retention.

Supportive care

Synergistic drug combinations and gaps between courses of drugs minimises drug toxicity, but even so, cancer chemotherapy cannot be used without extensive supportive care, which is as important to the patient's survival as the chemotherapy itself. Key components of such care are described in Box 8.

Box 8 Components of supportive care

1. *Control of infection.* Predictable periods of agranulocytosis from marrow failure may cause life-threatening infection. Patients are routinely placed in **reversed barrier nursing** conditions. They are usually given **broad-spectrum antibiotic** combinations at the first sign of infection. Granulocyte infusions are of limited use (colony-stimulating factors may be used; see Ch. 5).

2. *Awareness of thrombocytopenia.* Marrow failure predictably causes thrombocytopenia and a risk of severe bleeding. Intramuscular injections are absolutely contraindicated. Intravenous injections are safe (pressure can be placed on the bleeding). Platelet infusions may be valuable.

3. *Correction of anaemia.* Anaemia is often less of a problem because of the long half-life of red cells compared with platelets or white cells. However, transfusions are often needed. In the case of irreversible marrow failure induced by drugs and radiotherapy (e.g. in an attempt to cure certain leukaemias) bone marrow *transplantation* is often needed (usually from a related donor).

4. *Nausea.* This is often the worst symptom and requires aggressive management. Antiemetics are discussed in Chapter 11.

5. *Hair loss.* Though seemingly 'trivial' this may have a profound effect on morale. Patients must be warned if depilation is anticipated, and wigs should be made available.

6. *Terminal care.* This subject is beyond the scope of this book. Terminal care requires great medical and nursing skill, together with the appropriate use of drugs including analgesics (Ch. 7), antiemetics (Ch. 11) and laxatives (Ch. 11).

Self-assessment: questions

Multiple choice questions

1. Methotrexate:
   a. Is antagonised by folic acid
   b. Is antagonised by folinic acid
   c. Enters cells by an active uptake mechanism
   d. Is potentiated by intracellular metabolism
   e. Is potentiated by hepatic disease

2. At standard dosage, the following drugs commonly cause the adverse effects to which they are linked in the question:
   a. Bleomycin and bone marrow suppression
   b. Cyclophosphamide and bladder carcinoma
   c. Doxorubicin and cardiac failure
   d. Methotrexate and macrocytosis
   e. Vincristine and peripheral neuropathy

3. The following statements concerning anticancer chemotherapy are true:
   a. Normal cells are usually more sensitive to the effects of the drugs than is the malignant clone
   b. The drugs are best given continuously for as long as possible
   c. Resistance to anticancer drugs is a major problem
   d. Most patients manage chemotherapy without the need for complicated supportive care
   e. Anticancer drugs cannot be given orally

Case history question

A postmenopausal woman undergoes needle aspiration of a 3 cm lump in her breast. The aspirated cells are malignant, and she is admitted for segmental mastectomy and axillary lymph node sampling.

1. What are the two major roles of surgery here?

Thereafter she is offered six cycles of chemotherapy with fluorouracil–doxorubicin–cyclophosphamide.

2. By what mechanism might the tumour develop resistance to all these drugs?

She responds well to this cytotoxic regimen and is then started on tamoxifen, which is to continue for the next 5 years.

3. What is the most common adverse effect of tamoxifen that she should be warned about?

Short note question

Describe, giving examples, the mechanisms by which drugs used for cancer chemotherapy work. What adverse effects do the named drugs cause?

Self-assessment: answers

Multiple choice answers

1. a. **False**.
   b. **True**. Methotrexate is a competitive inhibitor of dihydrofolate reductase (Fig. 51), the enzyme that reduces dihydrofolate back to tetrahydrofolate. The latter is a cofactor in the conversion of uridylate to thymidylate. Folic acid therefore 'precedes' the inhibited step. Folinic acid can 'bypass' this by conversion to methylene tetrahydrofolate (Fig. 51).
   c. **True**. Methotrexate is taken up by the same system that imports preformed folate into the cell; the lack of this system in microorganisms explains the lack of antimicrobial effect of the drug.
   d. **True**. Within the cell methotrexate becomes attached to glutamic acid residues: the polyglutamated form of the drug has activity against thymidylate synthetase (Fig. 51).
   e. **False**. Methotrexate is cleared unchanged: it is potentiated by renal disease.

2. a. **False**.
   b. **True**. Transitional cell carcinoma, resulting from chronic inflammation of the mucosa, is a problem unless mesna is used.
   c. **True**. This is an avoidable cumulative effect.
   d. **True**. Inhibition of DNA synthesis in red cell precursors results in fewer divisions and larger circulating cells.
   e. **True**.

3. a. **False**. Normal cells recover more rapidly than the malignant clones.
   b. **False**. It is usual to give courses of treatment interspersed with gaps to allow tissues (such as marrow, mucosal surfaces and skin) to recover.
   c. **True**. Especially if drugs are given as monotherapy. The mechanisms of resistance lie outside the scope of this book but include 'pumping' mechanisms that remove drug from the cancer cell.
   d. **False**. Almost everyone on cytotoxic treatment requires support in the areas of infection, blood products and nutrition.
   e. **False**. There are many drugs that are routinely given by mouth.

Case history answer

1. a. To reduce the size of the malignant clone by many log-orders.
   b. To permit microscopic examination of axillary lymph nodes, thereby clarifying prognosis and permitting decisions about further treatment to be made.
2. Multidrug resistance (or MDR) is usually caused by expression of P-glycoprotein pumps on cell surfaces. These pumps permit drug efflux from the malignant cell. These pumps can be opposed by such drugs as the calcium antagonist verapamil (which is more commonly used for its cardiac and hypotensive actions).
3. Tamoxifen is usually well tolerated, but hot flushes are quite common.

Short note answer

Modes of action

Alkylating agents (e.g. cyclophosphamide and chlorambucil) transfer alkyl groups to nucleotide components of the DNA molecule. This results in misreading of the code, fragmentation of DNA and cross-linkage of DNA. Because alkylating agents interfere with transcription, their effects are not confined to rapidly dividing cells: any cell group may be affected.

Antimetabolites (e.g. methotrexate, 6-mercaptopurine) compete with the substrate for the enzyme and inhibit enzyme function. Methotrexate resembles dihydrofolate, the substrate for the enzyme dihydrofolate reductase. Methotrexate also binds to, and inhibits, thymidylate synthetase, another enzyme important in the synthesis of pyrimidine nucleotides. The net effect is inhibition of DNA synthesis. 6-Mercaptopurine is an analogue of the purine bases adenine and guanine; it inhibits the enzymes responsible for interconversion of purines and is probably also incorporated into DNA. Antimetabolite drugs are mainly effective against rapidly dividing cells.

Vinca alkaloids (e.g. vincrystine and vinblastine) bind to, and disrupt, the cytoskeleton (tubulin molecules). They produce arrest of mitosis and are effective mainly against rapidly dividing cells.

Antibiotics (e.g. daunorubicin) have been isolated from microbes (often fungi). They bind to DNA and block transcription and new DNA synthesis. They, therefore, have their effects on any cell, not just those which divide frequently.

Adverse effects

Suppression of bone marrow and mention the clinical consequences of this. All the above drugs, except the vinca alkaloids, produce marked marrow suppression.

Mucositis is produced by all the drugs to some extent, except the vinca drugs.

Nausea is produced by all the drugs (the vinca drugs to a lesser degree); mention its management briefly.

Alopecia occurs particularly with the antibiotics. *Specific organ toxicity* can occur:

- pneumonitis: 6-mercaptopurine, bleomycin, methotrexate, antibiotics
- heart muscle damage: doxorubicin
- cystitis: cyclophosphamide (mention mesna)
- neurotoxicity: vinca drugs in particular
- hepatitis: any of these drugs, but particularly methotrexate and 6-mercaptopurine.

16 Drugs and the skin

Overview

Skin conditions are common; they may be confined to the skin, may be part of a wider systematic illness or may be caused by an adverse drug reaction. Many treatments for skin infections can be applied topically. Common conditions include eczema, psoriasis and acne. Common treatments are emollients to help rehydrate the skin, topical corticosteroids for inflammatory conditions and antibiotics for acne.

16.1 Skin disorders

Learning objectives

You should:

- be able to list the major common skin diseases

- be able to describe appropriate treatments for each of these conditions

- know the major adverse effects of these drugs.

The skin normally forms a water-resistant barrier and prevents loss of fluid. It also generally prevents entry of drugs, although certain drugs are now specifically formulated to enter through the skin; this avoids first-pass metabolism and achieves direct entry into the systemic circulation. Sustained-release preparations are usually used with the drug contained in a reservoir held in place by an adhesive. Examples include glyceryl trinitrate, estradiol and progesterone, and nicotine (Chs 4 and 12).

The skin may suffer from a variety of conditions, usually not life threatening but perhaps disfiguring. The skin may also be secondarily involved as part of a systemic illness.

Emollients

In the treatment of skin diseases, simple emollients are very important and are generally underused. These are bland substances that sooth and hydrate the skin and reduce irritation; they are very useful in conditions where the skin is dry and scaly. These may be used as vehicles for drugs.

Examples include *aqueous cream* (water and oil emulsion) or *emulsifying ointment*. This is more greasy and less pleasant to use but more effective for chronic dry skin lesions. It can be used as a skin cleansing agent instead of soap.

Topical antiinfectives

For many bacterial skin infections, such as cellulitis or erysipelas, systemic antibiotics are more appropriate as the infection is deep seated. Topical antibacterials are generally avoided: they may promote colonisation with resistant organisms and cause sensitisation. Simple cleaning of a wound is often adequate. Exceptions are a staphylococcal infection of the skin (impetigo) or in the treatment of skin colonisation with multiresistant *Staphylococcus aureus* in health care professionals. *Mupirocin* is a suitable topical treatment here.

Antiviral and antifungal topical agents are discussed in Chapter 14.

Primary skin disorders

Eczema

Clinical sketch

A 21-year-old woman, who suffers from hay fever, reports that her skin is dry and irritated. This particularly bothers her on her face. She has had similar problems in the past, with no clear precipitant. She is particularly bothered now because the skin on her face is dry and flaking. She has had topical steroids in the past and wants them again now.

Comment: Topical glucocorticoids can cause striae and cutaneous atrophy, which would be disfiguring. It would be better to avoid the steroids and use an emollient for the dryness and possibly oral antihistamines for the itching (if she is not already taking one).

Eczema is an inflammatory response of the skin to either external or internal factors, acting either singly or in combination. These factors may be simple irritants, or there may be immunological mechanisms involved (there is an association of some forms of eczema with atopy). It may vary greatly in severity from dryness, scaling and itching, to severe itching with redness, formation of vesicles and perhaps exudation with crusting.

Treatment

An attempt should be made to identify and remove any causative irritants; dietary modification may occasionally help. If simple dryness of the skin and itching are present, an emollient to preserve the moisture of the skin may be adequate. In more severe cases, topical *glucocorticoid* creams and ointments are used in addition; a variety of such creams are available, of varying potency and strength (see Ch. 12 for their mode of action.) The weakest preparation compatible with successful treatment should be used because of the adverse effects of topical glucocorticoids, including cutaneous atrophy and striae (it is particularly important to use topical glucocorticoids very sparingly on the face where such skin changes would be quite disfiguring). When they are withdrawn, a rebound exacerbation of the condition may occur. Rarely, systemic absorption of high-dose or high-potency topical glucocorticoids leads to systemic adverse effects and hypothalamic–pituitary–adrenal axis suppression.

Examples. *Hydrocortisone* and *betamethasone* are both available as creams or ointments.

In acute severe eczema with extensive exudate, *potassium permanganate* soaks are used initially. Oral sedating antihistamines are sometimes useful to reduce the itching.

Psoriasis

Psoriasis is a chronic inflammatory reaction of the skin of unknown aetiology, although there is often a family history. A form of psoriasis can arise after a streptococcal infection. The affected skin appears as thickened scaling plaques, often on the elbows, knees and scalp, although any area may be involved.

Treatment

In mild cases, simple emollients may be adequate. Topical keratolytic preparations containing *coal tar* (e.g. coal tar shampoo) or salicylic acid are effective but not pleasant to use. They act by softening and removing hardened skin and also have an antiinflammatory effect. *Dithranol* acts in a similar manner and can be used for more severe disease; it is, however, irritant and can stain normal skin, so care must be taken to apply it only to the affected plaque. It is covered with a dressing for an hour and then washed off.

It was observed coincidentally that psoriasis improved in patients taking vitamin D. *Calcipotriol*, a vitamin D derivative, was developed for topical use in psoriasis. It has no effect on systemic Ca^{2+} balance but should nevertheless be avoided in patients with disordered Ca^{2+} metabolism. It is irritant, and local or generalised skin reactions can occur.

Specialist treatment. Ultraviolet light can improve psoriasis, and patients having this treatment may take a **psoralen** (a drug that increases the sensitivity of the skin) beforehand. This treatment needs careful supervision and is available in specialist centres only. Topical glucocorticoids are also used, but rebound of disease is a problem and they should be used only by specialists. In severe cases, systemic immune suppression may be necessary: methotrexate (Ch. 15) is used. This is clearly associated with increased risks, but in some patients there may be no alternative.

Acne

Acne is a chronic inflammatory condition that particularly affects the face and back, characterised by the presence of comedones (blackheads), papules, pustules and cysts. In severe cases it may cause permanent scarring. It arises with the activation of the sebaceous glands at puberty, causing increased greasiness of the skin, and tends to clear with age. There may also be colonisation of the skin and sebaceous glands by *Propionibacterium acnes*, a bacterium that breaks down fats in the sebum to form irritant fatty acids.

Clinical sketch

A 30-year-old man presents with red scaly lesions, most marked at his elbows and knees but also affecting his scalp and with some lesions on his trunk. The scalp is very itchy and the skin flakes readily. There is a family history of psoriasis, and he has had similar lesions for many years.

Comment: initial treatment with an emollient may be helpful but he may be helped by more specialist drug treatment.

Clinical sketch

An 18-year-old woman is distressed by the appearance of spots around her nose. She has blackheads and papules, and some pustules. She has been trying to hide these with cosmetics. She has some further lesions on her back.

Comment: this is a common problem of puberty. Benzoyl peroxide or a topical antibiotic treatment may help to clear the problem. Isotretinoin is teratogenic and so would not be a safe option in a girl of this age.

Treatment

Benzoyl peroxide kills the bacteria and peels the skin, unplugging the follicles: it can be irritant to the skin and a weak solution is applied to the face for a short period and then washed off; gradually, the duration of exposure and the strength of the preparation is increased. In moderate cases, long-term systemic or topical antibiotic treatment, usually with tetracycline or one of its derivatives or erythromycin, is effective.

In very severe cases, vitamin A derivatives such as *isotretinoin* can be used, given orally. Its adverse effects include hepatitis and altered serum lipids; most importantly, it is teratogenic and is usually given only to males, or to females who are using careful contraception (for at least a month before treatment and for at least 2 years afterwards, because isotretinoin concentrates in body fat and is only slowly cleared). Because of these hazards, isotretinoin can only be prescribed by hospital specialists. Tretinoin is a vitamin A derivative available for topical use, and the systemic adverse effects are avoided.

16.2 Skin and adverse drug reactions

Learning objectives

You should:

- be aware of the potential for skin disorders associated with drug therapy
- be aware of the seriousness of the reaction.

The skin is also a common site for manifestation of drug adverse effects, often allergic in nature. Rashes or itching can occur shortly after the drug is first taken, but sometimes not until 2–3 weeks later. Almost any type of reaction may occur, and these can mimic many skin conditions, including rashes, itching, photosensitivity, hair loss, purpura, blistering and pigmentation. A fixed drug eruption is a drug reaction that occurs in the same place on each exposure. Some reactions are particularly associated with certain drugs:

- morbelliform (measles-like): ampicillin, amoxicillin
- lichen planus-like: gold, antimalarials
- exfoliative dermatitis: penicillin, gold.

Clinical sketch

A newly diagnosed epileptic is prescribed carbamazepine for the first time. Two weeks later, he has developed ulceration in his mouth such that he has difficulty drinking. He is feverish and feels very unwell.

Comment: he is diagnosed as having Stevens–Johnson syndrome, a severe and unusual form of skin reaction to carbamazepine.

Most skin reactions are mild and self-limiting. Stevens–Johnson syndrome is a severe and usually fatal condition with skin blistering. It is associated with the use of some drugs such as fluconazole and carbamazepine.

Self-assessment: questions

Multiple choice questions

1. The following statements are correct:
   a. The skin prevents the entry of all drugs
   b. Topical corticosteroids may cause systemic adverse effects
   c. Psoriasis is treated with keratolytic agents or vitamin D derivatives
   d. Acne is treated with topical corticosteroids
   e. Vitamin A derivatives are teratogenic

2. The following statements are correct:
   a. Isotretinoin is used to treat herpes simplex
   b. Adverse drug reactions often affect the skin
   c. Methotrexate is used topically in severe psoriasis
   d. Eczema of the face is treated with high-potency fluorinated glucocorticoids
   e. Topical treatment is adequate for all skin conditions

3. The following drugs may be applied directly to the skin for systematic therapeutic effect (i.e. can affect the whole body)
   a. Hydrocortisone
   b. Oestrodiol
   c. Aspirin
   d. Glyceryl trinitrate
   e. Fucidic acid

Case history question

> An 18-year-old man presents with acne. This is moderately severe and has failed to respond to simple peeling agents used for some weeks.

1. What would you consider is the next line of treatment?

> There is some improvement on your second-line treatment but the condition does not resolve and there are some large inflamed areas. There is concern that these may go on to scar, since they are on the face.

2. What drug treatment would you consider now?
3. What precautions would you take and warning would you give before starting this treatment?

Extended matching items question

Theme: skin
Options

A. Isotretinoin
B. Hydrocortisone
C. Tetracycline
D. Emollient
E. Coal tar
F. Ciprofloxacin
G. Chlorpheniramine
H. Calcipotriol

Read 1–5 below and choose the most appropriate answer from options A–H. Each option can be used once, more than once or not at all.

1. A sedating antihistamine useful in itchy conditions
2. A drug with serious teratogenic effects if used in women
3. A vitamin D derivative used in psoriasis
4. An antibiotic used systemically in acne
5. An anti-inflammatory glucocorticoid used in skin conditions

Self-assessment: answers

Multiple choice answers

1. a. **False**. Many preparations take advantage of this.
   b. **True**. If used in very high dose.
   c. **True**. Keratolytics to reduce the scaling; calcipotriol's mode of action is unknown.
   d. **False**. Peeling agents and some antibiotics are used: corticosteroids would make things worse.
   e. **True**. So only given to women of child-bearing potential if they are using effective contraception.

2. a. **False**. Isotretinoin is used to treat acne and other skin disorders.
   b. **True**. A very common site of manifestation of adverse drug reactions.
   c. **False**. Used systemically.
   d. **False**. This would cause striae etc. on the face. Less potent steroids may be used with great care.
   e. **False**. For example, methotrexate, dapsone, etc.

3. a. **False**. Commonly used in dermatology for local effect but will not have a systematic effect. More potent corticosteroids may if applied in sufficient quantity have a systematic effect, as proven by adrenocortical suppression.
   b. **True**. Used in estrogen patches for systematic effect in the treatment of postmenopausal problems.
   c. **False**. Too irritant to use topically at all, although some salicylates are used in traditional rubefacients for relief of musculoskeletal pain. These do not have a systematic effect.
   d. **True**. Used in patches to treat angina.
   e. **False**. Although used topically to treat local infections, for instance in the eye.

Case history answer

1. Since topical peeling agents alone have been unsuccessful, it is time to consider systemic antibiotics. Topical antibiotics are generally less effective. Long-term oxytetracycline or erythromycin should be considered. It can take some weeks for this to have its maximum effect.
2. Since systemic antibiotics in addition to topical agents have failed to resolve the condition satisfactorily, it is time to consider vitamin A derivatives such as isotretinoin.
3. The potential adverse effects are hepatitis and altered serum lipids and teratogenicity. Fortunately, teratogenicity is not an issue in this male patient, but blood should be sent for serum lipids and for liver function tests before starting the therapy and intermittently during it. The patient should be warned of the major adverse effects. Because of these hazards and the need for careful monitoring, isotretinoin is usually only prescribed by hospital specialists.

Extended matching items answer

1. G. Chlorpheniramine is widely used to reduce the sensation of itchiness; warn the patient about the possibility of sedation.
2. A. Isotretinoin can be teratogenic in women: it must only be used in women of child-bearing age who are using effective contraception, and who will continue to use it for up to 2 years after stopping the isotretinoin. Isotretinoin may be retained for a long time in body fat.
3. H. Calcipotriol is used in psoriasis; it rarely has significant systemic vitamin D type activity.
4. C. Tetracycline or its derivatives are used in this way.
5. B. Topical hydrocortisone, as ointments and creams, is widely used as an effective antiinflamatory in skin disorders.

17 Drug overdose and poisoning

Overview

Drug overdose is one of the most common medical emergencies. In the majority of cases, it is deliberate, the result of social pressures or psychiatric illness, but accidental overdose by children remains common, despite 'child-proof' medicine containers. In an industrial setting, inadvertent acute poisoning can occur from a variety of non-therapeutic compounds, including heavy metals, insecticides and gases such as cyanide and carbon monoxide.

Management of overdose involves identifying the causative agent, assessing the dose involved, supportive care and minimising the adverse effects, with antidotes if possible.

17.1 The principles of supportive care

Learning objectives

You should:

- know the management of a poisoned patient, the principles of decontamination, acceleration of drug elimination, specific antidotes and supportive care

- understand the principles of supportive care

- know the main antidotes used and the drugs for which they are used

- be able to describe the principles underpinning the use of alkaline diuresis and haemodialysis/haemoperfusion for enhancing drug elimination.

Initial resuscitation and assessment of level of consciousness and vital signs should be followed by an attempt to discover:

- what drug(s) or toxin(s) were taken
- what dose(s) were taken (empty bottles can be very useful)
- roughly when did ingestion occur (though the patient's assessment of time lapse can often be unreliable).

Management comprises:

- Decontamination
- supportive care
- specific measures to reduce toxicity through the use of 'antidotes' or to enhance elimination.

The clinical sketches in this chapter illustrate the more common overdose/poisoning situations and their likely presentation.

Supportive care

Detailed consideration of supportive care is beyond the scope of this book, but the student should be aware of the principal ways in which poisoning can cause death and the measures by which death can be averted:

Coma. Death may result from obstruction of the airway by soft tissues, by aspiration of vomit or by depression of the 'respiratory centre'. It is essential that level of consciousness be monitored (e.g. using the Glasgow coma scale). Protection of the airway is critical: nursing in the 'recovery position' will usually be sufficient, but some patients need endotracheal intubation. Monitoring of arterial gases is critical in such severely ill patients: ventilatory failure necessitates mechanical ventilation.

Seizures. CNS excitation, resulting in seizures, can coexist with profound coma and can contribute to ventilatory failure. Antiepileptic drugs may be needed, and resistant cases may need to be paralysed and ventilated.

Cardiovascular toxicity. Toxins may cause arrhythmias (fast or slow), reduced stroke volume, vasodilatation or a combination of these: the resulting shock may prove fatal. In many cases acid–base and electrolyte imbalance are major contributing factors. Electrolyte/pH correction, temporary pacing, inotropic drugs and antiarrhythmics may all be needed in supportive care.

Renal failure. This is another common life-threatening problem.

An 18-year-old takes an impulsive paracetamol overdose. Thereafter, although he feels okay, he regrets his actions and is scared. He presents to hospital about 8 hours after drug ingestion. The doctors measure his plasma paracetamol concentration: it is above the 'treatment line', so N-acetylcysteine infusions are started. His clotting parameters and liver function tests remain normal and he makes an uneventful recovery.

Comment: patients are relatively asymptomatic between ingestion of the drug and development of liver impairment between 2 and 3 days thereafter. The insidious nature of this problem probably contributes to its mortality since patients can present too late for help. Prolonged prothrombin time and elevated transaminase levels are the first indication of impending illness; thereafter clinical features of acute liver damage develop. This young man was caught before clinically apparent liver damage was done.

Clinical sketch: salicylate

An 18-year-old patient takes an impulsive overdose of aspirin. She feels unwell almost at once with nausea, vomiting and tinnitus. She presents to A&E where she is found to be ill, tachypnoeic and dehydrated. Her arterial pH is 7.05 and her salicylate level is very high. Rather than rely on alkaline diuresis, the clinical team decides that haemodialysis is needed: she is moved to ITU.

Comment: metabolic acidosis is the commonest acid–base disturbance seen in adults after significant salicylate overdose. There is no specific antidote; management hinges on accelerating elimination of the drug. Alkaline diuresis (see text) increases the rate of elimination but haemodialysis is required in the most serious cases.

Clinical sketch: opiates

A young i.v. drug abuser is found unconscious. He has pinpoint pupils and is deeply cyanosed; his blood pressure is unrecordable. His arterial gases are as follows: pH 7.15, P_{CO_2} 10.5 kPa, P_{O_2} 6.5 kPa. The doctors gain i.v. access and give him i.v. naloxone. This improves his clinical features but he remains very ill: he is intubated and ventilated. The naloxone is repeated periodically in ITU.

Comment: this man has pronounced CNS depression causing type II respiratory failure and respiratory acidosis. He may have inadvertently taken too much heroin (street supplies vary in their purity); he may have taken more than one drug. Naloxone is a specific opiate antagonist; it has a very short half-life. Patients normally respond rapidly and completely if their only intoxication is with an opiate.

Clinical sketch: Tricyclic antidepressants

A 50-year-old man lost his wife a year ago and has been depressed ever since. His GP has prescribed amitriptyline, and this may have helped (he has been sleeping better). However, after leaving a suicide note, he takes a massive overdose of amitriptyline and is found by his daughter late that afternoon. A&E doctors find an unconscious man who starts to fit soon after arrival. He is transferred to ITU, where he dies of cardiac arrhythmias despite best efforts.

Comment: tricyclic antidepressants cause profound CNS depression, seizures, arrhythmias and shock. There are no accepted means of enhancing elimination, and no specific antidote is available; management is supportive.

Clinical sketch: iron

A 2-year-old child is attracted to her mother's iron tablets by their pretty colour. She swallows four 200 mg capsules of ferrous sulphate. Her worried parents take her to A&E with severe abdominal pain. Soon after arrival she develops signs of gastrointestinal bleeding. Her liver function tests deteriorate thereafter, and the prognosis is guarded.

Comment: this could well be a fatal dose without prompt treatment: gastrointestinal bleeding, coma and liver failure are the main features of severe poisoning. Decontamination is urgent: the amount of iron remaining in the stomach may be judged on abdominal radiograph. After gastric lavage, the chelator desferrioxamine (which is not absorbed) needs to be given orally (or down the lavage tube) to chelate as much of the unabsorbed iron as possible. Desferrioxamine also needs to be given parenterally to chelate the iron that has been absorbed.

Decontamination

Decontamination includes both removal of toxin from the skin and clothes in industrial accidents and removal of drug from the gastrointestinal tract (Box 9).

Box 9 Decontamination

1. Most drug overdoses are taken orally, and if the patient is seen soon after ingestion there may still be drug in the stomach. Some drugs, e.g. the tricyclics, delay gastric emptying; efforts to clear drug from the stomach may be useful up to 12 hours after ingestion.
2. Whatever measures are taken to remove drug from the stomach, *the airway must be secure*. If the patient

is unconscious, protection of the airway involves use of a cuffed endotracheal tube.

3. Syrup of ipecac (ipecachuana) is a useful emetic for conscious children and adults.

4. In unconscious patients, gastric lavage using a wide bore tube may be appropriate (see 2, above). Any anticipated benefits from such a procedure must be balanced against the risks.

5. Emetics and gastric lavage *are contraindicated* if the patient has ingested corrosive substances because of the risk of exacerbating oesophageal damage. Such substances include:

   - bleach and domestic alkali
   - mercuric salts.

6. *Activated charcoal* binds many drugs and toxins. It is mixed into a slurry with water and either swallowed or left in the stomach tube after lavage.

7. *Decontamination of the skin*, e.g. after an industrial accident, involves:

   - removal of contaminated clothes
   - copious washing.

Specific antidotes

Specific antidotes are available for some drugs/toxins (Table 3).

Table 3 Specific antidotes

Drug/toxin	Antidote
Paracetamol	*N*-acetylcysteine is a specific antidote
Opiates	Naloxone is an antagonist
Benzodiazepines	Flumazenil is an antagonist
Iron	Desferrioxamine chelates
Copper	Penicillamine chelates
Lead	Edetate (EDTA) chelates
Mercury, arsenic	Dimercaprol chelates

Methods of enhancing elimination

Manipulation of urinary pH

Some drugs become unionised at urinary pH and may be reabsorbed in the distal tubule. Relatively small changes in urinary pH produce relatively large changes in the fraction of drug unionised (see Ch. 1 for the Henderson–Hasselbach equation, which describes this relationship) and alter renal clearance. This is of practical value with overdoses of:

- salicylates
- phenobarbital.

In both cases, sodium bicarbonate is given as i.v. infusions. This increases urinary pH. Such **alkaline diuresis** is often 'forced' by administration of i.v. fluid together with loop diuretics.

Forced alkaline diuresis implies large fluid volumes. This may precipitate pulmonary oedema and close monitoring is mandatory:

- central venous pressure (CVP) may need to be measured.
- urinary pH needs to be measured by pH meter.

Haemodialysis and haemoperfusion

Drugs with relatively small apparent volumes of distribution (VD) are largely restricted to the plasma, whereas those with large VD are extensively distributed to the tissues. Drugs of small VD may be removable by haemodialysis (the extracorporeal pumping of blood across a large surface area of semipermeable membrane) or haemoperfusion (the pumping of blood through a column of adsorbent material, such as charcoal).

Factors influencing the utility of these measures for a particular drug include molecular weight, water solubility and protein binding.

Haemodialysis may be valuable for:

- salicylate
- aminophylline
- lithium

Haemoperfusion may be valuable for:

- phenobarbital
- Carbazamepine.

17.2 Specific drugs

Learning objectives

You should:

- be able to describe the clinical syndromes that are commonly encountered after overdoses of paracetamol, salicylate, opiates, benzodiazepines, stimulants, tricyclic antidepressants, heavy metals and Organophosphates.

Many patients overdose with more than one drug.

Paracetamol

In therapeutic doses, paracetamol is principally metabolised to non-toxic, water-soluble conjugates. However, in overdose, conjugation becomes saturated and 'excess' drug is oxidised to a toxic metabolite. The toxin forms covalent bonds with proteins, both structural and enzymic, thereby denaturing them. Cells employ glutathione as a defence against such toxins: it forms non-toxic conjugates with the toxin. However, intracellular glutathione 'stores' are soon exhausted after significant paracetamol overdose.

Glutathione cannot be used as an antidote because of its inability to enter cells. *N*-acetylcysteine is a glutathione precursor. Although very safe, *N*-acetylcysteine is not without risk (allergy) and should not be used indiscriminately.

Risk of liver damage correlates well with plasma paracetamol concentration, and this measure is used to guide therapy. Because drug absorption may not be complete within the first 4 hours after ingestion, measurement of plasma paracetamol should not be done within this period. Thereafter, patients with a plasma concentration above the 'treatment line' (see the British National Formulary) should be given *N*-acetylcysteine (as an i.v. loading dose, followed by i.v. infusion).

Beyond 14 hours after paracetamol overdose, the benefits of *N*-acetylcysteine are less clear, though many units would still try using it even in late presenters.

Established acute liver failure needs to be treated in specialist centres and carries a high mortality rate; transplantation may be required.

Methionine, an amino acid given orally, can also be used to regenerate glutathione stores but is less effective than *N*-acetylcysteine.

Salicylate

Aspirin has several metabolic effects: it stimulates the respiratory centre, interferes with carbohydrate and lipid metabolism and is itself a relatively strong acid. Stimulation of the respiratory centre, which causes hyperventilation, results in early **respiratory alkalosis**. To compensate for this, there is renal loss of bicarbonate ions, which reduces buffering capacity; higher salicylate concentrations then induce **metabolic acidosis** readily (both directly and by changes in carbohydrate and lipid metabolism).

Salicylate poisoning gives symptoms soon after drug ingestion: abdominal pain, nausea, tinnitus, deafness, vertigo and hyperpnoea. If the overdose is large, fever, dehydration, metabolic acidosis, renal impairment and cardiovascular collapse may follow.

Severity of poisoning can be assessed by measuring plasma salicylate concentration: plasma salicylate over 750 mg/l, 6 hours after drug ingestion, confirms severe poisoning (though better guidance is given by serial measurements to establish whether concentrations are rising).

Rehydration is an important part of general care. Drug elimination can be enhanced by alkalinisation of the urine or, in severe cases, by haemodialysis.

Opiates

Sedation, cough suppression and respiratory depression occur as a direct consequence of stimulation of opioid μ-receptors. This results in deep coma with pin-point pupils, hypotension and hypothermia.

Patients with **ventilatory failure** should receive the specific antidote *naloxone* as an i.v. injection. This opioid receptor antagonist causes prompt improvement in the level of consciousness unless other sedative drugs have been taken. Naloxone's duration of action is very short, and it may need to be given frequently.

Buprenorphine, a synthetic opiate, may not be reversed by naloxone.

Benzodiazepines

The GABA agonist action of the benzodiazepines causes CNS depression. However, benzodiazepines have a relatively flat dose–response curve and do not induce surgical levels of anaesthesia even after overdose. They are consequently safer than the barbiturates in this setting. However, patients may still vomit and aspirate, and those with chronic pulmonary disease are still at risk of ventilatory failure.

Flumazenil (a specific benzodiazepine antagonist) is very expensive and can precipitate seizures in patients addicted to benzodiazepines; its use is therefore restricted to:

- making a diagnosis
- patients in unrousable coma, particularly where arterial gases show evidence of ventilatory failure.

Flumazenil has a short duration of action and may need to be repeated frequently.

Tricyclic antidepressants

Tricyclic antidepressants have complex pharmacological effects (Ch. 6) including inhibition of reuptake of noradrenaline into neurones, anticholinergic actions and quinidine-like antiarrhythmic effects:

- combined effects on the CNS cause agitation at lower concentration but result in profound CNS depression and seizures at higher levels
- anticholinergic effects cause tachycardia
- quinidine-like action results in QT prolongation and ST changes in the ECG and reduced stroke volume (hence reduced cardiac output).

Early features may include blurred vision, retention of urine, dry mouth and agitation.

Features of severe poisoning include coma, seizures, arrhythmias and shock.

Because anticholinergic effects delay gastric emptying, emesis (or gastric lavage) can be indicated even beyond 12 hours after ingestion.

Tricyclic antidepressants have very large volumes of distribution. Consequently, measures such as haemodyalisis are of no value (there is simply too little drug in the plasma for any impact to be made). With no accepted means of enhancing elimination, and no specific antidote, management hinges on supportive care.

Stimulants (e.g. 'Ecstasy')

Ecstasy (see Ch. 18) is an amfetamine derivative, *methylenedioxymetamfetamine*. It is widely available to young people and taken orally. Its use is entirely illicit, i.e. it is not made by reputable manufacturers; therefore, quality control is poor and tablet contents may vary.

Clinical effects include vomiting, tachycardia, hyperthermia and hypo/hypertension. Rhabdomyolysis (destruction of skeletal muscle), renal failure and disseminated intravascular coagulation (a blood clotting disorder) may be seen.

Death is usually caused by cardiac arrhythmias.

There is no specific antidote and neither haemodialysis nor haemoperfusion are beneficial. Management is supportive.

Heavy metals

Iron. Desferrioxamine chelates iron (see the clinical sketches). The symptoms of iron poisoning evolve over several days:

phase 1 is characterised by gastrointestinal features and may involve severe ulceration; it evolves over about 6 hours

phase 2 between 6 and 24 hours, comprises resolution of symptoms—most patients have no further problems

phase 3 12 to 48 hours after serious poisoning: a minority of patients develop shock, acidosis and renal/hepatic failure

phase 4 comprises late complications (2 to 6 weeks after poisoning) from high intestinal or pyloric strictures.

Lead. Lead poisoning can present with encephalopathy and peripheral neuropathy. *Chelators* include EDTA, penicillamine and calcium edetate.

Mercury. Mercury poisoning can present with tremor, encephalopathy and renal impairment. *Chelators* include dimercaprol and penicillamine.

Organophosphates

These insecticides are widely used in farming. They are extensively absorbed from the skin and inhibit acetylcholinesterase.

The main acute effects of massive exposure are respiratory muscle paralysis and coma.

Atropine is used to oppose the excessive acetylcholinergic activity in the autonomic nervous system. Praloxidime is used to help regenerate acetylcholinesterase.

Self-assessment: questions

Multiple choice questions

1. Poisoning with benzodiazepines:
   a. Causes seizures
   b. Causes respiratory depression
   c. Should be reversed with flumazenil in all cases
   d. Is more severe in the presence of respiratory disease
   e. Can be reversed by haemodialysis

2. In the case of iron poisoning:
   a. Gastric lavage causes oesophageal damage
   b. Oral desferrioxamine is adequate to chelate the fraction of the dose that has been absorbed
   c. Oral desferrioxamine is useless
   d. Patients may be discharged within 24 hours of poisoning
   e. Serum iron concentrations give a good idea of prognosis

3. Following paracetamol poisoning:
   a. Symptoms and signs develop quickly
   b. Serum paracetamol levels should be estimated as soon as possible after poisoning
   c. Estimation of the International Normalised Ratio is the most useful guide to severity of poisoning in patients who present late
   d. N-acetylcysteine works by chelating paracetamol
   e. N-acetylcysteine should be given to all patients irrespective of their drug concentrations

Case history questions

Case history 1

> A man takes a deliberate overdose of amitriptyline, but 4 hours later regrets this and presents to hospital.

1. How essential is it to measure drug concentrations?
2. Should he be given any prophylactic drugs?

> Gastric lavage is done, and he is sent to the ward. His plasma potassium is 2.9 mmol/l (reference range 3.5–5.0 mmol/l). His heart rate is 140 beats/min, regular, and his blood pressure is 110/60 mmHg.

3. Should anything be done at this stage?

> Later, he becomes unconscious, has a series of generalised fits and his pulse rate rises to 180 beats/min with blood pressure of 100/60 mmHg. The doctor gives him physostigmine for the coma and convulsions.

4. Why physostigmine?
5. Is this drug of first choice for convulsion in a tricyclic overdose?
6. Should an antiarrhythmic drug be given?

Case history 2

> A 20-year-old i.v. drug abuser is admitted comatose after a probable opiate overdose. She is given naloxone i.v. and her level of consciousness improves. Gastric lavage is performed and she is admitted and sent to the ward.

1. What else must be done?

Short note questions

1. Consider the following model illustrating volume of distribution (VD): 1 g each of two compounds A and B are added simultaneously to a small glass beaker, of unknown volume. The beaker is filled with water and has some black powder (looks like charcoal) in the bottom. We lack the means to measure the volume of the beaker directly but can measure the concentrations of A and B: that of A is about 1 g/l, that of B is about 0.001 g/l.

   a. What are the VD values of A and B?
   b. What is the probable explanation for the difference?
   c. What does the charcoal represent in this model?
   d. If the relative VD values of two drugs are the same in vivo, as A and B in this model, which is more amenable to removal by dialysis in the event of overdose?

2. Write short notes on the clinical features and management of severe aspirin poisoning.

Self-assessment: answers

Multiple choice answers

1. a. **False**. Benzodiazepines cause sedation, and seizures are very uncommon.
   b. **True**. Respiratory depression is rarely severe enough to threaten life.
   c. **False**. Flumazenil should be given where there is diagnostic difficulty and where there is respiratory failure (arterial partial pressure of O_2 (Po_2) less than 8.0 kPa).
   d. **True**. Precipitation of respiratory failure is more likely in patients whose blood gases are usually poor.
   e. **False**. Benzodiazepines have very large volumes of distribution.

2. a. **False**. Gastric lavage is contraindicated for corrosive substances (such as bleach) but not iron.
   b. **False**. Desferrioxamine is not absorbed; it must be given parenterally to chelate absorbed iron.
   c. **False**. When desferrioxamine is given into the stomach, it chelates unabsorbed iron.
   d. **False**. The symptoms of serious iron poisoning evolve over several days.
   e. **True**. Serum iron >90 mmol/l indicates the need for parenteral desferrioxamine. Though desferrioxamine is safe, adverse reactions to it include anaphylaxis, hypotension and visual/hearing impairment.

3. a. **False**. Most patients remain asymptomatic until they develop hepatic necrosis (takes about 24 hours to become apparent).
   b. **False**. Estimates made in the first 4 hours after ingestion are not reliable because drug absorption is still in progress.
   c. **True**. Clotting abnormality is a sensitive indicator of developing liver damage.
   d. **False**. *N*-acetylcysteine is a glutathione precursor that forms adducts with reactive paracetamol metabolites.
   e. **False**. *N*-acetylcysteine does cause anaphylaxis occasionally and should be reserved for those patients with drug concentration above the 'treatment line' on the standard graph.

Case history answers

Case history 1

1. There is no antidote for tricyclics, and no means of increasing their clearance, so knowing drug concentrations will not alter management. All cases of tricyclic poisoning should be admitted, and most physicians would want to observe for 48 hours because of the tendency for late complications.
2. No. Vital signs should be observed, and electrolyte concentrations should be measured.
3. He is hypokalaemic: this predisposes to tachyarrhythmias and should be corrected using an i.v. infusion of potassium chloride diluted in 0.9% saline or 5% glucose. His tachycardia is currently insignificant, and his blood pressure is well maintained: antiarrhythmic drugs are not indicated. A cardiac monitor should be used, and the patient should be nursed in a high-dependency area (such as a coronary care unit).
4. Tricyclic drugs have marked antimuscarinic properties, which may cause coma and fits. Physostigmine is an anticholinesterase (Ch. 8) that potentiates acetylcholine; furthermore, it crosses the blood–brain barrier.
5. The effects of physostigmine are short lived, and it is not considered first-line therapy; i.v. diazepam is probably preferable to terminate fits, and if coma becomes a problem (through respiratory failure) ventilation is indicated.
6. His blood pressure is still well maintained, so the arrhythmia is unlikely to be life threatening at the moment. However, an ECG should be done and the arrhythmia should be identified. Acidosis, if present, needs to be corrected. Antiarrhythmic drugs should be reserved for life-threatening arrhythmias; their early use will often make the situation worse. Lidocaine, beta-blockers and phenytoin are most often employed.

Case history 2

Naloxone has a very short duration of action, and repeat doses may be needed: ward doctors should be warned of this, and close observations made of the level of consciousness. Opiates like dihydrocodeine and dextro-propoxyphene are formulated in compound tablets with paracetamol, and patients often take more than one type of pill: unless paracetamol concentrations are measured this poisoning may go un-noticed until liver failure ensues. Salicylate concentrations should also be measured, given the ready availability of this drug, to judge whether alkaline diuresis is required.

Short note answers

1. a. For compound A, VD = 1 g ÷ 1 g/l = 1.0 litres. For compound B, VD = 1 g ÷ 0.001 g/l = 1000 litres.
   b. The likeliest reason for the difference is that compound B binds avidly to the charcoal.
   c. In this model, charcoal represents the tissues.
   d. The drug with the smaller VD will be more readily removed from the body.

2. Make the following points.
   a. Discuss pertinent pharmacokinetics:
      • aspirin has a small volume of distribution
      • much of the drug is eliminated unchanged in the urine
      • aspirin is an acid, and tubular reabsorption of aspirin can be reduced if the urine is made alkaline
      • Mention also that salicylate pharmacokinetics become zero order at high concentration and that the protein binding of the drug can be saturated at high plasma concentration (so the unbound drug fraction rises; explain the importance of this).

   b. State that management is heavily influenced by plasma salicylate concentrations. Mention that salicylate concentrations often need to be measured more than once (in case absorption is slow).
   c. Decontamination of the gut (lavage or emesis) is indicated for several hours after ingestion.
   d. Activated charcoal may reduce drug absorption.
   e. Supportive care is important and comprises:
      • Rehydration
      • Correction of hypokalaemia, hyperglycaemia and severe acidosis.

   f. Drug clearance is increased by alkalinisation of the urine if plasma salicylate exceeds 750 mg/l:
      • 1.4% sodium bicarbonate is infused i.v., giving 225 μmol over 3 hours to achieve a urine pH between 7.5 and 8.5
      • loop diuretics are often needed if urine output does not match the infusion rate of bicarbonate.
      • input/output balance and central venous pressure should be measured.

   g. In severe poisoning (plasma salicylate >1000 mg/l), or poisoning complicated by renal failure, haemodialysis may be required.

18 Substance dependency and abuse

Overview

Substance use is very common. Depending on the substance used and the extent of its use, this may be very harmful. This chapter reviews some of the issues around substance abuse, the commonly abused substances, including alcohol and tobacco, and the treatments available. The success rate for maintaining abstinence in many forms of substance abuse is low but this should not discourage repeated attempts.

18.1 Drug use

Learning objectives

You should:

- be able to define key terms related to substance abuse
- be aware of general issues which apply across many forms of substance abuse.

A wide variety of legal and illegal drugs and substances can be used to create a sense of well-being or to escape from an unpleasant situation. Most societies have legal restrictions on the use of such drugs. There are a number of risks associated with drug use:

- overdose
- direct physical or mental damage from a drug, e.g. cirrhosis with alcohol abuse
- inappropriate behaviour and legal difficulties, e.g. driving while drunk
- distortion of perception and response to environment: self-neglect, drift into criminal subculture (perhaps to finance illegal drug use)
- exposure to unknown substances: users of illicit drugs may not know what they are using; adulteration is common

- spread of disease, e.g. hepatitis B or HIV disease by sharing needles between injecting drug abusers
- drug dependency.

Definitions

Drug dependency (**addiction**) is a compulsion to continue taking a drug, either because of its pleasant effects or, more commonly, because of fear of drug withdrawal. Dependency is sometimes described as *physical*, where there is a clear physical withdrawal syndrome, or *psychological*, where the drug is used for pleasure or as support and there is no clear withdrawal syndrome. Drug dependency may be stable if the patient has an easily obtainable supply but may have severe detrimental effects on the individual and society if the supply is difficult; when the patient may resort to criminal behaviour to obtain the drug.

Tolerance occurs if the body adapts to the continual presence of a drug so that greater doses are required to achieve the same effect. This occurs with many drugs of abuse and may occur because of increased metabolism of the drug (alcohol, barbiturates) or because of altered receptor sensitivity (opioids).

The range of substances that can be used is enormous. What is being used at any time and in any place is a matter of popular culture. Some of the more commonly used substances are described below. Relapse rates despite treatment are high for most forms of substance abuse. Simultaneous abuse of multiple drugs is common.

18.2 Substances abused

Learning objectives

You should:

- know the major commonly abused substances and their effects
- be able to describe the medical treatment of abuse.

Tobacco

Tobacco is usually smoked. One of its many components is nicotine, which is a CNS stimulant. The user may, therefore, feel more alert, calmer and more in control. Nicotine is addictive and there is a withdrawal syndrome that encourages continued use. Tolerance to its effects tends to occur. The kinetics of nicotine after smoking are almost the same as after i.v. use: very rapid absorption, leading to the desired CNS effects. Nicotine itself increases blood pressure and in larger doses cause CNS toxicity, but much of the harm from smoking comes from the associated tars and gases inhaled from the burning tobacco. These cause lung cancer and cancer of the tongue and are associated with bladder cancer. They cause chronic lung damage, and usually manifest as **emphysema** or **chronic bronchitis**. They also precipitate **ischaemic heart disease**. Smoking tobacco is, therefore, a major public health problem.

Treatment

Patients can be weaned off smoking onto nicotine replacement therapy. This can be taken as a spray, as a chewing gum or as a transdermal patch. The aim is to reduce the dose received gradually and withdraw the drug completely. This obviously does not avoid the harmful effects of nicotine but does avoid the other effects of smoking.

Amfebutamone (Buproprion). This is an SSRI (selective serotonin reuptake inhibitor) antidepressant that is used for the treatment of smoking in reducing doses over 7 weeks. It reduces the compulsive behaviour involved in smoking and the urge to smoke. It can be used with nicotine replacement therapy.

Alcohol (ethanol)

Alcoholic drinks contain from 4% (weak beer) to 45% (whisky, brandy) ethanol in water. It is the most widely abused drug and a major cause of drug dependency (alcoholism).

Clinical pharmacokinetics

Ethanol is rapidly absorbed after ingestion, although this may be slowed by food. It is metabolised in the liver to acetaldehyde by two pathways: a specific alcohol dehydrogenase and the less specific microsomal enzymes. These microsomal enzymes are inhibited by acute ethanol intake but induced by chronic intake; this is a possible source of drug interactions. The acetaldehyde is then broken down further by aldehyde dehydrogenase. Small amounts of ethanol are excreted unchanged in urine and in the breath. The metabolism is saturable, i.e. at high doses, alcohol exhibits zero-order metabolism and the clearance of alcohol is not exponential but is at a steady rate (see Ch. 1). Women are in general less tolerant of the acute and long-term effects of alcohol than men.

Psychological effects. Alcohol is a depressant and causes disinhibition and relaxation, with slowing of mental function. Aggression and confusion may occur. Tolerance and drug dependency may develop with prolonged use.

Physical effects. These can be considered in the short term, overdose, and over a longer term if taken at high dosage.

- short term (overdose)
  — incoordination
  — injury because of intoxication
  — unconsciousness
  — death
- long term (high doses)
  — hypertension
  — peripheral neuropathy
  — damage to the cerebrum, partly caused by vitamin deficiencies
  — cirrhosis
  — nutritional deficiencies (especially vitamins)
  — cardiomyopathy.

Withdrawal. On withdrawal, delirium tremens (DTs) may occur; the patient becomes tremulous, anxious and confused and may suffer hallucinations, convulsions, coma and death.

Treatment

In the acute stage of alcohol withdrawal, sedatives such as *chlordiazepoxide* or other benzodiazepines are used for

---

Clinical sketch

A patient is brought to the A&E department by ambulance having been found collapsed in the street. On examination, the patient seems to be intoxicated; he is confused and uncoordinated. He smells of alcohol. The patient seems to be complaining of chest pain and a chest radiograph reveals several fractured ribs.

Comment: Drunkenness is common and patients who have been injured while drunk occupy much of the time of staff in the A&E department. Fractured ribs are particularly common—often caused by falls where the patient has made little effort to protect himself.

The patient sobers up and gives a history of heavy alcohol abuse over some months. The patient agrees not to drink again and is allowed home. Two days later the patient is readmitted in a delirious state complaining of visual hallucinations.

Comment: Alcohol is a CNS suppressant: as with any CNS suppressant that is withdrawn suddenly, the brain may, in effect, become overactive. This may manifest by confusion, delirium and hallucinations. In alcohol abuse, this state is known as delirium tremens and can progress to fitting. It is potentially fatal and should be treated as a medical emergency with sedatives such as benzodiazepines. The patient probably also needs high-potency vitamin B_1 (thiamine) to avoid the development of Wernicke's encephalopathy. This deficiency of vitamins is the result of chronic malnutrition since the patient may have been deriving most of his calorie intake from alcohol.

short periods (2–7 days) to avoid convulsions and other withdrawal symptoms. (Clomethizole should *not* be used any more.) The patient may also have nutritional deficiencies, particularly vitamin B_1, and should receive supplements to prevent serious CNS or cardiac effects.

Disulfiram inhibits aldehyde dehydrogenase; as a result, the acetaldehyde accumulates with toxic effects. It is used to dissuade alcoholics from taking alcohol, as if they drink while taking it, they will experience unpleasant adverse effects, with nausea and vomiting and flushing; severe cases may be fatal. It is useful in a small number of alcoholics who are determined to stop drinking.

Acamprosate reduces the compulsion to drink and so may be useful in maintaining abstinence in combination with counselling and other support.

Sedatives/hypnotics

Benzodiazepines

The potential for benzodiazepines (see Ch. 6) to cause tolerance and dependence was not recognised by doctors for many years. As a result, doctors unwittingly caused many cases of dependence by overprescribing of these drugs. These drugs are also abused illegally, either alone or in combination with other drugs. They may be taken orally, or the tablets may be crushed and dissolved in water or other solvents and then injected. Temazepam is a widely used hypnotic that is particularly favoured by injecting drug abusers.

The psychological effects are similar to those of alcohol. The physical dangers are less, although injury may occur. Overdose, accidental or deliberate, is rarely fatal unless there is underlying cardiac or respiratory disease or other drugs are abused simultaneously. The withdrawal syndrome consists of increased anxiety, insomnia and sometimes convulsions.

Barbiturates

Barbiturates (Ch. 6) were widely used as hypnotics and sedatives before the benzodiazepines were available. They are now rarely used for medical purposes and hence are not readily available as drugs of abuse. Their effects are similar to those of alcohol. Barbiturates are metabolised by the liver and are liver enzyme inducers. Tolerance, therefore, occurred in regular use. Barbiturates are particularly dangerous in overdose, when coma and cardiovascular collapse may occur. Withdrawal often caused severe confusion, agitation and convulsions.

Cannabis

Cannabis is widely used as a relaxant and mild intoxicant. The dried leaves of the cannabis plant may be smoked or eaten (marihuana). A more concentrated form is the resin from the plant, compressed into blocks (hashish). There are several active compounds in cannabis; Δ^9-tetrahydrocannabinol is thought to be the most important. There are specific cannabinoid receptors in the brain, although their physiological function is at present not clear.

Psychological effects. Relaxation, talkativeness and increased awareness of sensation occur. Concentration and coordination are impaired. Occasionally, a user will experience anxiety and paranoia, and even a toxic psychosis. The long-term effects of the drug are debated; many claim it has none, others point to evidence of brain damage in some users. Users of cannabis are more likely to use other drugs. A mild withdrawal syndrome is described in heavy users. Cannabis is under investigation for possible use in multiple sclerosis and some other neurological conditions.

Amfetamines

Amfetamines are stimulants and indirect sympathomimetics, i.e. they stimulate the release of endogenous catecholamines and so activate the sympathetic nervous system. Initially, they were used for the treatment of depression and as appetite suppressants; now they are used very rarely in medicine to treat narcolepsy. Amfetamines are widely abused; most amfetamines are now made in illegal laboratories. They may be taken orally, sniffed or injected.

Effects. The physiological and psychological effects are similar to those of adrenaline: hypertension, tachycardia (sometimes reflex bradycardia) and mydriasis; in large doses, cardiac arrhythmias, angina or sudden death may occur. The user may become exhilarated, energetic, lose his appetite and feel that his physical and mental abilities have been expanded; with long-term use, anxiety and irritability may occur. In high doses, confusion and psychosis may be seen. The amfetamines postpone fatigue rather than prevent it and, after use, many users feel exhausted. On withdrawal, depression is common, and amfetamines are said to be psychologically but not physically addictive. Tolerance occurs with chronic use.

Methylenedioxymethamfetamine (MDMA, Ecstasy) is an amfetamine derivative that has, in addition to the effects of amfetamines, hallucinogenic properties (see below).

It has become particularly widely used in recent years and has caused a number of deaths as a result of cardiac arrhythmias or as a result of myolysis and subsequent renal failure.

Cocaine

Cocaine is derived from the coca leaf. It is an indirect sympathomimetic and a membrane stabiliser and is still used by ear, nose and throat surgeons as a local anaesthetic (see Ch. 8). Cocaine hydrochloride is a white powder that can be injected but more commonly is sniffed and absorbed through the nasal mucosa. In this form, cocaine has been an expensive drug popular with wealthy users. Cocaine freebase is powder treated with alkali to form nuggets ('crack'), which can be smoked. It is said to give very rapid effects and has been sold relatively cheaply.

Effects. The effects are similar to amfetamines: exhilaration, loss of appetite and fatigue, occasionally anxiety, panic or psychosis. After inhalation, the effects last for about 15–30 minutes and repeated doses are usually used. After-effects include fatigue and depression. Physical effects include tachycardia and hypertension, and possibly angina, acute myocardial infarction, cardiac arrhythmia and sudden death. Cocaine sniffing will cause intense vasoconstriction of the nasal mucosa and may cause necrosis of the nasal septum. Cocaine is said to be psychologically rather than physically addictive.

Opioids

Opioids (see Ch. 7) can all be abused; the partial agonist drugs (*pentazocine, buprenorphine*) were developed in an unsuccessful attempt to produce an analgesic with no abuse potential. Raw opium was widely smoked in the Far East. The refined alkaloids *morphine* and *codeine* are taken orally, injected or smoked. *Diamorphine (heroin)* is a potent morphine derivative that is particularly widely available and abused.

Effects. When injected, the user experiences a 'rush' or sensation of intense pleasure. The chronic user, in contrast, mainly uses it to avoid the unpleasant effects of withdrawal. In large doses, sedation is more prominent. Overdose can occur with respiratory depression and death. Tolerance occurs quickly. Physical dependence also occurs within a few weeks of regular use and a severe withdrawn syndrome occurs within a few hours of the last dose: muscle aches, sneezing and rhinorrhea, and yawning, progress on to chills and piloerection ('going cold turkey'). There is also psychological dependence. Abuse by injection is associated with the infectious hazard outlined above. Sniffing or inhaling the fumes of heroin ('chasing the dragon') is increasingly common. Chronic users of opioids often abuse them with other drugs in an attempt to regain the 'rush'.

Methadone is an opioid with a long half-life, active after oral administration. It is used to avoid the withdrawal symptoms in opioid users, its advantages being that it can be given once per day under supervision. The dose can be gradually reduced over a period of a few weeks or months until total withdrawal is achieved. Many patients are maintained indefinitely on it. *Buprenorphine* is also used as maintenance treatment: its partial agonist/antagonist effects may limit the effects of other opioids if taken in addition. *Naltrexone*, an oral pure opioid antagonist, is under investigation as a maintenance treatment.

Hallucinogens

LSD (lysergic acid diethylamide) is a synthetic ergot derivative and a hallucinogen that is widely used. It acts largely by blocking 5-HT receptors. Users report intensification of all the senses and synaesthesia (merging of the senses, e.g. seeing music or feeling colours). Distortions of the senses occur and users may see pseudohallucinations (which they know to be false) or true hallucinations. Some users describe mystical experiences, others severe anxiety, disorientation or acute psychosis. Rarely LSD users may harm themselves or others during the 'trip'. Many users experience 'flash-backs' where they may reexperience the effects of LSD without having taken any. Occasionally long-term psychotic reactions may occur in LSD users. Physical effects do not occur, nor does physical dependence.

Other hallucinogens. Many other naturally occurring alkaloids can act as hallucinogens, including *atropine*, *muscarine* and *psilocybin* from fungi or *mescaline* (from a cactus).

Solvents

Many organic solvents can be inhaled to produce effects similar to those of alcohol: disinhibition, euphoria, dis-orientation and dizziness leading to stupor. These can be found in glues, dry cleaning fluids, paints, nail varnish remover and many other household substances. They are commonly put into a plastic bag from which the user inhales. Because organic solvents are lipid soluble, the acute effects clear quickly when the use is stopped. Solvents are particularly abused by children. The adverse effects in short-term use are injury and occasionally sudden death caused by sensitisation of the myocardium to catecholamines by the solvent. In the long term, the adverse effects include poor concentration, liver and kidney damage and possibly permanent brain damage.

Self-assessment: questions

Multiple choice questions

1. The following statements are correct:
   a. Drug dependency describes a compulsion to continue taking a drug
   b. Tolerance means that an increased dose of the drug has no effect
   c. Alcohol is associated with a physical withdrawal syndrome
   d. Alcohol is mostly excreted unchanged in the urine
   e. Disulfiram is used to treat alcohol dependency

2. The following statements are correct:
   a. Benzodiazepine abuse is common
   b. Tolerance occurs to benzodiazepines
   c. Benzodiazepines may cause liver enzyme induction
   d. Barbiturates are safe in overdose
   e. Physical withdrawal syndromes are seen with benzodiazepines

3. Amphetamines:
   a. Cause catecholamine release from nerve endings
   b. May cause angina
   c. May cause weight gain
   d. Withdrawal may cause rebound depression
   e. Are usually diverted from legal medical use

4. The following statements are correct:
   a. Cocaine is a local anaesthetic
   b. Sniffing cocaine may destroy the nasal septum
   c. Dependency only occurs after i.v. use
   d. Withdrawal syndrome includes constipation, drowsiness and miosis
   e. Methadone is a long-acting opioid used to treat dependency

Case history questions

Case history 1

> A 24-year-old man is found unconscious in a public toilet and is brought to a casualty department. There are no signs of injury and blood sugar is normal. He has needle track marks on his arms and is noted to have small pupils and slow, shallow respiration.

1. What is the likely diagnosis?
2. What treatment should be given immediately?

> The patient recovers consciousness initially but an hour later becomes unconscious again.

3. What has happened?
4. What are the effects of sudden withdrawal of the drugs to which this patient is addicted?
5. What other drugs are commonly abused intravenously?

Case history 2

> A 60-year-old man is found to have hepatomegaly. He admits to drinking a bottle of whisky a day.

1. What is the likely cause of the hepatomegaly?
2. What is considered a 'safe' maximum weekly intake of alcohol?
3. Will the patient's capacity to metabolise drugs be increased or decreased?
4. What drugs are synergistic with alcohol in affecting the CNS?
5. What antibiotic should be avoided in such a patient?

Case history 3

> A 60-year-old man has ischaemic heart disease. He has smoked 40 cigarettes per day for 45 years and has attempted to stop on many occasions unsuccessfully. He has been put on a waiting list for coronary artery surgery but has been told that if he does not stop smoking, the operation will be worthless. He comes to you again to ask for help.

1. What pharmacological treatments are available?
2. Are there any concerns about their use in this case?
3. What other support should the patient be offered?

Short note questions

Write short notes on:

1. Treatment of alcoholism.
2. Treatment of opiate addiction.
3. Illicit misuse of prescribed drugs.

Extended Matching items question

Theme: drug abuse
Options

A. Cirrhosis
B. Heroin
C. Cocaine
D. Hepatitis A
E. Disulfiram
F. HIV
G. Pethidine
H. 'Cold turkey'
I. Barbiturates
J. Tolerance
K. Hepatitis B
L. Dependency
M. Ecstasy
N. Benzodiazepines
O. Thiamine
P. Methadone
Q. Delirium tremens
R. Naloxone

For each of the following case histories answer the questions from options A–R. Each option may be used once, more than once or not at all.

1. A 40-year-old man comes to his GP complaining of unsteadiness when he walks and is noted to have an enlarged liver. On questioning, he admits to drinking about half a bottle of whisky per day as well as wine and beer.
   i. Choose one liver complication caused by alcohol abuse.
   ii. What vitamin deficiency is likely in heavy drinkers?
   iii. What may happen to a heavy drinker who suddenly stops drinking?
   iv. What drug might be used to diminish the severity of the withdrawal syndrome?

2. A 24-year-old man comes to the dentist requesting treatment. He is generally dishevelled, and the dentist notes marks on the patient's left forearm that the patient says were caused by a cat scratch. The patient also has small pupils. On examining the oral cavity, the dentist finds dental caries and candidiasis.
   i. Choose one drug which this patient could be abusing.
   ii. Choose one infectious complication of drug abuse which the dentist should consider in this patient.
   iii. Patients on such drugs often require escalating doses to achieve the desired effect; What is this phenomenon called?
   iv. What drug is used to try to avoid a withdrawal syndrome and maintain such addicts?

Self-assessment: answers

Multiple choice answers

1. a. **True**. A distinction is sometimes made between dependency and addiction but we consider this spurious.
   b. **False**. Tolerance means that an increased dose is needed to achieve the same effect.
   c. **True**. This may be very severe.
   d. **False**. Mostly metabolised.
   e. **True**. By inhibiting alcohol dehydrogenase, toxic metabolites of alcohol are formed.

2. a. **True**. Often iatrogenic.
   b. **True**. Tendency to increase the dose occurs, even in therapeutic use.
   c. **False**. No effect.
   d. **False**. On the contrary, one of the most dangerous of overdoses.
   e. **True**. Including insomnia, anxiety, etc.

3. a. **True**. The definition of an indirect sympathomimetic.
   b. **True**. May cause tachycardia and hypertension.
   c. **False**. May cause loss of appetite and weight loss.
   d. **True**. Hence a psychological compulsion to continue taking the drug.
   e. **False**. Amphetamines have few medical uses today.

4. a. **True**. Still used by ENT surgeons.
   b. **True**. Because of intense vasoconstriction.
   c. **False**. Although obvious, this is a common misunderstanding by opioid users.
   d. **False**. These are all opioid effects: the withdrawal syndrome is, therefore, the opposite of these.
   e. **True**. It has relatively little potential for abuse itself and avoids the withdrawal syndrome in well-motivated users.

Case history answers

Case history 1

1. Opiate (probably heroin) toxicity.
2. Intravenous naloxone.
3. Naloxone has a short half-life, unlike many commonly abused opiates: the naloxone has probably been cleared, allowing the opiate effects to reappear.
4. Muscle aches, sneezing and rhinorrhoea, yawning, mydriasis, progressing on to chills and piloerection ('cold turkey').

5. Drug abusers may abuse many drugs intravenously and often use mixtures of drugs. Commonly used are a variety of opioids, benzodiazepines, amphetamines and cocaine.

Case history 2

1. Alcoholic hepatitis, fatty infiltration of the liver or cirrhosis (with regeneration). Patients with cirrhosis are at risk of hepatomas also.
2. Roughly 21 units per week for men and 14 for women (a unit is half a pint of beer, a short of spirits or a glass of wine—about 15 g alcohol).
3. Alcohol acutely inhibits liver enzyme drug metabolism but in the long term is a liver enzyme inducer; this is the likely condition in this patient when he is not acutely drinking.
4. Any CNS depressant, especially benzodiazepines.
5. Metronidazole; this has a disulfiram-like effect.

Case history 3

1. This patient could be given nicotine replacement therapy (or could buy it over the counter himself) or *amfebutamone*, or both.
2. Amfebutamone can cause a range of adverse effects including gastrointestinal upsets and anxiety. Nicotine may stimulate angina, by causing tachycardia and hypertension. So should he be given nicotine replacement therapy? Again this is a question of balancing risk and benefit: the balance would seem to favour giving the nicotine replacement.
3. The effectiveness of both of these drugs is greatly enhanced if the patient is part of a well-defined support programme to monitor and encourage the patient. This should be part of the 'contract' made with the patient before prescribing either of these drugs. It would be worth defining why previous attempts have failed.

Short note answers

1. This should consider immediate detoxification with benzodiazepines and vitamins. Psychological treatments rather than pharmacological treatments have a major role to play in treating alcohol abuse. Acamprosate is used in selected patients to reduce the desire to drink. Clomethiazole should be avoided as a sedative in the early stages, since patients may substitute an alcohol addiction for a clomethiazole addiction.

2. Patients should be transferred from illicit opiates to oral methadone or buprenorphine. Only doctors with special licences may legally prescribe any other drug for the treatment of opioid addiction. The replacement could either be gradually reduced until the patient is weaned off the drug, which would be the ideal, or be used as maintenance treatment with no dose reduction. This is clearly less desirable than total withdrawal and might be considered damage limitation in that it will avoid the patient needing to seek illegal supplies of opioids with all of the attendant risks of injection, illegal activity, etc. Unfortunately, some patients continue to misuse illicit drugs in addition to their methadone. Naltrexone is under study as a treatment for opioid addiction in the hopes of reducing patients' craving for the drug.

3. This needs to consider the therapeutic drugs which have psychotropic effects and potential for abuse. The single largest group of these are the benzodiazepines. These are over used in medicine especially in long-term treatment. Illicit benzodiazepines are almost all diverted from medical use and their abuse could be largely eliminated with better prescribing. Barbiturates are rarely used in medicine now and are rare as drugs of abuse. Opiates might also be abused, especially such drugs as dihydrocodeine or buprenorphine. Again, better prescribing is the key. Drugs such as diamorphine are almost never diverted from medical use. In addition to considering the potential drugs in this answer, it is also important to consider what we mean by better prescribing: this means only issuing these drugs for short-term use, explaining this carefully to the patient, and so avoiding the potential for abuse. Many patients are on such drugs long term already and may need to be weaned off them—changing this culture is very difficult but essential.

Extended matching items answer

1. i. A. Cirrhosis is common. Alcoholic hepatitis may occur, but not hepatitis A or B, which are infections.
   ii. O. Thiamine deficiency is common and may cause serious neurological and cardiac problems.
   iii. Q. This is confusion, agitation, and fitting in some cases. In severe cases, it may be fatal.
   iv. N. Diazepam or other benzodiazepines are used to diminish the risks of sudden withdrawal.

2. i. B or G. This patient is using an injected opioid—probably heroin (diamorphine), but pethidine is also possible.
   ii. F and/or K. Hepatitis B and HIV are often spread between drug abusers who share needles and other injecting equipment. Medical and paramedical staff may be at risk because of their contact with blood and other body fluids. The presence of oral candidiasis is strongly suspicious of HIV disease in this patient.
   iii. L. Users need to increase the dose to achieve the same effect as the number and sensitivity of opioid receptors is decreased (downregulation).
   iv. P. Methadone has a long half-life and can be given orally once per day under supervision. It is useful to avoid withdrawal symptoms in patients who are opioid dependent. Some argue against its use since some addicts will use methadone with other illicit opioids, or they may become addicted to the methadone.

Drugs in pregnancy, breast-feeding, children and the elderly

Overview

Prescribing for certain groups of patients requires particular care. This is because, by virtue of a physiological state, their response to drugs and their vulnerability to adverse drug reactions are altered. The groups considered here are pregnant and breast-feeding women (where the major concerns are of harm to the fetus or the child), and children and the elderly (where the major concerns are around pharmacokinetic and pharmacodynamic differences in drug response compared to the young adult).

19.1 Pregnancy and breast-feeding

Learning objectives

You should:

- be aware of the hazards of prescribing to women at different stages of pregnancy
- understand which drugs can be safely given to breast-feeding mothers.

Drug use in pregnancy is now limited by doctors' and patients' awareness of the possible harm that may be done to the fetus. This was brought home by the thalidomide disaster of the 1960s, when thalidomide used as a sedative by pregnant women caused deformities of the limbs in the fetus. Despite the risks, some medical conditions require drug treatment during pregnancy and the benefits and risks of this need to be carefully weighed. A broad principle, however, is to avoid drugs in pregnancy as much as possible. This might also be taken to apply to women of child-bearing age—who might after all be pregnant at the time you write a prescription, or become pregnant while taking a drug prescribed by you.

Drugs and the fetus

Drugs may adversely affect development of the fetus and cause deformities (teratogenic), particularly during the first trimester of pregnancy when the major organs and limbs are being formed. The list of teratogenic drugs is long: some such as cytotoxics might be anticipated; others may be unexpected and found during animal testing (although this is not completely reliable—thalidomide had not been identified as a teratogen in animal studies, partly because it had been tried only in rodents) or found tragically by chance. It must be remembered that 1–2% of all births are of a child with a malformation of some kind, and it is important not to over- or underestimate the potential of a drug to cause deformity. Not all exposures to a teratogenic drug will cause a malformation, e.g. warfarin causes deformities in only about 5% of cases. A teratogenic drug may be taken by a woman before she realises that she is pregnant; in some cases, the risks of using a teratogenic drug may be outweighed by the benefits, e.g. warfarin in a patient with a prosthetic heart valve.

> *Some teratogenic drugs:*

- phenytoin: craniofacial and limb abnormalities
- carbamazepine: craniofacial and limb abnormalities
- sodium valproate: neural tube abnormalities, spina bifida
- ACE inhibitors: abnormalities of the skull
- alcohol: growth retardation and cranial abnormalities
- stilbestrol: adenocarcinoma of the vagina in the daughters of women exposed during pregnancy.

After the first trimester
The second and third trimesters are mainly stages of growth and development, and drugs taken by the mother may still affect the fetus. Antithyroid drugs may lead to goitre or hypothyroidism in the fetus. Tetracyclines may interfere with bone and teeth formation. There are many other drugs that may have adverse effects on the fetus; a full list should be consulted before prescribing for a pregnant woman.

Drugs in the pregnant mother

The pharmacokinetics of drugs may be altered in pregnant women.

Absorption. Gastrointestinal motility is slowed, which increases absorption of poorly soluble drugs such as digoxin.

Distribution. Plasma volume and extracellular fluid increase up to 50% and this will reduce the plasma concentration of drugs with a small volume of distribution for a given dose. Changes in albumin also occur: this falls by around 20% while α_1-acid glycoprotein, to which basic drugs bind, increases by about 40%. This will mean increased free drug for a given concentration for acidic drugs (phenytoin, valproate), while for basic drugs (propranolol, chlorpromazine), the free fraction will fall for a given plasma concentration. This may be of importance if therapeutic drug monitoring is undertaken.

Elimination. Renal plasma flow increases but this is important only for a few drugs, such as ampicillin, where larger doses may be needed. For most drugs, renal elimination is relatively unaltered. Liver metabolism is induced by progesterone in pregnancy and so the clearance of drugs metabolised by the liver may be enhanced.

Some common chronic conditions in pregnancy

Epilepsy

There is an increased incidence of congenital deformities in the children of pregnant epileptic women, probably largely because of the use of anticonvulsant drugs. Although most anticonvulsants are teratogenic, the risks to the mother and to the fetus of uncontrolled epilepsy outweigh any risks of teratogenesis, and so pregnant epileptic women are advised to continue their medication. *Carbamazepine* is probably the least likely to cause deformities, although little comparative evidence is available.

Altered pharmacokinetics may make drug treatment for epilepsy difficult in pregnancy; total anticonvulsant concentrations tend to fall because of increased volume of distribution and enhanced metabolism, although this may be slightly countered by decreased protein binding. Measurement of plasma concentrations at frequent intervals is advised during pregnancy for drugs such as *phenytoin*, with dosage adjustment as necessary. It is not usually possible to measure free drug, and so to compensate for this, it is common practice to keep the plasma concentration at the lower end of the therapeutic range; however, as in all therapeutic drug monitoring, the well-being of the patient and not the plasma concentration is the major measure.

Infections

Urinary tract infections in particular are common in pregnancy, and appropriate drug treatment must be determined by sensitivity testing. Suitable drugs include penicillins, cephalosporins and nitrofurantoin.

Antimicrobials to avoid in pregnant women:

- tetracyclines: teeth and bone deformities in fetus; hepatitis is more common in pregnant women
- metronidazole: possibly teratogenic
- trimethoprim: folate antagonism, possibly teratogenic
- quinolones: may damage growing cartilage
- isoniazid, rifampicin: use with great care because of the risk of hepatitis
- aminoglycosides: 8th nerve damage in the fetus.

Clinical sketch

A woman is 20 weeks pregnant. She develops frequency and dysuria and urine testing shows blood and leucocytes. The doctor thinks about what antibiotics might be prescribed.

Comment: Urinary tract infections are common in pregnant women and should always be treated vigorously since they may give rise to pyelonephritis or premature delivery. At 20 weeks, the risk of developing fetal malformation is small, since we are now in the second trimester. However, the appropriate antibiotics need to be considered carefully. The best choice would be a cephalosporin or co-amoxiclav. Nitrofurantoin would also be safe for lower urinary tract infections.

Diabetes mellitus

Diabetes mellitus may become unstable in pregnant women and some pregnant women may develop gestational diabetes for the first time. All such women need careful specialist monitoring and very tight control of the diabetes. Some diabetic women may be adequately controlled on diet, but many will require insulin. Oral hypoglycaemic drugs should not be used.

Hypertension

Pregnant women may develop hypertension with proteinuria as part of toxaemia of pregnancy, in which case fetal loss is high. Alternatively, they may have hypertension as an incidental problem. Few antihypertensive drugs have been evaluated in pregnancy. *Methyldopa* has been established by long usage to be safe, as has *labetalol* and *hydralazine*. Diuretics and ACE inhibitors are not suitable. The role of other beta-blockers or calcium-channel blockers has been questioned as, although effective in treating hypertension, they do not seem to improve the fetal prognosis. Some such as *atenolol* seem to lead to low birthweight. Bed rest is also important in the management of hypertension in pregnancy. Occasionally, hypertension is sufficiently severe to require early delivery of the fetus.

Hyperthyroidism

Carbimazole can cross the placenta and cause hypothyroidism and goitre in the fetus. The lowest possible dose of carbimazole should, therefore, be used, along with beta-blockers to control symptoms.

Breast-feeding

Although many drugs taken by the mother may be detectable in breast milk, in many cases the concentrations are low and the dose to the child is clinically unimportant.

Drugs that can be given safely to mothers who are breast-feeding:

- penicillins, cephalosporins
- theophylline or beta-agonists
- glucocorticoids (although high doses may affect the fetus and cause adrenal suppression)
- anticonvulsants
- tricyclic antidepressants
- neuroleptics such as chlorpromazine
- antihypertensives such as methyldopa, hydralazine
- warfarin or heparin.

Drugs to be avoided in mothers who are breast-feeding:

- aspirin
- ergotamine
- sulphonamides, ciprofloxacin, tetracyclines, chloramphenicol
- benzodiazepines
- lithium
- antithyroid drugs or iodine
- sulphonylureas
- antineoplastic drugs.

Drugs that inhibit lactation:

- bromocriptine
- oestrogens and progestogens (high doses)
- thiazides.

Clinical sketch

A 30-year-old woman gives birth to a normal child but develops a deep vein thrombosis (DVT) immediately afterwards. She is breast-feeding the child.

Comment: Treatment of the DVT will require heparin (unfractionated or low-molecular-weight forms) followed by warfarin for a period of 6 to 12 weeks. Warfarin does appear in breast milk in very low concentrations but should not be harmful to the child. It is, therefore, reasonable for her to continue breast-feeding.

19.2 Children

Learning objectives

You should:

- be aware of the pharmacokinetic and pharmacodynamic factors that are distinct to children and will affect drug levels
- understand the issues in prescribing for children.

Half of all children visiting GPs' surgeries will be issued with a prescription, usually for short-term medication, especially antibiotics. Using drugs properly in children requires an understanding of the alterations in pharmacokinetics and pharmacodynamics that occur, especially in neonates (age up to 1 month) and infants (age up to 4 years).

Pharmacokinetics

Distribution. Children and neonates have a higher body water/fat ratio than adults, which will result in relatively higher concentrations of water-soluble drugs. Lipid membranes may be more permeable in neonates: in particular, the blood–brain barrier will not be effective. Protein binding will be reduced in neonates.

Metabolism. In neonates, this will be reduced: in older children, it may be relatively greater than in adults. For instance, children may need relatively higher doses of theophylline or phenytoin than adults (based on a dose per unit body weight) to attain therapeutic concentrations.

Excretion. Neonates have diminished glomerular filtration rate and tubular excretion compared with adults: this decreases the clearance of such drugs as *penicillin*. Older children have renal function similar to that of adults.

Pharmacodynamics

Some drugs will demonstrate a reduced effect in neonates compared with adults or older children (e.g. *digoxin*), while some have an increased effect (e.g. CNS depressants). This is sometimes the result of altered pharmacokinetics (for instance, the volume of distribution of lipid-soluble CNS depressants); in other cases, there are alterations in tissue sensitivity.

Clinical sketch

A 7-year-old child with severe asthma is prescribed an inhaled corticosteroid. The mother is concerned that this may give rise to impaired growth.

Comment: Systemic corticosteroids can give rise to impaired growth in children. High-dose inhaled

---

corticosteroids may have a sufficient systemic effect also to impede growth. However, far more likely to impede growth is uncontrolled disease, such as asthma. As always, the benefits of therapy must be weighed against the risks and in severe childhood asthma the inhaled corticosteroid is appropriate.

Adverse effects

Adverse effects may differ slightly from those seen in adults; for instance, long-term *glucocorticoid* use may lead to impaired growth, while *theophylline* may lead to overactivity and learning difficulties. *Aspirin* may cause Reye's syndrome (hepatic failure).

Dosage in neonates and children

Altered pharmacokinetics and pharmacodynamics make determination of doses difficult in children. Doses are sometimes calculated on the basis of body weight; the use of square metre of body surface area is better, usually derived from nomograms of height and weight. However, effective doses with minimal adverse effects are often determined only by experience. It is vitally important to consult an appropriate source of doses related to age etc., before prescribing for young children.

Drug licensing and children

A common problem in prescribing for children (affecting about 40% of all drug use in children) is that the drug has not been adequately evaluated in children and so is not licensed in this age group. This requires 'off-label' prescribing, i.e. prescribing outside the terms of the product licence and labelling. A manufacturer may not seek a licence for use in children: the necessary trials would be expensive and difficult, and there would be little commercial return on this investment. Licensing agencies are increasingly aware of this problem and encourage or even require companies to submit data on children.

Where possible, a licensed product should be prescribed. Where not possible and where 'off label' use is necessary, it is important that the prescribing should be as evidence based as possible, i.e. supported by randomised clinical trials and with good information on the pharmacokinetics and dynamics of the drug in children.

19.3 The elderly

Learning objectives

You should:

- be aware of the physiological and pathological factors common in elderly people that may influence drug effects
- be aware of the effect of coexisting medical problems on drug effects
- know the likely drug interactions that can occur in this group.

Drugs are widely used in the elderly: the elderly (over 65 years) account for about 15% of the general population but about 40–45% of prescriptions. The elderly are prone to many chronic degenerative diseases, which may influence drug effects and which promotes prescribing. They may have several medical problems that may lead to multiple drug therapy (polypharmacy) (Fig. 52).

Often there are difficulties of diagnosis in the elderly, and doctors may be excessively enthusiastic in their desire to treat symptoms. Some complaints may be inappropriately treated with drugs, e.g. dizziness caused by age-related loss of postural stability might be treated with *prochlorperazine*, which may lead to parkinsonism and further treatment. Many problems of the elderly are psychosocial and cannot be expected to respond to drugs. Often, drugs are started in the elderly and not discontinued although the original indication for the drug has long since resolved.

Adverse drug reactions

Adverse reactions are more common in the elderly and may result in one in ten admissions of elderly patients to hospital. The adverse drug reactions are largely related to increased drug action (type A, see Ch. 21), rather than the idiosyncratic adverse effect (type B). There are several reasons:

- *increased use* of drugs makes adverse reactions more likely, and *polypharmacy* increases the risks of drug interactions

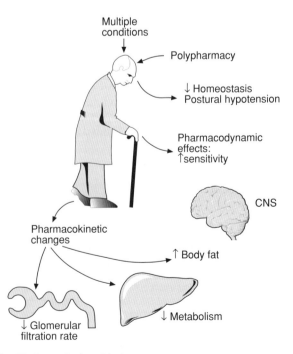

Fig. 52 Drugs in the elderly.

A 75-year-old woman comes to ask for a repeat prescription for her usual medicines: nifedipine 20 mg twice per day, bendroflumethiazide (bendrofluazide) 2.5 mg, ranitidine 150 mg twice per day, Slow K tablets one three times per day, diclofenac 50 mg three times per day, and allopurinol 300 mg per day. The case notes contain the diagnoses of hypertension, dyspepsia and gout. She feels reasonably well but complains with a smile that she rattles as she walks! Her blood pressure is unsatisfactory at 180/100 mmHg.

*Comment: This patient states that she has no complaints. But is there really no problem? She may suffer from hypertension, dyspepsia and gout, but she definitely has one other problem: **polypharmacy!** Careful analysis and monitoring will reveal whether the patient really needs all these drugs.*

How did she end up on all of these drugs? The sequence of events was that she was noted at a routine health check to have a blood pressure of 170/102 mmHg. Her doctor prescribed nifedipine 20 mg twice daily. A month later, her blood pressure was 120/60 mmHg and she complained of dizziness, dyspepsia and swollen ankles. Her doctor added in bendroflumethiazide 2.5 mg per day, and ranitidine 150 mg twice per day. Another month passed and her ankles remained swollen: her serum potassium was 3.2 mmol/l. Her doctor increased the dose of bendroflumethiazide to 5 mg per day and added in potassium supplements, two tablets twice per day. Two weeks later, she had her first ever attack of gout and was treated with diclofenac 50 mg three times per day. Allopurinol was later added in, while the diclofenac was continued. A month later her blood pressure was 180/100 mmHg.

Look up the adverse effects of nifedipine, diuretics and non-steroidal anti-inflammatory drugs!

- *altered pharmacokinetics*: many drugs have not been adequately studied in the elderly
  — absorption may be slower in the elderly
  — distribution may be altered because of decreased serum albumin concentrations and a relative increase in body fat and decrease in body water; lipid-soluble drugs may have an increased volume of distribution, which, coupled with reduced elimination, may prolong the duration of their effects
  — elimination of many drugs in the elderly is reduced: glomerular filtration rate and tubular secretion will be reduced, which may increase adverse reactions from drugs such as *cimetidine* or *digoxin*; liver size and hepatic blood flow and hence enzyme metabolism will also be reduced in the elderly—this is particularly important for

drugs that undergo first-pass metabolism, which will have greater bioavailability in the elderly, e.g. *propranolol* or *verapamil*

- *altered pharmacodynamics*, with increased organ or receptor sensitivity: this applies to many CNS depressants, such as *benzodiazepines*, for reasons that are not entirely clear, and to other drugs such as antihypertensives
- *diminished homeostatic reserve*: as a result many drugs that affect homeostasis in vital organs have a disproportionate effect in elderly patients, e.g. antihypertensives may lead to postural hypotension because of reduction of the normal reflex responses
- *the disease state* may influence the response to drugs; for instance, patients with rheumatoid arthritis may be more prone to suffer gastrointestinal bleed after NSAIDs.

Compliance

Compliance with prescribed drugs may be poor or sporadic in the elderly, especially where several drugs are prescribed together. This may be the result of poor understanding by the patient and poor explanation by the doctor of the purpose of the prescription.

Recommendations for prescribing in the elderly

1. Assess the clinical situation carefully, considering other drugs, previous history and the need to prescribe at all.
2. Keep the drug regimen as simple as possible and treat only major problems.
3. Start with the lowest effective dose (often 50% of the usual adult dose) and build up the dose gradually as necessary. Consider carefully the choice of drug in the elderly and work from a limited range of drugs with which the prescriber is very familiar.
4. Explain carefully to the patient the proposed therapy, its purposes, administration and its adverse effects. Verbal explanation may need to be supplemented with written material. Issue a clear prescription for the pharmacist.
5. Avoid inappropriate and overenergetic treatment: consider the patient as a whole and not as a collection of symptoms or diseases.
6. Review medication and compliance frequently and be alert for adverse drug reactions, which may mimic other disease or present in a non-specific manner in the elderly.

Self-assessment: questions

Multiple choice questions

1. The following drugs may be safely given to a pregnant woman in the first trimester:
   a. Carbamazepine
   b. Prednisolone
   c. Ciprofloxacin
   d. Co-trimoxazole
   e. Etretinate

2. In pregnant women:
   a. The plasma volume decreases
   b. The free portion of acid drugs rises
   c. Plasma drug concentrations monitoring is accurate
   d. Carbimazole may cause fetal goitre
   e. Sulphonylureas may be used to manage gestational diabetes mellitus

3. In prescribing for children:
   a. Children are basically small adults
   b. Doses for children are best calculated on a simple body weight basis
   c. Adverse drug reactions may occur of a type that are not seen in adults
   d. In a child aged 5 years, the liver metabolism of drugs is proportionately less than that of an adult
   e. Children have relatively high water to fat ratios

4. In prescribing for the elderly:
   a. Pharmacokinetic alterations may occur compared with younger patients
   b. Increased sensitivity to doses of benzodiazepines is an example of pharmacodynamic changes
   c. Polypharmacy is common
   d. Homeostatic mechanisms are well maintained
   e. Compliance with prescribed drugs is variable

Case histories

Case history 1

> An epileptic woman becomes pregnant, while taking phenytoin.

1. Is she at an increased risk of having a child with a congenital defect?
2. Concerned about the safety of her child, she wishes to discontinue her antiepileptic medication; what do you advise her?
3. If her dose remains unchanged, how will the pregnancy affect the total and free plasma phenytoin concentration?
4. Is this of clinical significance?
5. Can she breast-feed without risk to the child?

Case history 2

> A 75-year-old man is diagnosed as hypertensive and the doctor wishes to institute drug treatment with a water-soluble beta-blocker.

1. Is this patient in general more likely to suffer adverse drug reactions than a younger patient?
2. Will the clearance of the drug prescribed be affected by the patient's age?

> The patient subsequently complains of falling episodes and is found to have postural hypotension.

3. What should the doctor do?
4. The patient later develops Parkinson's disease and is given levodopa and selegeline, and later still digoxin because of atrial fibrillation. What problems might the use of so many drugs pose?

Short note questions

Write notes on:

1. Polypharmacy in the elderly.
2. Pharmacokinetic and other differences between children and adults.
3. Drug treatment of epilepsy in a pregnant woman.

Self-assessment: answers

Multiple choice answers

1. a. **False**. It may cause fetal abnormalities but nevertheless it is the anticonvulsant of choice in pregnancy, as it seems to be the safest of the antiepileptic drugs.
   b. **True**. As generally used. Very high doses for long periods might be harmful.
   c. **False**. There is a theoretical risk of damage to fetal cartilage.
   d. **False**. Risk of teratogenesis as trimethoprim is a folate antagonist.
   e. **False**. A vitamin A derivative and highly teratogenic.

2. a. **False**. Substantially increased.
   b. **True**. As albumin binding is proportionately decreased.
   c. **False**. Although free drug levels remain much the same, total drug (which is what is measured in therapeutic drug monitoring) is altered because of changes in protein binding.
   d. **True**. Also neonatal hypothyroidism.
   e. **False**. Insulin therapy must be instituted.

3. a. **False**. This is a common but potentially dangerous mistake. Children should be considered quite separately from adults.
   b. **False**. The best way is probably on a dose per body surface area basis.
   c. **True**. For example, Reye's syndrome on aspirin, or stunted growth on glucocorticoids.
   d. **False**. Children have relatively well-developed liver drug-metabolising enzyme systems.
   e. **True**. Hence they may need lower doses than predicted of many water-soluble drugs.

4. a. **True**. For example reduced clearance etc. If this were an essay question could you discuss it with examples?
   b. **True**. Again, a slight change to this question would make it suitable for an essay or short answer.
   c. **True**. Because of increased illness and perhaps poor prescribing. Around 75% of elderly patients have taken a therapeutic drug within the preceding 2 weeks compared with 33% of younger patients.
   d. **False**. These become increasingly impaired with time.
   e. **True**. Often poor, especially if the patient is required to take a complex drug regimen:

occasionally too good, with the patient taking excessive drug.

Case history answers

Case history 1

1. Yes, probably from both the epilepsy and the drugs. Harelip deformities are associated with phenytoin.
2. It would have been desirable to have this patient on carbamazepine before she became pregnant. Now, however, the risks to her and to her child of stopping therapy outweigh those of continuing.
3. The total plasma phenytoin will fall because of the increased volume of distribution, and because of the reduction in serum albumin. However, the free phenytoin will remain roughly the same.
4. The free drug is active, and since this remains largely unchanged, the change in total drug is of little clinical consequence. However if a doctor measures total plasma concentrations and finds them low, he may mistakenly increase the dose of the drug.
5. Yes.

Case history 2

1. In general yes, for many reasons: the most important of which is increased drug use in this age group.
2. Yes: water-soluble beta-blockers are cleared by the kidney through glomerular filtration and this will fall with advancing age. The dose of beta-blocker used should be low initially and titrated for effect. The use of a low starting dose is advisable for other reasons also, such as increased sensitivity to the effects of drugs.
3. There are many factors that need to be considered in causing postural hypotension in the elderly, but a reasonable first step would be to stop the beta-blocker. It might be worth trying another antihypertensive (e.g. a thiazide). However, if the patient shows a poor tolerance for such drugs, even if he is hypertensive off treatment, it may be best to leave the hypertension untreated.
4. There may be an increased risk of drug interactions and of poor drug compliance.

Short note answers

1. The issues to be considered are:

   • possible inappropriate responses to multiple symptoms
   • inappropriate treatment of adverse effects of some medications with other medication

- increased risk of adverse reactions and interactions in the elderly
- problems with poor patient concordance and adherence to prescribed medication
- need to take holistic overview of the patient's condition to avoid polypharmacy.

2. A comparison of adults and children in pharmacology should cover:
   - need to consider different relative distributions of fat and water between adults, children and neonates
   - appropriate dosing regimens, based on milligrams or unit dose per body surface area
   - decreased renal function in neonates relative to adults and children
   - relatively well-preserved hepatic function in children compared with adults
   - Different patterns of adverse reactions in children compared with adults, e.g. theophylline causing hyperactivity and attention deficit disorders, sedatives causing paradoxical excitation, etc.

3. Key elements are:
   - the need to maintain control of the epilepsy, which if uncontrolled would be more harmful to the fetus and the mother than any drug.
   - choice of appropriate drug or least harmful drug before the woman becomes pregnant (most often carbamazepine)
   - potential misleading plasma concentration levels in pregnancy because of changed body water and plasma protein levels
   - possible prenatal diagnosis of such potential drug effects as spina bifida, which may allow the woman to decide to abort a malformed fetus if tested early enough.

20 Effects of disease state on drug response

Overview

For the majority of drugs, clinically serious interindividual variation in response is not a frequent problem – most have fairly reproducible effects. However, certain diseases alter drug response predictably, necessitating dose alteration to avoid either toxicity or therapeutic failure. Disease may affect either pharmacokinetic factors (absorption, distribution, metabolism or excretion) or pharmacodynamic factors (concentration–response relationships).

You should be familiar with Appendix 2 and 3 of the British National Formulary. These give warnings and recommendations concerning dosing in hepatic and renal disease, which are the two most commonly encountered disease states of relevance.

20.1 Pharmacokinetic factors

Learning objectives

You should:

- know the pharmacokinetic mechanisms whereby disease may alter drug response
- be able to give clinically relevant examples of disease-related changes to the processes of absorption, distribution, metabolism and excretion
- be able to describe the important features of drugs likely to be affected by changes in liver function (be aware of Appendix 2 in BNF)
- Describe the important features of drugs likely to be affected by changes in renal function (be aware of Appendix 3 in BNF).

Disease states can affect:

- absorption
- distribution
- metabolism
- excretion.

Absorption

Absorption can be altered by **blood flow**:

- reduced blood flow to the gut: this rarely compromises drug absorption
- reduced muscle blood flow: the i.m. route of administration is prone to slow absorption if muscle blood flow is reduced, as it can be in shock.

Altered transit time. Acute gastrointestinal infections, both viral and bacterial, may increase motility, reducing transit and hence drug absorption. The severe chronic diarrhoea often seen in AIDS patients may reduce the absorption of anti-tuberculosis drugs.

Clinical sketch: drug absorption

The victim of a road traffic accident is in great pain from multiple injuries. His blood pressure is 80/30 mmHg. The emergency team's doctor is happy to use diamorphine, and gives it i.m. at the roadside, but it does not seem to work.

Comment: there are many reasons why diamorphine would often be contraindicated in such circumstances (head injury, for example). However in this hypothetical case, it has been given by the wrong route. Muscle blood flow is reduced in shock, and the drug will not be reliably absorbed.

Distribution

Plasma protein binding

Drugs are transported in the plasma bound to plasma proteins, mainly albumin and α_1-acid glycoprotein. Diseases that change plasma protein concentrations alter drug effect by increasing or decreasing the drug concentration unbound in the plasma water. The concentration of α_1-acid glycoprotein rises in acute infection, inflammation or infarction. Albumin concentrations may be markedly reduced by chronic liver disease and nephrotic syndrome. (See the clinical sketches on protein binding and drug distribution, p. 224.)

A 50-year-old man with insulin-dependent diabetes has been on phenytoin for epilepsy for many years. He develops peripheral oedema and notices foamy urine. Shortly thereafter he develops severe ataxia, and presents acutely to hospital.

Comment: phenytoin has serious concentration-dependent adverse effects, including ataxia and sedation, which are dependent on its unbound fraction and so are potentiated by hypoalbuminaemia. It sounds like this man has developed nephrotic syndrome (probably a complication of his diabetes). He probably has hypoalbuminaemia, and this is the likeliest cause of his phenytoin toxicity.

Clinical sketch: protein binding and drug distribution

Patient A has cerebral malaria and is treated with quinine: the peak drug concentration is 20 µg/ml.
   Patient A recovers uneventfully. In contrast *patient B*, who is healthy, takes an overdose of quinine (his mother's prescription—she was given it for night cramps). On admission, his peak drug concentration is also 20 µg/ml. *Patient B* develops bilateral blindness, which never fully recovers.

Comment: concentrations of α_1-acid glycoprotein are low in health but rise in some diseases, because it is an acute-phase reactant. Although the total quinine concentrations in patients A and B are identical, the free drug levels are markedly different because of the variation in the level of α_1-glycoprotein to bind drug: hence the marked difference in response.

Clinical sketch: tissue distribution

A patient with meningococcal meningitis is treated with high doses of i.v. benzylpenicillin. As he recovers, and can take drugs by mouth, ampicillin is started in place of benzylpenicillin. From this point, his improvement falters: repeat lumbar puncture suggests inadequate treatment.

Comment: this would be unusual management—it is produced here to illustrate a point. The penicillins are polar compounds that do not readily cross the blood–brain barrier. In meningitis, this barrier becomes inflamed, allowing greater partition of the antibiotic into the CNS. The danger comes as meningitis resolves, because care must be taken that CNS drug concentrations are maintained to achieve full resolution.

Tissue distribution

Most drugs have their effects in specific tissues, diffusing out of the plasma to reach effective local concentrations. Inflammation of membrane barriers and changes in local pH may affect this process (see the clinical sketch on tissue distribution).

Metabolism

Alteration in drug metabolism is among the most commonly encountered causes of disease-induced changes in drug response. Predictably, the drugs concerned:

- are extensively metabolised to inactive derivatives
- have serious concentration-dependent toxicity
- have narrow therapeutic indices.

Most drugs are metabolised in the liver. This organ has tremendous reserve, and changes in drug effects may not be seen until there is loss of much of the parenchyma. Even so, caution is recommended in both acute and chronic liver disease. Both first-pass metabolism and systemic metabolism may be reduced.

Clinical sketch: drug metabolism

An alcoholic patient develops decompensated liver failure as a result of pneumonia. He is given pethidine because of pleuritic chest pain.

Comment: this is extremely dangerous. Even 'weak' analgesics such as codeine may precipitate coma.

Clinical sketch: drug metabolism

A man with known alcoholic cirrhosis is seen in clinic. He smokes, and complains of wheeze. He is already taking salbutamol, and the doctor starts aminophylline.

Comment: he is at risk from aminophylline toxicity. This drug has a narrow therapeutic range and is eliminated by hepatic metabolism.

Clinical sketch: drug metabolism

An alcoholic patient takes a paracetamol overdose and presents to the A&E department about 6 hours thereafter. His paracetamol level is below the 'normal treatment line' but he is given N-acetylcysteine nevertheless.

Comment: alcohol is an inducer of the CYP450 enzymes that metabolise paracetamol to its toxic metabolite. Such patients are at increased risk of severe liver damage. Patients taking liver enzyme inducers should be treated at lower plasma concentrations of paracetamol.

Excretion

Drugs that cause concern in patients with renal impairment usually fulfil the following criteria:

- they are excreted unchanged
- they cause serious concentration-dependent toxicity
- their therapeutic indices are small.

Both acute and chronic renal failure reduce drug excretion rate in proportion to the reduction in glomerular filtration rate. Major examples include:

- aminoglycosides
- digoxin
- sulphonylureas.

BNF Appendix 3 lists many others.

Clinical sketch: drug elimination

An elderly woman with impaired renal function is treated with digoxin for new-onset atrial fibrillation. She presents to the A&E department 6 months later in complete heart block, and her digoxin level is found to be greatly above the therapeutic range.

Comment: digoxin concentrations ought to have been measured and the dose adjusted.

Clinical sketch: drug elimination

A young man is admitted with extensive burns and develops Gram-negative septicaemia. He is treated with antibiotics, including gentamicin. His renal function has not been as closely monitored as it should have been. Gentamicin concentrations have been measured during the admission but, towards the end of the New Year bank holiday weekend, he complains of tinnitus, deafness and vertigo.

Comment: this man was always at high risk of renal failure, and frequent monitoring of renal function and gentamicin concentrations is mandatory. Ototoxicity is not unusual with the aminoglycosides, which may also cause worsening renal function.

20.2 Pharmacodynamic factors

Learning objectives

You should:

- be able to classify the influences of disease states on drug response
- understand the pharmacodynamic mechanisms that explain both reduced and increased drug responses
- be able to outline some clinical examples of such altered drug response.

Reduction in drug effect

Less responsive 'target'

Disease may compromise the function of target organs or alter their receptor status. For example, insulin-dependent diabetes mellitus cannot be treated with sulphonylureas because the disease state results from the loss of pancreatic beta-cells. Since much of the response to sulphonylureas results from increased insulin secretion, their activity is much diminished. In contrast, of course, sulphonylureas are routinely used in the treatment of non-insulin-dependent diabetes where peripheral insulin resistance is involved.

Clinical sketch: less responsive 'target'

An elderly man presents with pulmonary oedema caused by a myocardial infarction. The A&E doctor gives him 80 mg furosemide (frusemide), puts in a catheter and waits for diuresis to reduce the pulmonary oedema. The patient's dyspnoea diminishes a little, but there is only a sluggish diuresis. Meanwhile, some blood results have come through: haemoglobin 8.6 g% (86 g/l; normochromic and normocytic), urea 90 mmol/l, creatinine 400 µmol/l.

Comment: this man probably has chronic renal impairment, judging by his haemoglobin. If so, the relative lack of response to the loop diuretic is understandable. The initial reduction in his breathlessness might have been a result of the vasodilatation caused by furosemide.

Clinical sketch: less responsive 'target'

An opiate addict is admitted with a fractured humerus. He is given diamorphine for his pain, but it does not seem to work well.

Comment: there is downregulation of opiate receptors in opiate addicts, and response to a given dose is lower than expected. However, common-sense suggests other reasons why the patient may be asking for a larger dose: clinical judgement is required here.

The presence of endogenous ligands

If the disease allows the accumulation or increased synthesis of endogenous compounds with the opposite effect to that of the drug, the drug will be rendered less efficacious. For example, phaeochromocytomas are catecholamine-secreting tumours (usually benign; usually in the adrenal cortex). They present with hypertension (often accelerated

---

Clinical sketch: endogenous ligands oppose drug action

A man with chronic renal failure is being treated for chronic duodenal ulcers. These seem remarkably 'resistant' to treatment with ranitidine.

Comment: the gastric hormone gastrin is normally metabolised in the kidneys and accumulates in patients with chronic renal failure, opposing the effects of H_2 blockers such as ranitidine.

hypertension). Use of beta-blockers in patients with phaeochromocytomas may cause a rise in blood pressure because the high concentration of circulating catecholamines binds readily to α-adrenoceptors, causing vasoconstriction (and hence an increase in peripheral resistance), while the beta-blockers may decrease the vasodilatation previously experienced by the patient.

Enhanced drug effect

More responsive 'target'

Disease may already 'mimic' the desired drug effect, so that addition of the drug causes unexpectedly marked response. The 'interactions' between chronic liver disease and anticoagulant/antiplatelet drugs are commonly encountered in this regard. Clotting factors are synthesised in the liver, and parenchymal liver disease often prolongs tests of intrinsic and extrinsic clotting cascades. Consequently, the effects of warfarin and aspirin are more pronounced than in health.

Clinical sketch: more responsive 'target'

A patient is admitted with pleuritic chest pain and a normal chest radiograph. Ventilation perfusion scanning suggests a 'moderate' probability of pulmonary embolism. D-dimers are raised. Warfarin is started using a standard dosing regimen. The first INR performed, 4 days later, is 8.0; liver function tests become available at the same time and suggest liver disease.

Comment: use of warfarin in patients with unrecognised liver disease may cause uncoagulable blood, and tests of coagulability should always be done before starting treatment.

Clinical sketch: More responsive 'target'

A man with chronic pancreatitis presents with atrial fibrillation and is put on warfarin. The first INR performed, 4 days later, shows an INR of 6.0.

Comment: clotting factors II, VII, IX and X are dependent upon vitamin K, a lipid-soluble vitamin, for their synthesis. Pancreatitis often manifests with maldigestion/malabsorption of fat. This man may well be vitamin K deficient.

Clinical sketch: more responsive target

An elderly woman, on long-standing diuretics for congestive cardiac failure, is started on an angiotensin converting enzyme (ACE) inhibitor. After the first dose, upon rising from the seated position, she collapses and is found to be hypotensive.

Comment: homeostatis is often poorly maintained by the elderly. This problem is exacerbated here by the naturesis induced by her diuretic. Such patients should be started on extremely low ACE inhibitor doses.

Clinical sketch: more responsive target

An elderly woman suffers diarrhoea from villous adenomas of the large bowel: she has refused surgery. She presents with atrial fibrillation and is started on digoxin (but not warfarin for fear of haemorrhage from the adenomas). Six months later she is admitted with complete heart block, at which time her potassium is 2.8 mmol/l.

Comment: villous adenomas can cause profound hypokalaemia, which, in turn, increases the response to digoxin (see Ch. 4).

Idiosyncratic responses are more likely in some disease states

The mechanisms underlying idiosyncratic (type B) adverse drug reactions are often poorly understood. Certain diseases seem to render patients more likely to such reactions.

Clinical sketch: increased risk of idiosyncratic adverse reactions

A man with advanced AIDS takes co-trimoxazole as prophylaxis against *Pneumocystis carinii*. He develops a severe rash, which is attributed to the sulphonamide.

Comment: HIV disease seems to predispose towards frequent reactions to sulphonamides. The mechanism is unclear, but impaired cell detoxification of chemically reactive drug derivatives has been suggested as the cause.

Self-assessment: questions

Multiple choice questions

1. Response to the following drugs is affected adversely by the disease state:
   a. Morphine and hepatic failure
   b. Propranolol and phaeochromocytoma
   c. Gliclazide and renal failure
   d. Sulfinpyrazone and renal failure
   e. Aminophylline and cirrhosis

2. The following statements are correct:
   a. The only determinant of the effect of liver disease on response to a drug is the degree to which it is cleared by hepatic metabolism
   b. The only determinant of the effect of renal disease on response to a drug is the degree to which it is cleared, unchanged, by the kidney
   c. Heart failure has little impact on drug response
   d. Aminoglycosides should be avoided in myasthenia gravis
   e. Digoxin should be avoided in pre-excitation syndromes (such as Wolff–Parkinson–White syndrome)

Case history questions

Case history 1

A middle-aged man with alcoholic chronic liver disease is given phenytoin for generalised tonic/clonic seizures. His liver function tests are as follows (normal range in parentheses):

albumin 37 g/l (32–42), bilirubin 14 mmol/l (2–17), gamma-glutamyltransferase 230 mg/l (<50), prothrombin time 32 seconds (control 13 seconds).

The plasma phenytoin concentration is closely watched for 3 years thereafter: the concentration remains within the therapeutic range and seizure frequency declines. He becomes lost to follow-up. The patient is admitted to hospital 5 years later with severe ataxia. His plasma phenytoin concentration is well above the therapeutic range and his liver function tests are as follows:

albumin 17 g/l, bilirubin 50 mmol/l, gamma-glutamyltransferase 350 mg/l, prothrombin time 125 seconds (control 13 seconds).

1. Comment on the case: what are the likely mechanisms of the adverse reactions, and in what ways might they have been avoided?

Case history 2

An elderly woman develops atrial fibrillation, and is given digoxin to control her ventricular rate. Relevant blood results at the time are (normal values in parentheses):

Na^+ 140 mmol/l (135–145), K^+ 3.9 mmol/l (3.5–5.4), urea 14 mmol/l (2.5–7.0), creatinine 140 mmol/l (50–130).

Two years later she develops peripheral oedema and nocturnal breathlessness. Her doctor diagnoses congestive heart failure, starts a thiazide diuretic and later adds an angiotensin-converting enzyme (ACE) inhibitor. Her symptoms improve. Two years later, she is admitted to hospital in complete heart block with the following blood results: Na^+ 138 mmol/l, K^+ 1.4 mmol/l, urea 45 mmol/l, creatinine 360 μmol/l.

1. Comment on the case: what are the likely mechanisms of the adverse reactions and in what ways might they have been avoided?

Self-assessment: answers

Multiple choice answers

1. a. **True**. Morphine may precipitate fatal coma.
   b. **True**. Phaeochromocytoma is a rare cause of hypertension, in which a tumour secretes catecholamines. The main effect is an increase in peripheral vascular resistance caused by noradrenaline. Paradoxically, beta-blockers may worsen blood pressure control by opposing β_2-effects and by preventing the binding of noradrenaline to β_1-adenoceptors, thereby increasing its binding to α-adrenoceptors.
   c. **True**. Gliclazide is a sulphonylurea hypoglycaemic agent that is mainly excreted unchanged; it produces profound hypoglycaemia in patients with renal failure.
   d. **True**. Sulfinpyrazone is a uricosuric used in gout (Ch. 9). For the drug to work, there must be adequate renal function; furthermore, sulfinpyrazone clearance is reduced by renal failure.
   e. **True**. Aminophylline clearance is reduced in chronic liver disease.

2. a. **False**. Hepatocellular disease may cause hypoalbuminaemia: drugs extensively bound to albumin may, therefore, be more potent. Such patients have impaired clotting, increasing the effect of anticoagulants and antiplatelet drugs (such as aspirin).
   b. **False**. The accumulation of metabolic waste in patients with renal failure occupies binding sites on albumin and other plasma proteins: some protein-bound drugs may, therefore, be potentiated.
   c. **False**. Severe heart failure reduces the volume of distribution of some drugs (notably lidocaine).
   d. **True**. Aminoglycosides may cause a degree of non-depolarising blockade at the motor end plate. This is usually of no consequence, but in myasthenia gravis, aminoglycosides may worsen weakness.
   e. **True**. Digoxin slows the rate of conduction across the atrioventricular (AV) node and may encourage aberrant conduction in WPW syndrome: this may cause ventricular tachycardia.

Case history answers

Case history 1

The lack of linearity between the dose of phenytoin and its plasma concentration (i.e. zero-order pharmacokinetics) should be covered. The extensive binding of phenytoin to plasma proteins should be mentioned and the fact that phenytoin is largely cleared by hepatic metabolism. This man had impaired liver function to start with, but during his loss from follow-up, the situation worsened: he probably continued to drink. The liver function tests give good guidance of this worsening status. Clearance of phenytoin is almost certainly lower and, given the low albumin, its free fraction is probably higher (you should discuss the importance of free drug fractions at this point). This man's problems might have been avoided had regular follow-up been undertaken, but he defaulted. You may want to discuss the problem of giving potentially toxic drugs, like phenytoin or warfarin, to patients who are likely to default.

Case history 2

It should be stressed at the start that digoxin is cleared almost entirely by renal excretion and that its effects are potentiated by hypokalaemia (the mechanism of this should be presented). This old woman had renal impairment to start with and probably had a low digoxin clearance. Her renal function deteriorated, however (possibly caused by the ACE inhibitor), and this, together with the thiazide-induced hypokalaemia, caused severe toxicity. She should have been followed more closely, with estimations of renal function, K^+ and plasma digoxin concentration.

21 Adverse drug reactions and drug interactions

Overview

Adverse drug reactions are a common cause of iatrogenic morbidity and mortality. They may affect as many as 20% of patients in some form. Simple measures may prevent some of these. You should report all serious or novel adverse drug reactions to the appropriate drug licensing agency.

Drug interactions may be kinetic or dynamic. They may be useful or harmful. Certain drugs and certain patients are particularly likely to be involved in adverse interactions and we should be aware of these.

21.1 Adverse drug reactions

Learning objectives

You should:

- be aware of the importance of adverse drug reactions in causing illness
- understand the simple classification of adverse drug reactions
- understand some of the mechanisms of adverse drug reactions
- understand the importance of reporting adverse drug reactions and know how to do it.

Any drug has the potential to cause an adverse drug reaction (ADR). ADRs can be defined as any unintended harmful effect of a drug. Before prescribing, the potential risks of any drug must be weighed against the possible benefits; doctors should only prescribe when the benefits outweigh the risks. ADRs are very common. It is estimated that ADRs occur in 10–20% of all patients prescribed drugs and are the cause of up to 10% of all GP consultations, 4% of all hospital admissions and about 1 in 1000 deaths. ADRs may mimic natural disease and are generally underdetected by doctors.

Classification

A useful classification of ADRs is as follows.

Type A: the **augmented** effects. These are dose related and are where the ADR is caused by an excessive response to the drug and may result from pharmacokinetic or pharmacodynamic problems. These ADRs are predictable from the known effects of the drug and are dose related, e.g. hypotension in patients taking antihypertensives, or excessive sedation in a patient taking carbamazepine. Such effects are very common but are often not severe. Type A ADRs can be managed often by dose modification.

Clinical sketch

An elderly patient is prescribed benzodiazepines for inability to sleep after a recent bereavement. Two days later the patient crashes his car. Although not badly injured he has no recollection of the event leading up to the crash.

Comment: This is probably a type A reaction to benzodiazepines: increased sedation or incoordination if the patient is not used to such sedative drugs. Such adverse events are more likely to occur in the elderly, who are more sensitive to benzodiazepines. The patient should have been warned not to drive while taking the drug, or at least not drive until it was clear to what extent it would cause such sedation.

Clinical sketch

A patient is given carbamazepine to treat epilepsy. Within 2 weeks of starting therapy the patient develops severe mucosal ulceration.

Comment: This is Stevens–Johnson syndrome, a type A reaction to carbamazepine. It was unpredictable (provided it had never happened to the patient before) and the patient should avoid carbamazepine thereafter.

Type B: the **bizarre** effects. These is not predictable from the known effects of the drug and are not dose related. These often have an immunological basis: as such, there is often no clear relationship to the dose of drug. Such ADRs are relatively rare but are disproportionately important because the ADR is often very serious, e.g. anaphylaxis with penicillin, or agranulocytosis with carbimazole. Withdrawal of the drug is necessary.

Type C: effects of **chronic** administration. These effects are caused by adaptation, change in receptor sensitivity, etc. For example, the on–off phenomenon with levodopa.

Type D: **delayed** effects. These are the long-term effects such as carcinogenesis or effects on reproduction, e.g. stilbestrol (Ch. 19).

Type E: **end of use** or **withdrawal** reactions. These occur if there have been changes such as receptor up-regulation, e.g. rebound angina on withdrawal of beta-blockers.

Type F: *unexpected* **failure** *of therapy.* These are common and dose related. They are sometimes caused by drug interactions, e.g. failure of the oral contraceptive in a woman prescribed the enzyme inducer carbamazepine.

Drug testing

Premarketing testing of a new drug will involve its administration to an average of about 2000 humans (this number continues to rise as drug testing becomes more rigorous). This will show up many common ADRs, especially type A. However, type B reactions may be relatively rare, perhaps with an incidence of only 1 in 10 000 prescriptions, or less, and so are unlikely to be seen in trials. These may only become apparent after the drug is launched and the numbers of humans treated with it rises. Likewise the late type C and D effects are

---

Clinical sketch

In the course of a trial of a new drug, a patient develops hepatitis. No other patient on the trial has developed such an effect. The manufacturer wonders whether this is an adverse drug reaction or a naturally occurring disease.

Comment: This is a fairly common situation. Hepatitis can occur naturally in the general population but this could also be the manifestation of a very rare adverse drug reaction. Prelicensing clinical trials are usually not large enough to detect such adverse reactions reliably, which may be confused with naturally occurring disease. This case would prompt the company to undertake very intensive investigations of liver functions and risk of hepatitis. It would also prompt closer observation after licensing and drug launch of the possible adverse effects on the general population who might be prescribed the drugs.

---

only likely to be seen after the drug has been available for some years. It may be difficult to connect an adverse event with the drug, especially if the ADR resembles other disease. For example liver damage was seen in those prescribed perhexilene, an antianginal drug now withdrawn. The drug caused histological changes identical to those resulting from alcoholism and was not recognised as an ADR initially.

It is important, therefore, when new drugs are prescribed that doctors observe closely for any possible adverse effects and report them to the proper authorities. In the UK, the Committee on Safety of Medicines (CSM) is the statutory body responsible for collecting this data and reports to CSM can be made on special yellow cards, which are widely available. This system has been responsible for identifying many previously undescribed and serious ADRs. The CSM is particularly keen to have reports of all serious reactions to any drug and of any reaction to new drugs, identified in the advertising and the British National Formulary by a black triangle ▼.

In addition, specific postmarketing safety surveillance is often carried out on new drugs by the manufacturer, using computerised records from hospitals and primary care.

Clinical sketch

A patient is prescribed a new highly effective antibiotic. Five days later the patient presents to her GP complaining of severe dizziness and drowsiness. The doctor wonders if the antibiotic might be responsible. This possible reaction is not described in the drug information supplied by the manufacturers

Comment: The doctor should report this potential adverse reaction to the Committee on Safety of Medicines. Every year, one or more drugs are withdrawn because new adverse effects appear shortly after the drug has been launched. The fact that such an adverse effect is not included in the initial drug literature should not deter doctors from making reports. Such reporting is essential for the public health and a key cornerstone in drug safety.

Patients particularly at risk of adverse reactions

- The elderly: little physiological reserve and altered phamacokinetics and pharmacodynamics
- The very young
- Patients with renal disease
- Patients with liver disease
- Genetically predisposed patients, e.g. with glucose 6-phosphate dehydrogenase deficiency who may get haemolysis when treated with many drugs such as

sulphonamides or antimalarials such as primaquine, or patients with acute intermittent porphyria, who may get exacerbations if given many drugs that are metabolised by the liver and interfere with haem breakdown, such as estrogens. There are many other genetic variations which alter both the response to drugs and the risks of adverse reactions.

Ways to avoid adverse drug reactions

Prescribe drugs only when necessary, and for the shortest time in the lowest dose possible. Try to prescribe only drugs with which you are familiar—this is one of the virtues of using a limited drug formulary. Warn the patient of any common or major adverse reactions. Genetic variation is now being explored and will in the future allow us to tailor therapy to a patient more carefully.

21.2 Drug interactions

Learning objectives

You should:

- understand the mechanisms of drug interactions

- be aware of the drugs and patients most likely to be involved in such adverse reactions.

Drug interactions may be harmful or beneficial. Not all interactions are of clinical importance, and, like ADRs, they may not occur in every patient. Constant vigilance is, therefore, required to avoid drug interactions and to spot them when they do occur. Many lists of possible drug interactions are available. Rather than learn lists, it is better for the most part to consider which patients are at risk, which drugs are most likely to be involved and what the possible mechanisms are. Some common or dangerous interactions are mentioned but the list is not complete: check carefully if there is any doubt before prescribing. Many general practitioners now prescribe using computers and many pharmacies also use computers in their dispensing: suitable software is available to aid the detection of potential interactions.

Patients who are at risk of interactions

- The elderly (see Ch. 19): polypharmacy, poor homeostatic mechanisms, etc.
- Severely ill patients: for similar reasons and also because a drug interaction may be difficult to distinguish from the natural history of the disease,

e.g. heart failure treated with diuretics may be exacerbated by NSAIDs, which cause fluid retention
- Patients who depend on prophylactic therapy for disease suppression, e.g. epileptics, patients on immunosuppressants or oral contraceptives
- Patients with liver or renal disease
- Patients with more than one doctor, when confusion may arise over what drugs the patient is taking
- Patients who take non-prescribed drugs, e.g. those bought 'over the counter' such as theophylline, pseudoephedrine in decongestants and, of course, ethanol; always ask the patient about such drugs— many patients do not think of such drugs when asked about what medicines they are taking.

Drugs at risk

Some drugs are particularly likely to be involved in serious interactions:

- Drugs with a narrow therapeutic index (Ch. 1), e.g. warfarin, digoxin, cytotoxics, lithium, aminoglycosides, theophylline
- Drugs with a steep dose–response curve (Ch. 1), where a minor change in plasma concentration may make a major change in effect, e.g. oral hypoglycaemics, warfarin
- Drugs with a major effect on a vital process such as clotting (warfarin)
- Drugs where a loss of effect may lead to disease breakthrough, e.g. antiepileptics
- Drugs that may induce or inhibit mixed function oxidase enzymes and so may decrease metabolism of other drugs, and drugs that depend on these enzymes for their metabolism (e.g. theophylline, warfarin, phenytoin, oral contraceptives, cyclosporin and many others).
- Drugs that affect cardiac conduction: many drugs cause prolongation of the QT interval on the ECG, a marker of altered intracardiac conduction as a result of effects on ion channels in cardiac cells; such drugs may cause cardiac arrhythmias, especially if combined, e.g. the antihistamine terfenadine and the prokinetic agent cisapride.

Mechanisms

Drug interactions may be pharmacodynamic or pharmacokinetic.

Pharmacokinetic mechanisms

This is where the interaction causes a change in the plasma concentration of one or other drug leading to a greater or lesser effect.

Absorption. Drugs such as colestyramine may bind to other drugs (e.g. digoxin, thiazides) in the gastrointestinal tract and prevent their absorption. Some drugs (e.g. opiates) may slow transit time and so may slow absorption, but the total amount absorbed may be unchanged. Some drugs depend on enterohepatic circulation, e.g. they are excreted in a conjugated form in bile, the conjugation is broken down by bacteria in the gastrointestinal tract and the free drug is reabsorbed, enhancing drug effect, e.g. oral contraceptive estrogens. If this is prevented, for example by amoxicillin altering gut flora, the drug may lose its effect.

Metabolism. Enzyme inducers (e.g. phenytoin, carbamazepine, rifampicin) will decrease the effects of many drugs; since enzyme induction requires synthesis of new protein, it may take 2–3 weeks to reach its maximum effect. Enzyme inhibitors (erythromycin, ciprofloxacin, isoniazid, cimetidine, sodium valproate, metronidazole, allopurinol, dextropropoxyphene, sulphonamides and many others), however, are effective very rapidly. Problems may arise, therefore, when a patient stable on a drug is prescribed either an enzyme inducer or inhibitor. Problems may also arise if a patient is stabilised on a drug while receiving an enzyme inducer or inhibitor, which is then withdrawn.

Distribution. Only free drug is pharmacologically active, but many drugs are heavily protein bound, e.g.

warfarin to albumin. If another drug with a high affinity for protein is prescribed, the result may be a displacement of warfarin from the protein-binding sites, increasing the free drug and its effects (but this is transient, see Ch. 1). This may cause confusion if therapeutic drug monitoring is used, because this usually measures total rather than free drug.

Excretion. Drugs can interfere with excretion, for example thiazides and NSAIDs interfere with the excretion of lithium. This effect can sometimes be beneficial, e.g. reducing the clearance of penicillin by giving probenecid.

Pharmacodynamic mechanisms

Pharmacodynamic mechanisms are, in general, more common but are predictable from the known effects of the drug, e.g. two antihypertensives may be used to lower the blood pressure more than either alone. Alternatively, the actions of diuretics are opposed by NSAIDs, which may cause fluid retention, or the effects of oral hypoglycaemics may be opposed by thiazides. Other pharmacodynamic interactions can arise from the effects of drugs on electrolyte or fluid balance, e.g. diuretic-induced hypokalaemia enhances digoxin toxicity.

Self-assessment: questions

Multiple choice questions

1. Adverse drug reactions:
   a. Are a common source of morbidity
   b. Type A reactions are rare
   c. Type B reactions are often serious
   d. Type B reactions will generally have been identified before a drug is marketed
   e. Serious adverse reactions to all drugs should be reported to the CSM

2. Drug interactions:
   a. May result from altered metabolism
   b. May be caused by plasma protein displacement
   c. Are always harmful
   d. Are more likely in the elderly
   e. Are more likely in patients with ischaemic heart disease

3. The following drugs may interact:
   a. Glibenclamide and rifampicin
   b. Heparin and phenytoin
   c. Erythromycin and theophylline
   d. Co-proxamol and warfarin
   e. Benzodiazepines and ethanol

Case history questions

Case history 1

A 68-year-old woman with non-insulin-dependent diabetes is treated with glibenclamide. She is found unconscious one evening, and taken to hospital. Her blood sugar is found to be low.

1. How would you classify this adverse reaction?

When she has been treated and has recovered, she describes how she was given fluconazole for a fungal infection the day before.

2. Is this relevant?

She is prescribed amoxicillin instead for the infection but develops bronchospasm for the first time in her life.

3. What class of adverse reaction is this?

4. Will decreasing the dose be adequate to prevent such an adverse effect?

Case history 2

A 35-year-old woman with epilepsy is prescribed ciprofloxacin for a urinary tract infection. She is currently taking carbamazepine. Five days later she has her first fit in 5 years.

1. What is the likely cause of the fit?
2. What would have been an appropriate antimicrobial choice in this patient?

Short note questions

Write short notes on:

1. The distinction between type A and type B adverse drug reactions
2. The key means to identify adverse drug reactions

Extended matching items questions

Theme: adverse drug reactions
Options

A. Glyceryl trinitrate
B. Benzylpenicillin
C. Verapamil
D. Trimthoprim
E. Teratogenicity
H. Immune-mediated toxicity
I. Drug accumulation
J. Carcinogenicity
K. Phenoxymethylpenicillin
L. Exaggeration of the therapeutic effect
M. Mutagenicity
N. Atenolol
O. Placental damage

For each of the following case histories 1–4, choose the most appropriate answer from the options A–O. Each option may be used once, more than once or not at all.

1. A 40-year-old cigarette smoker consults his doctor about episodic chest pain: the doctor finds the patient's feet are a little cold, and that his chest is a little wheezy, but otherwise there are no positive signs. The ECG is abnormal, suggestive of ischaemic heart disease, and the doctor diagnoses the chest

pain as angina pectoris: a drug is started. Two weeks later the patient sees the GP again: he is very wheezy, indeed he can hardly talk, and for the past 2 weeks he has been unable to walk because of severe pain in his calves.

Which drug did the GP give for the angina?

2. A young woman presents with severe dysuria. Dipstick testing of her urine reveals 'protein +++, blood +++': the doctor diagnoses a urinary tract infection. He prescribes a drug, but 2 days later the woman returns with a florid rash.

   i. Which drug was prescribed?
   ii. What is the likely mechanism?

3. A 20-year-old man has a very severe psoriasis and is under the care of a team of dermatologists. They have tried him on a number of regimens without success and eventually start him on methotrexate. This drug seems to work, and so the man doubles the dose without seeking medical advice; he also defaults from clinic for a month. When he next presents to clinic he is not well: he has a sore throat, conjunctivitis and a temperature of 40 °C. His total white cell count is found to be very low at 1.0×10^9 cells/l; he is anaemic with a haemoglobin of 9.5 g% (95 g/l).

   The methotrexate has caused this problem, but by what mechanism?

4. A 30-year-old woman is given an antibiotic by i.v. injection for pneumonia. Five minutes later, she is found collapsed with profound hypotension, a generalised rash and is dyspnoeic with wheezing.

   i. What antibiotic is she likely to have been given?
   ii. What is the mechanism of this reaction?

Theme: adverse effects of drugs

Options

A. Nausea
B. Dyspepsia
C. Rash
D. Bleeding
E. Agranulocytosis
F. Constipation
G. Headache
H. Dizziness
I. Ankle swelling
J. Sedation
K. Diarrhoea
L. Cold hands
M. Drug interactions
N. Peptic ulceration

For each of the drugs in 1–4 below, select the two or three most serious adverse effects from the options A–N about which you would wish to warn patients for whom you are prescribing. Serious is taken to mean frequent or severe. Options can be used once, more than once or not at all.

1. Amlodipine
2. Carbimazole
3. Warfarin
4. Diclofenac

Self-assessment: answers

Multiple choice answers

1. a. **True**. For instance, in the elderly, adverse reactions may cause between 10–20% of hospital admissions (less commonly a cause in younger patients).
   b. **False**. These are related to the expected pharmacological effects of a drug and are common.
   c. **True**. Often immunological in origin and generally more serious and unpredictable than type A.
   d. **False**. Given their relatively low frequency and the small numbers of patients treated before a drug is marketed, it is less likely that type B reactions will be seen before marketing.
   e. **True**. Also all adverse reactions (serious or not) with new drugs.

2. a. **True**. For example, liver enzyme induction or inhibition.
   b. **True**. These are not usually of major importance, because the body clears free drug and a temporary increase in free drug because of protein displacement will be followed by increased clearance to restore free drug concentrations.
   c. **False**. For example, penicillin and probenecid, ACE inhibitors and diuretics.
   d. **True**. Because of polypharmacy, because of increased susceptibility to the harmful effects of drugs and because of altered pharmacokinetics and dynamics.
   e. **False**. More likely in patients with congestive cardiac failure, liver or renal disease.

3. a. **True**. The metabolism of glibenclamide and other sulphonylureas is increased because of enzyme induction by the rifampicin and the result may be hyperglycaemia.
   b. **False**. But phenytoin does interact with warfarin.
   c. **True**. Concentrations of theophylline may rise and cause serious adverse effects.
   d. **True**. Co-proxamol is a combination of paracetamol and dextropropxyphene (a drug-metabolising enzyme inhibitor) and so may increase warfarin concentrations and cause bleeding.
   e. **True**. A pharmacodynamic interaction leading to increased drowsiness.

Case history answers

Case history 1

1. At first glance, this seems to be type A (augmented effect) adverse drug reaction. Given its severity, the doctor should report it to the CSM.
2. Now it seems more likely to be a drug interaction, caused by liver enzyme inhibition by the fluconazole.
3. This is a type B (bizarre, not predictable from the pharmacological action of a drug) adverse drug reaction.
4. No: the offending drug must be withdrawn.

Case history 2

1. Ciprofloxacin inhibits some liver enzymes but not those involved in the metabolism of carbamazepine. It is, therefore, unlikely to have had a pharmacokinetic interaction with carbamazepine. Even if it did inhibit the metabolism of carbamazepine, one would have anticipated that this would cause increased drowsiness and ataxia through raised carbamazepine concentrations rather than loss of control. Ciprofloxacin and other 5-quinolones can inhibit the inhibitory effects of GABA (gamma-aminobutyric acid). This can lead to overactivity of the CNS, e.g. vivid dreams or hallucinations, confusion in the elderly and a lowering of the fitting threshold. In this patient, the quinolone has probably lowered the fitting threshold to the extent that it is no longer adequately controlled by the carbamazepine, leading to the fit.
2. Trimethoprim would have been a more appropriate choice with no risk of either kinetic or dynamic interactions with the carbamazepine. The quinolone was contraindicated in an epileptic.

Short note answers

1. The distinct features of type A and B adverse drug reactions are:
   - type A: common, usually not severe, predictable, dose related, augmented effect of the drug
   - type B: rare, often severe, often immunological in origin, unpredictable from the known pharmacology of the drug.

2. This should include prelicensing testing in drug trials, which will mainly reveal type A adverse reactions, postlicensing surveillance (either formal postmarketing surveillance or specific cohort or case-control studies), case reports in medical literature, and yellow card reporting to licensing authorities. These are not discreet; for instance, an increase in yellow card reports may prompt the undertaking of a cohort study or specific prescription event monitoring.

Extended matching items answers

Theme: adverse drug reactions

1. i. N. These are classical adverse reactions to beta-blockers (even relatively cardioselective ones like atenolol), although rarely seen in such a severe form. This patient was clearly at risk of developing these reactions, and atenolol was a bad choice.

2. i. D. The most likely drug here is trimethoprim.
   ii. H. The mechanism is immune mediated. (The other antibiotics are not commonly used for urinary tract infections, although all might cause a rash.) This is a type B or bizarre reaction and was not predictable unless the patient had previously had a similar effect.

3. L. Methotrexate inhibits the conversion of folic to folinic acid and interferes therefore with purine and ultimately DNA formation. Hence it is used in conditions with a high cell turn over, like some malignant conditions, psoriasis and some inflammatory conditions. What has happened here is predictable from the pharmacology of the drug and is an exaggerated pharmacological effect (type A adverse drug reaction), so that the methotrexate is now affecting the blood precursors.

4. i. B. The antibiotic is probably penicillin.
   ii. H. This is classical anaphylaxis. The mechanism is immune mediated, through IgE. The patient may have had a history of previous penicillin exposure, and possibly previous adverse effects.
   iii. Supplementary question: how would you treat this patient? See Chapter 10 for the answers.

Theme: side effects of drugs

1. Best answers are I, G and H. Amlodipine causes vasodilatation and as such may cause ankle swelling and headache. It sometimes causes relaxation in the smooth muscle of the gastro-oesphogeal junction and causes dyspepsia. In some patients, postural hypotension and dizziness may be a concern.

2. Best answers are E and C. Carbimazole can cause agranulocytosis, a rare but potentially fatal adverse effect. Patients must be warned to look out for any evidence of infection, such as a sore throat; if there is such evidence then a full blood count measuring white cells needs to be undertaken. If carbimaxole does cause agranulocytosis, withdrawal alone is usually adequate to restore white cell numbers. A much more common adverse effect of carbimazole, however, is rash. If this occurs it may be necessary to discontinue the carbimazole and try propylthiouracil instead.

3. Best answers are D and M. Warfarin inhibits the formation of the clotting factors II, V, VII and IX. In excess, therefore, it is prone to cause bleeding. Warfarin is probably the drug most commonly involved in serious adverse drug interactions as drugs which potentiate the warfarin (e.g. by inhibiting its metabolism), which reduce the tendency to clotting in other ways (e.g. antiplatelet effect) or which cause a risk of bleeding (e.g. by peptic ulceration) may all interact with warfarin. Patients need to be carefully warned about alerting their doctor or pharmacist before taking any prescribed or over the counter medicines while on warfarin. If in any doubt of the safety of a drug in combination with warfarin seek advice from the British National Formulary or your local drug information centre.

4. Best answers are N, B and C. Diclofenac like most non-steroidal anti-inflammatory drugs can cause dyspepsia (a direct effect of the acidic drug in the stomach) or peptic ulceration (inhibition of cyclo-oxygenase inhibiting maintenance of the gastric mucosa). Dyspepsia is not a reliable warning of the peptic ulceration. These drugs should clearly be avoided in patients with a previous history of peptic ulceration. Diclofenac has a range of other adverse effects, of which the most common is probably rash. However, it can also cause headache and drug interactions (for instance with diuretics its effects may be inhibited, leading to undercontrol of hypertension or to heart failure).

22 New drugs and clinical trials

Overview

This chapter considers the process of developing new drugs: where they come from and how they are tested. The basic issues in designing a clinical trial are considered.

22.1 New drugs

Learning objectives

You should:

- be able to explain the stages of new drug development
- be aware of the likely sources for new drugs.

New drugs are developed and marketed, and the drugs learnt by a doctor as a medical student will almost certainly be obsolete within his professional career. The doctor must understand where new drugs come from, how they are developed and licensed and how their value in therapy should be assessed.

How are new drugs found?

In the past, therapeutics was empirical, and drugs were natural substances or their derivatives and found by chance and experience to be valuable, e.g. digitalis. With the development of the chemical industry, new synthetic chemicals were produced and screened for activity in various animal models or diseases, e.g. benzodiazepines. Existing drugs were purified to extract the active component and ensure more consistent quality, e.g. digoxin. These were slow and cumbersome processes and are less common today.

As our understanding of the pathophysiology of diseases grew, drugs were developed to imitate or replace naturally occurring compounds e.g. levodopa. Later still, the ability developed to design drugs to attach to an important receptor in the pathophysiology of the disease, e.g. β-adrenoceptor agonists or antagonists. Some drugs are enzyme inhibitors (e.g. angiotensin-converting enzyme (ACE) inhibitors, proton pump inhibitors). New targets for drugs are identified as a result of better understanding of the pathophysiology of a condition and of how the body works. In the future, these targets might be identifying and replacing a single gene to produce an altered gene product within the body, e.g. in therapy for inborn errors of metabolism.

Where do new drugs come from?

Almost all new drugs are the result of research conducted by the pharmaceutical industry, based on extensive work to understand the mechanisms behind the disease. Drug development involves a considerable commercial risk—less than 1 in 1000 molecules studied reach clinical trials and less than 1 in 100 drugs that enter trials are ever marketed. On average, it costs £150–200 million to develop a novel drug, and it can take anything from 8–15 years.

22.2 Testing new drugs

Learning objectives

You should:

- be able to explain the advantages of the randomised controlled trial design for a new drug evaluation
- be able to explain drug licensing and its significance.

Promising molecules undergo tests initially in animals (but increasingly in in vitro systems to reduce the numbers of animals involved) to detect their pharmacokinetics, pharmacodynamics and toxicity, including teratogenicity and carcinogenicity. However, animal studies, although essential, do not always predict effects in humans. Drugs that show a likelihood of therapeutic benefit and acceptable toxicity will be subsequently tested in humans.

Testing in humans is generally divided into four phases, but the exact duration and size of these studies will be determined by the nature of the drug and its proposed uses. For instance, an antihypertensive that will be taken for many years needs to be more carefully evaluated in humans and to be less toxic than a cancer chemotherapy drug, which will be used for short periods in patients with a poor prognosis.

Clinical trials are usually considered in four phases.

Phase I. Small studies of the basic clinical pharmacology of a drug involving 50–100 healthy volunteers. These trials will examine pharmacodynamics and pharmacokinetics and will involve the use of various doses.

Phase II. The early clinical investigations to determine if the drug has the intended therapeutic effect in patients. A group of 50–300 patients will be studied, looking at efficacy and also at pharmacokinetics, pharmacodynamics and adverse effects using various doses.

Phase III. If the early trials show promise, advanced clinical investigations will follow. These will involve 300–5000 patients with the relevant condition and will look at efficacy and adverse effects. They may compare the new drug with existing treatments. Study of special patient groups, e.g. elderly, patients with renal disease, etc., will also be undertaken.

Licence application. If all of these studies show that the drug is effective and relatively safe compared with existing therapies, the company may apply for a licence to market the drug. The evidence will be considered by the licensing authority and if considered satisfactory, a licence will be granted. The drug may then be marketed for specific indications, but testing does not end yet.

Phase IV. The average number of humans studied before a new drug is marketed is approximately 3000; it is clear that common adverse effects will, therefore, have been identified at this stage, but rarer effects, for instance with an incidence of 1 in 10 000, may not. After marketing, the number of patients who use the drug will rise rapidly, and previously undetected adverse effects may appear. It is imperative, therefore, that trials continue after marketing: these test the drug as it is used in the real world but focus more on adverse effects (**post marketing surveillance**) and less on efficacy. They may involve 2000–10 000 or more patients. Other trials exploring other uses of the drug will also continue.

Design of clinical trials

The design of clinical trials is complex but of great importance, since poorly designed trials delay progress and waste resources. There are many possible designs depending on the drug and the nature of the condition to be treated. Some features are essential.

A clear question to be answered should be established in advance. A trial should be designed to answer a specific hypothesis. For example, the question 'What happens if we give drug X to hypertensives?' is too vague, with no clear focus of what is being sought— how will you know when you find it? The question 'Drug X will not lower blood pressure by 5 mmHg in hypertensive patients' is clearcut. A hypothesis is usually stated as a negative ('the null hypothesis') and then the trial is designed to disprove the hypothesis. This double negative may seem perverse but it makes the trial much more rigorous than a positive hypothesis. Most trials can really only answer the one question for which they were designed ('hypothesis testing'): too often, trials are badly designed with multiple ill-defined endpoints and end up with no useful information or, even worse, misleading information. Sometimes people try to extract answers other than to the original question from trials. This is unreliable, since a trial will rarely provide a definitive answer to any other question; however, it may raise questions that can be answered in further trials ('hypothesis generation').

Comparison with other treatments. Where there is an effective treatment already in existence for the condition in question, it is inadequate simply to compare the new drug with placebo: rather it should be compared with the best current treatment.

The subjects of the trial. These should be appropriate. For example, if the drug for heart failure is to be used mainly in elderly patients, then it should be tested in such patients and not in younger patients. The trial should also include enough subjects to allow the question posed to be answered.

The duration of the trial. The trial should be of an appropriate duration. For example, for antibiotics a few days may be appropriate, but for an antihypertensive, trials should be measured in months or years.

The trial should be analysed statistically. The statistical analysis of the trial is of vital importance and should be clearly established before the trial is performed. This needs to address questions such as the size of the trial (is it large enough?). How will the results be analysed? In any treatment with any drug, some patients will do well and some will do badly. If you conduct a trial, you could get an unfavourable result by chance. Think about tossing a coin: imagine that heads is a good outcome and tails a bad outcome. You would expect to get an equal number of heads and tails (unless the coin is biased). Now toss a coin 10 times—how many heads and how many tails? By chance you may have hit a streak of heads or of tails. Similarly, in a trial, an unfavourable or favourable result might have arisen by chance. How do you know whether your result is correct or not? One way is to increase the size of your trial (the more times you toss the coin, the closer the ratio of heads to tails becomes). In clinical trials this is expensive and may expose more patients to adverse events. So we test the probability of a trial to give us accurate results, and report the results as statistically significant or not. Statistically significant by convention means that the result we got was only likely to occur by chance 1 time in 20 (also known as the 5% significance level). You may have hit on the 1 in 20 chance of course, but we have to draw a line somewhere. The results of a trial analysed in this way are therefore *probably* accurate—there is little absolute certainty in medicine. Finally, we need to distinguish statistical significance from clinical significance: a statistically significant result could be so small that it may mean nothing in terms of benefit to patients.

The ethics of the trial should be considered. Trials should be designed so as to minimise any possible harm to the patients who participate. The patients should be made fully aware that they are participating in a trial and consent to this. To protect both patients and themselves, investigators should have the protocol considered by an expert ethical review committee. However, trials that are poorly designed are also unethical even if they are unlikely to harm patients—poor science is a waste of time and resources, and of patients' goodwill. In any trial there are risks (of adverse effects) and benefits (that a potential treatment will be found effective or ineffective and so we do not need to waste anymore time or money on it). A poorly designed study that cannot provide the benefits of answering these key questions exposes the patients to the hazards of a new treatment for no good reason: the balance of risks and benefits is firmly against the study.

Clinical sketch

A doctor is asked by a pharmaceutical company to enter the next five depressed patients he sees into a clinical trial in which they will be given a new drug. There is a payment for each patient he enters. The doctor agrees.

Comment: This sounds like a 'seeding' study, an attempt to get the doctor used to prescribing the new drug so that he will continue it later. The payment per patient could be interpreted as an out and out bribe. A non-comparative study of this kind sounds scientifically useless. The doctor needs to be clear on the aims and design of the study and its ethical approval. He also needs to inform patients they are taking part in a clinical trial and obtain their consent.

Placebo

Investigators must consider the placebo effect whereby patients may seem to improve when given any treatment, effective or not. Trials are often placebo controlled, i.e. patients are divided at random into two groups, half are given a placebo and half the active drug; the difference in response between the two groups gives a measure of the effectiveness of the drug. If there is an effective treatment already available for a disease, then a placebo-controlled trial may be unethical: the comparison should be the standard treatment. Alternatively, if the new treatment is an add-on to existing treatment rather than a replacement for it, the patients in both arms could receive the standard treatment and then, in addition, half new drug, half placebo.

Blinding

Often trials are conducted in a double-blind fashion whereby neither the patients nor the investigator seeing the patients and measuring the effects of the drug know which patients are taking which drug or placebo; this reduces the possibility of bias on the part of either the patient or the investigator. Blinding is not always possible, depending on the circumstances, but if not included in the trial protocol, the reasons why not should be carefully justified.

Randomisation

One problem in trials is ensuring that the patients receiving the trial drug and the comparator are similar, so that any difference between the treatments can be confidently attributed to the treatments and not to the selection of patients. For example, if all the smokers or all the women went into the placebo arm of a trial of a new drug for airways obstruction, would that bias the results? Quite probably, but there are other areas where the bias might not be so apparent or even where we just do not know what other factors might influence the outcomes. To get around this we randomly select patients into the different arms of the trial. In this way, we hope that any unknown factors that might bias the results will appear in equal numbers in both arms of the trial and will cancel each other out, leaving us able to attribute any difference in outcome to the treatments studied.

Size of trial

A common design fault is to include too few subjects in a trial. This may cause an indeterminate result when the trial is analysed statistically—a waste of effort. Conversely, a trial should not include so many subjects that it is impossible to complete nor should it expose an excessive number of patients to unknown risks. A statistician should be consulted to calculate the optimum size for a trial likely to give a definite result in favour of or against new therapy.

Drug licensing

Drugs are licensed for sale according to the evidence presented to the licensing authority. In the UK, the licensing authority is the Secretary of State for Health, guided by the Medicines Control Agency and one of its committees, the Committee on the Safety of Medicines (CSM). Increasingly, drug licensing takes place at a European level where the agencies are the European

Medicines Evaluation Agency (EMEA). Factors considered in the licensing process are the quality of the drug (is it well and safely manufactured?), its efficacy (does it work in the condition for which the licence is sought?) and its relative safety (is it as safe as the existing therapy or, if not, does its greater efficacy justify its greater toxicity?). Note that the efficacy of the drug relative to existing drugs is not generally considered, only its relative toxicity.

The CSM is also responsible for monitoring reports of adverse drug reactions and reviewing new knowledge that may allow an extension or a reduction in the terms of the licence of a drug, or even its withdrawal.

Drug licensing is mainly concerned with drug safety: many countries now have separate agencies that advise on not just whether a drug may be prescribed but whether it should be prescribed from the point of view of its effectiveness or value for money.

22.3 Prescribing new drugs

Learning objectives

You should:

- be able to explain the principles of being a good prescriber

- be able to list sources of information for updating knowledge in therapeutics.

The true role of any new drug in therapeutics and its adverse effects is often unclear at first and may only become apparent with time. Comparative data with existing drugs are often inadequate. Very few new drugs are true innovative advances, and the majority are minor variations on existing drugs ('me-too' drugs). In general, doctors should prescribe new drugs only when they are sure that the new drug is an improvement on existing therapy, in terms of efficacy, safety or cost, and never simply because they are new. New drugs should be prescribed with particular caution (see Ch. 21) and any adverse effect reported to the CSM.

Where do doctors get their information about new drugs?

Many of the most commonly used drugs today were not available at the time that many doctors were medical students. Doctors must, therefore, keep up to date in pharmacology and therapeutics, since existing knowledge may rapidly become obsolete. The most common source of information about new drugs for doctors are the pharmaceutical companies and their representatives; however, doctors must be aware that companies aim to sell their products and that the information they supply may, therefore, be biased. Doctors should be capable of critically reviewing the evidence presented and should use independent evaluations of new drugs, such as those in the *Drugs and Therapeutics Bulletin* or in peer-reviewed journals. There are several other sources of information about drugs in general and not just new drugs.

The British National Formulary **(BNF)** is updated every 6 months and distributed free to doctors in the UK. It lists drugs by their therapeutic uses and provides information on indications for the drugs, formulations and doses, and adverse effects. It also has useful sections on prescribing in general, prescription writing, drugs in the elderly and in children, and in renal and liver disease, as well as drug interactions. It is a most valuable source and prescribing doctors should always carry one and refer to it regularly.

Drug information services are pharmacist operated and sited in regional health authorities. They are available for consultation by letter or telephone (telephone numbers are in the BNF). Many produce local drug information bulletins.

A 'summary of product characteristics' or drug data sheet is produced by the pharmaceutical industry, together with other extensive material, much of which is more promotional than informational.

Clinical sketch

A drug company representative comes to see a GP and tells him of the highly effective new antidepressant produced by his company. This drug is claimed to be effective in 95% of patients and to have no significant adverse effects. This is supported by a large amount of literature, which the drug representative gives the doctor. The doctor is impressed and prescribes the drug to the next depressed patient who consults.

Comment: Doctors should not depend on drug company promotional activities as their only source of information about new drugs but should seek out independent sources as well. These will often take a rather more jaundiced view of the company's product. Experience with other antidepressants tells us that no drug is effective in such a high percentage of patients: it would take very strong evidence to convince doctors that the new drug will be substantially different in this area. Such a high percentage response rate may be a consequence of careful patient selection before entry to the trial or a placebo effect, and it is unlikely to be reflected in clinical practice. Similarly, adverse drug reactions are often not well identified in clinical trials and new drug monographs often report few adverse drug reactions in comparison to those for older drugs. With experience, more adverse effects will appear! Doctors should, therefore, be extremely cautious in prescribing new drugs and report all adverse drug reactions. Do not think that such promotional activities of companies will not affect you!

Marketing

Drug companies survive by selling their product and must make a profit both to fund further research on new products and to remain in business. Companies, therefore, spend large amounts—at least £400 million a year in the UK—promoting their products to doctors, but the enthusiasm of a company for its products sometimes exceeds the critical opinion of an independent reviewer of the value. Doctors should, therefore, exercise particular care in considering promotional material and always seek independent evidence.

Prescribing

Prescribing may be defined as the practical everyday use of drugs. It is, therefore, based on the clinical pharmacology of a drug but also includes factors such as the diagnosis, the patient's previous medical history, as well as other sociological and medical factors. Doctors often prescribe for reasons other than the pharmacological effects of the drug, although this might be deplored. Other reasons include the placebo effect, meeting patient demand, maintaining the vital relationship with the patient or even terminating the consultation. Prescribing for these reasons may be wasteful and harmful to the patient.

Good prescribing is:

- appropriate (is a drug needed at all?)
- effective and safe (given the diagnosis and consideration of patient factors, which drug is best and in what dosage?)
- cost effective (takes due account of the costs of drugs: where efficacy and safety are equal then the least expensive drug is the most appropriate; however, more expensive drugs may be justified for a better effect or because they are safer); doctors should bear in mind that money spent unnecessarily on inappropriate or unnecessary drugs is wasted and deprives other patients of essential care.

Doctors must consider all prescribing as an experiment, in which the outcome may be beneficial or harmful to the patient. In each case, the risks and benefits must be weighed and a drug administered only if the expected benefits outweigh the risks.

How to be a good prescriber

- Stay up to date with information from independent sources.
- No one can know all about the 5000 preparations in the BNF. Use a limited range of drugs with which you are familiar. Most doctors do 70–80% of their prescribing from a personal formulary of about 50 drugs. Drugs should be added to or subtracted from this only after careful consideration and review of evidence. Most hospitals have written formularies for their staff to use, and increasingly GPs are developing their own formularies as a useful way to rationalise drug therapy.
- Prescriptions should be written with the generic name of the drug and not its proprietary name where possible.
- Prescribing for individual patients should be reviewed regularly, and unnecessary drugs stopped; communication between doctors in hospitals and in general practice is particularly important.
- If in any doubt about dose or any other details of a drug, look it up in the BNF or other appropriate resource; be especially careful when prescribing new or unfamiliar drugs.
- Individualise prescriptions, do not prescribe in a routine manner: consider the patient, the disease, the choice of drug and formulation, the dose, other possible interacting diseases or drugs (including drugs that a patient might buy themselves over the counter without prescription). Consider also patient convenience, and keep drug therapy as simple as possible to minimise interactions and adverse effects.
- Educate the patient. Drugs may not be the most appropriate way of managing a problem. The patient should know what they have been prescribed and why, how they are to use the medication, and for how long, and what the possible adverse effects are.

In long-term treatment, patients on average take only about 60–70% of prescribed drugs: this is particularly so when patients are unsure of points mentioned above, or when the drug regimen is complex. Both of these may represent failure on the part of the doctor. We must help our patients to make best use of their medicines in any way we can.

Self-assessment: questions

Multiple choice questions

1. The following statements are correct:
   a. Phase I trials involve large numbers of patients
   b. Phase IV trials are completed before a drug is marketed
   c. Drug licensing considers efficacy, safety and cost
   d. New drugs are superior to older drugs and so should be widely prescribed
   e. New drugs may be designed for effect at specific receptors

2. Trials:
   a. That are double blind means that neither the doctor nor the patient know what drug the patient is taking at a particular time
   b. that are placebo controlled are appropriate to show that a new drug is more effective than existing therapy
   c. Should be reviewed by an ethics committee before being undertaken
   d. Results that come from several small but similar trials are inevitably more reliable than the results of a single large trial
   e. that are analysed statistically can prove that a new drug is effective

3. The following statements are correct:
   a. The BNF contains up to date information about drugs, doses and formulations
   b. 'Me-too' drugs generally have little advantage over existing drugs
   c. Comparative data on efficiency between new and existing drugs is essential before a new drug gets a licence
   d. All prescribing is an experiment
   e. Drugs should be prescribed by brand name

4. A good prescriber:
   a. Stays up to date
   b. Usually prescribes new drugs
   c. Uses a wide range of drugs to treat all conditions
   d. Never looks anything up
   e. Communicates well with colleagues and patients

Case history question

A drug manufacturer wishes to trial a new antihypertensive drug and compare its efficacy with an existing drug. It decides to conduct the study in primary care and seeks to recruit GPs to help.

1. What will the GP need to know about the drug before agreeing to take part?
2. What will the GP need to know about the kind of patient required?
3. What reassurances would a GP need that the study was scientifically sound?

Short note question

Compare and contrast the criteria for drug licensing with those for good prescribing.

Self-assessment: answers

Multiple choice answers

1. a. **False**. Usually involve normal subjects or small numbers of patients if the drug were considered too toxic to give to normal subjects, e.g. anticancer agents.
   b. **False**. These are postmarketing surveillance studies.
   c. **False**. Cost may not be considered by law.
   d. **False**. Despite what drug company advertising might have you believe.
   e. **True**. For example, sumatriptan as a serotonin analogue.

2. a. **True**. It is usually possible to break a code to find out what the patient is taking in case of emergency.
   b. **False**. The comparison should be against the best existing therapy (although this is often not the case in advertising).
   c. **True**. To protect both the patient and the investigator.
   d. **False**. Many trials are too small to show a genuine significant clinical effect: a single trial of adequate size is generally superior.
   e. **False**. Statistics can only give a probability, never certainty, especially at commonly used levels of significance such as $P < 0.05$. Statistical significance is also not the same as clinical significance.

3. a. **True**. The best available source and should be carried by all prescribing doctors.
   b. **True**. Again, a drug company may not like to admit this and will go to great lengths to demonstrate a minor or supposed advantage as a selling point.
   c. **False**.
   d. **True**. An important attitude for safe prescribing.
   e. **False**. There are, however, exceptions such as some fixed drug combinations or slow-release preparations.

4. a. **True**. Using reliable independent sources.
   b. **False**. A good prescriber will use new drugs where appropriate, i.e. where there is evidence of a clear therapeutic or other advantage.
   c. **False**. In general, good prescribers will work from a formulary of drugs (written or not) with which they are familiar.
   d. **False**. This attitude smacks of arrogance.
   e. **True**. An essential component.

Case history answer

1. The GP would need to know the likely adverse effects of the drug, their likely frequency compared with existing therapies and what evidence there was, to date, in small studies of the drug.
2. The GP would need to know exactly what the entry criteria are, since it may be that the practice will, in fact, have few patients who meet the entry criterion, or who fall out because the exclusion criteria are so strict. In general, there always seem to be lots of suitable patients—until you go to look for them!
3. The GP would need to be reassured that the study has been approved by an ethics committee which takes account not only of the likelihood of patient harm, and this harm is outweighed by the likelihood of patient benefit, but also that the study is scientifically sound and will add useful information to medical knowledge. The key factors the ethics committee will have to consider are the design of the study, randomisation, duration, entry and exclusion criteria, suitability of comparator, size and analysis of the trial. These factors are complex and probably beyond the ability of the average doctor to interpret. It is important, therefore, that the doctor ensure that such matters have been considered by an ethical review board, such as an ethics committee.

Short note answer

Drugs are licensed on the basis of their efficacy, their safety and their quality of manufacturer. Good prescribing must be effective: this is not quite the same as efficacy, which may be based on a surrogate marker, e.g. lowering blood pressure rather than preventing strokes. Effectiveness is also a measure of what the drug will actually do in the real world rather than in the idealised circumstances of the clinical trial. The trial regimen may be such that it is impossible to apply in practice.

Safety. The doctor must select the patients carefully. It is unlikely he would be able to select in exactly the same way as using the clinical trial and, therefore, the risks and benefits of the drug may vary. Also for a new drug the doctor may prefer to wait until there is more experience available.

Appropriate. A key question for a doctor is, is the drug better than the one already being used? If not, the doctor should carry on with the current prescription and reserve a new drug for very occasional use or not use it at all. Prescribing should be cost-effective. If a drug is no better than existing therapy and if it is more expensive than existing therapy then it should not be used.

Index

Q indicates a topic mentioned in a question to which the reader will find more detailed mention in the answer. Abbreviations: COPD, chronic obstructive pulmonary disease.